Simplified Drugs
and Solutions
for Health Care
Professionals

Simplified Drugs and Solutions for Health Care Professionals

Norma Dison, PhD, RN
Professor Emeritus
College of Nursing and Health Sciences
Winona State University
Winona, Minnesota

ELEVENTH EDITION

with 307 illustrations

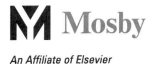

An Affiliate of Elsevier

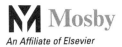
An Affiliate of Elsevier

Publisher: Nancy L. Coon
Editor: Jeff Burnham
Developmental Editor: Linda Caldwell
Associate Developmental Editor: Lisa P. Newton
Project Manager: Mark Spann
Production Editor: Beth Hayes
Manufacturing Manager: Karen Boehme
Designer: C. J. Petlick

A NOTE TO THE READER:
The author and publisher have made every attempt to check dosages and nursing content for accuracy. Because the science of pharmacology is continually advancing, our knowledge base continues to expand. Therefore we recommend that the reader always check product information for changes in dosage or administration before administering any medication. This is particularly important with new or rarely used drugs.

ELEVENTH EDITION
Copyright © 1997 by Mosby, Inc.

Previous editions copyrighted 1957, 1960, 1964, 1968, 1972, 1976, 1980, 1984, 1988, 1992

All rights reserved. No part of this publication may be reproduced, stored in a retrieval system, or transmitted, in any form or by any means, electronic, mechanical, photocopying, recording, or otherwise, without prior written permission from the publisher.

Permissions may be sought directly from Elsevier's Health Sciences Rights Department in Philadelphia, USA: phone: (+1)215-238-7869, fax: (+1)215-238-2239, email: healthpermissions@elsevier.com. You may also complete your request on-line via the Elsevier Science homepage (http://www.elsevier.com), by selecting 'Customer Support' and then 'Obtaining Permissions'.

Printed in the United States of America
Composition by Graphic World, Inc.
Lithography by Graphic World, Inc.
Printing/binding by Malloy Lithographing

Mosby
11830 Westline Industrial Drive
St. Louis, MO 63416

Library of Congress Cataloging-in-Publication Data

Dison, Norma.
  Simplified drugs and solutions for health care professionals / Norma Dison. — 11th ed.
    p. cm.
  Rev. ed. of: Simplified drugs and solutions for nurses, including mathematics. 10th ed. c1992.
  Includes index.
  ISBN 0-8151-2505-4
  1. Pharmaceutical arithmetic. 2. Drugs—Dosage.
3. Pharmaceutical arithmetic—Problems, exercises, etc. 4. Drugs—Dosage—Problems, exercises, etc. I. Dison, Norma Simplified drugs and solutions for nurses, including mathematics. II. Title.
  [DNLM: 1. Drugs—administration & dosage. 2. Mathematics. QV 16 D611s 1996]
RS57.N37 1996
615'.4'01513—dc20
DNLM/DLC
for Library of Congress   96-10794
                                                                                            CIP

04 05 06 07 08 / 9 8 7 6 5 4 3

Reviewers

Kathleen Dolin
Nursing Instructor
Practical Nursing Program
Monroe County Area Vocational Technical School
Bartonsville, Pennsylvania

John Martel, BA, BPE
Professor, Health and Biology
St. Clair College
Windsor, Ontario

Marilyn M. Mohr, RN, MSN
Instructor
Missouri Baptist Medical Center
School of Nursing
St. Louis, Missouri

Donna S. Thomas, RN, BSN, MSN
Nursing Instructor
Lutheran Medical Center
School of Nursing
St. Louis, Missouri

Mary Wellhaven, RN, PhD
Assistant Professor
College of Nursing and Health Sciences
Winona State University—Rochester Center
Rochester, Minnesota

Teresa A. Zayac, BSN, RN
Instructor
Practical Nurse Program
Canton City Schools
Canton, Ohio

Preface

Accurate calculation of medication dosages is critical to the delivery of safe, competent patient care. Yet many students and beginning health care professionals struggle to master this essential skill. Some need to improve their understanding of basic math before they can apply math skills to drug calculation. *Simplified Drugs and Solutions for Health Care Professionals* is designed to ensure that all students can learn to competently and confidently calculate medication dosages. Explanations throughout the book are clear and concise; examples reinforce and clarify the discussions. Many explanations have been rewritten and expanded. Key concepts are highlighted for emphasis and easy retrieval.

Students can assess their math abilities by taking the math pretest at the beginning of the book. For those needing further study, Unit I provides an extensive review of the basic processes of arithmetic. New content in this unit guides students in calculating percentages. Unit II discusses systems of weights and measures. Emphasis is placed on the metric/SI system and commonly used equivalents. Two methods of converting temperature are included in the unit. Tables summarizing equivalent units are printed on the inside covers of the book for quick reference. A list of common medication abbreviations can also be found on the back pages of the book. Pretests have been added to Units II and III for preliminary skill assessment.

Unit III, Dosages and Solutions, has been extensively revised to enhance learning and to reflect changes in clinical practice. Three methods for solving problems—two variations of ratio and proportion and the *"desired" over "have" times "quantity"* formula are presented. Students are encouraged to select the method with which they feel most comfortable and use that method consistently. Discussions of various types of dosage calculation include all three methods.

Many new practice problems are included in this edition. To help students prepare for what they will encounter in clinical practice, reproductions of actual drug labels and illustrations of syringes accompany the problems. The larger page size and additional space between problems enable students to work out solutions on the book pages. Answers to all problems are provided at the end of the book. Many new tables and figures have been added. Each chapter in Unit III contains questions to encourage the student to ✤THINK CRITICALLY about some aspect of dosage and solutions. These chapters present patient situations that require solutions. Other new content includes examples of medication administration records (MAR), additional examples of physician order forms, instruction on the reading of orders for intravenous therapy, information on the strength and tonicity of intravenous solutions, and more tables and figures. Practice problems have been added to the chapter on geriatric dosages. A new chapter, Home Care

Considerations, has been added. A comprehensive posttest, new to this edition, is included at the end of the book.

Parts of Chapter 15 and all of Chapters 16 and 17 were co-authored with my good friend and colleague, Mary Ellen Kitundu M. Ed, RN, Assistant Professor, College of Nursing and Health Sciences, Winona State University, Winona, Minnesota.

Many of the changes in this edition were based on comments from students and faculty. Any suggestions for future editions would be deeply appreciated.

Acknowledgments

I would like to thank the following companies for allowing the reproduction of actual drug labels and medical equipment in the book.

> Abbott Laboratories
> Apex Medical Corporation
> Apothecon
> Baxter Healthcare Corporation
> Burroughs Wellcome Co.
> Ciba-Geigy Corporation
> CompuMed, Inc.
> Du Pont Merck
> Du Pont Pharma
> Eli Lilly and Company
> Fujisawa USA, Inc.
> Glaxo Wellcome
> IMED Corporation
> Johnson & Johnson
> Marion Merrell Dow Inc.
> Mayo Clinic
> Medic Alert Foundation United States
> Novo Nordisk Pharmaceuticals Inc.
> Ortho Pharmaceutical Corporation
> Pfizer Inc.
> Roche Products, Inc.
> Roxane Laboratories, Inc.
> SmithKline Beecham
> The Upjohn Company
> Upsher-Smith Laboratories, Inc.
> Warner-Lambert Company
> Wyeth-Ayerst Laboratories

Norma Dison

Contents

Introduction

Unit One   **Basic Arithmetic**   1
Pretest   2

1. **Roman Numerals and Arabic Numbers**   9
   Combination of Basic Roman Numerals   10

2. **Fractions**   13
   Types of Fractions   14
   Expressing Fractions in Higher or Lowest Terms   14
   Changing Improper Fractions to Mixed Numbers   17
   Changing Mixed Numbers to Improper Fractions   18
   Comparing the Size of Fractions   19
   Adding Fractions   22
   Subtracting Fractions   26
   Multiplying Fractions   28
   Dividing Fractions   30

3. **Decimals**   33
   Rounding Decimals   34
   Adding Decimals   38
   Subtracting Decimals   39
   Multiplying Decimals   40
   Dividing Decimals   43
   Comparing the Value of Decimals   45

4. **Percentage**   47

5. **Fractions, Decimals, and Percentages**   51

6. **Ratio and Proportion**   55
   Ratio   55
   Proportion   58
   Unit One Posttest   60

Unit Two   **Systems of Weights and Measures**
Pretest   65

7. **Weight and Volume: Metric/SI and Apothecaries' Systems**   69
   Metric/SI System   69
       Changing Greater Units to Lesser Units   71
       Changing Lesser Units to Greater Units   72

Apothecaries' System 76
  Approximate Equivalents: Metric/SI and Apothecaries' Systems 79

8 Household Measures 83

9 Linear Units of Measure 89
Metric/SI System 89
Metric/SI-English Conversions 93

10 Temperature Conversion: Celsius (Centigrade) and Fahrenheit 96
Formulas Using Decimals 97
Formulas Using Fractions 98
Unit Two Posttest 101

Unit Three Dosages and Solutions
Pretest 107

11 Interpretation and Implementation of Physician's Order 123
Legal Aspects of Drug Therapy 124
Medication Orders 124
  Types of Medication Orders 126
  Drugs Supplies and Storage 127
  Medication or Identification Cards 133
  Interpreting Medication Orders 134
  Components of Medication Orders 135
  Times of Administration 136
  Twenty-Four Hour or Military Time 138
  Transcribing Orders 140
  Checking the Transcribed Order 141
Reading Medication Labels 142
  Preparing the Dose Ordered 144
Administering the Drug 144
  Documentation and Observation 146
Patient Education 151
Storage and Control of Drugs 152

12 Computation of Oral Dosages 156
Review of Ratio and Proportion 156
Checking Calculations 157
Oral Tablets and Capsules 158
Dosage Calculations Using the Same Units of Measure 159
Methods of Calculation 159
  Method 1: Using 2 Ratios Established by Drug Label and Prescribed Dose 160
  Method 2: Dosage Formula 161
  Method 3: Using 2 Ratios Established According to Size 161
Assess Whether the Answer is Reasonable 162
Using Different Size Units of Measure in the Metric/SI System 170
Using Two Sizes of Tablets or Capsules 173
Using Different Systems of Measurement 178

13 Computation of Dosage from Solutions: Oral, Injectable, and Diluted 181
Oral Solutions of Drugs 182
Intramuscular and Subcutaneous Injections: Prepackaged Sterile Solutions 188

Reconstitution and Dosage of Crystalline and Powdered Drugs: Oral and
    Injectable *193*
    Injectable Solutions *193*
    Oral Solutions *195*
Preparing External Solutions from Stronger Drugs *199*

14 Insulin Dosage *202*
Hypoglycemia and Hyperglycemia *202*
Sources of Insulin *204*
Strength of Insulin *204*
Insulin Syringes *204*
Insulin Labels *206*
Activity Time Spans *206*

15 Intravenous Fluids and Medications *213*
Reading Orders for Intravenous Therapy *214*
    Computerized Orders *217*
Calculating the Rate of Flow *221*
    Calculating the Rate of Flow in Milliliters/Hour *223*
    Calculating the Rate of Flow in Drops *224*
    Using the Rate of Flow when Milliliters/Hour is Known *224*
Estimating the Rate of Flow *227*
Increasing the Rate of Flow by a Specified Percent *228*
Keep Open Rate of Flow *231*
Intravenous Medications *232*
    Compatibility of Medications with Each Other and Intravenous Solutions *233*
    Intermittent Administration of Medications *235*
    Volume Control Chambers *236*
    Heparin Lock *237*
    Flushing Intravenous Lines *238*
Determining Flow Rate for Administering Specific Amount of Drug in a Specified
    Amount of Time *238*
Determining the Amount of Drug that has been Administered in a Particular
    Amount of Solution *239*

16 Heparin Dosage and Administration *240*
Heparin Administration *240*
    Measurement of Heparin *241*
Calculations for Intravenous Administration of Heparin *241*

17 Critical Care Dosages *245*

18 Pediatric Dosages *251*
Calculation of Dosage Based on Weight in Kilograms *251*
Calculation of Dosage Based on Body Surface Area *257*
    Formula for Estimating BSA in m^2 *257*
Estimating Body Surface Area Using the West Nomogram *259*
Clark's Formula *260*
Young's Formula *260*

19 Geriatric Dosages *261*
Physiologic Factors *261*
Drug Interactions *261*
Drug Compatibility *262*

Contents

    Older Adults' Compliance with Drug Therapy *262*
    Nursing Interventions that Reduce Drug Therapy *265*
    Storage of Medicines *265*
    Disposal of Drugs that are No Longer Needed *265*
    Computation of Geriatric Dosages *265*

20 **Home Care Considerations** *269*
    Teaching the Patient and Family Members About Drug Therapy at Home *269*
    Psychology of Medicating *270*
    Basic Medication Information that the Patient Should Know *271*
    Remembering and Complying with Medication Schedule *274*
    Safeguarding the Welfare of Patients *276*
    Over-the-Counter Drugs *277*
    Obtaining Medications *278*
    Home Storage of Medications *278*
    Unit Three Posttest *280*
    Comprehensive Posttest *283*
    Answers to Problems *294*

Introduction

Considerable responsibility accompanies the preparation and administration of medications. This responsibility includes giving the right drug, in the right dose, at the right time, to the right person. The health care professional can administer medications only as prescribed by the physician. However, the health care professional is legally responsible for the administration of drugs. This means that health care professionals must be familiar with their patients' medical conditions. They must also know how the prescribed drugs are expected to affect the patient, the usual range of dosage for the medication, the route of administration, precautions to be followed preceding and following the administration of the medication, and the signs and symptoms of side effects.

The health care professional assumes legal, moral, and ethical responsibilities when administering drugs. The patient and the family must be instructed about medications that are given. If the medications are to be continued at home, the health care provider is responsible for helping the patient develop a reasonable schedule for taking each drug. The provider must make sure the patient understands the accompanying information and precautions for the drug being taken. Teaching patients and their families about medications requires knowledge, patience, willingness to repeat information, and the ability to individualize instructions. The provider must allow opportunity for the patient to practice administering the medication.

The health care professional uses the basic arithmetic of daily living that is taught in elementary school in calculating dosages and in mixing solutions. Review and practice facilitates skill in the basic processes used in solving the problems of drugs and solutions. Unit I of this book reviews basic arithmetic, Unit II presents different systems of measurement and conversion from one system of measurement to another, and Unit III covers types of problems that may be encountered in clinical practice. When problems are worked that require converting from one system of measurement to another, answers that differ from each other by as much as 10% may result. An amount greater than this is certain to be in error. In problems that do not require conversion from one system of measurement to another, no margin of error is permitted. It must be remembered that an answer is either right or wrong when working problems that involve drugs and solutions.

In addition to having considerable knowledge about the particular drugs and patients, health care professionals also recheck the orders, drug preparations, and doses carefully before administration, and check again whenever patients question whether a medication is the correct one. These practices help ensure the safety of patients. If the health professional has doubts or questions about a medication, dose, or a calculation, it is wise to ask an appropriate health professional or the supervisor to also check. The pharmacist is an excellent resource person to consult when questions arise about medications, and the physician should be consulted when there are questions about the order for medications.

Agency policies concerning administration of medications vary. Those agencies that have in-service training for new employees may not allow health professionals to administer medications until they have completed the unit on medications and have undergone appropriate orientation and supervision.

Unit One

Basic Arithmetic

Skill and accuracy in basic arithmetical processes are essential when computing dosages. Completing the arithmetic pretest will allow assessment of student mastery of knowledge in basic arithmetic.

Basic arithmetic processes are reviewed in this unit. Roman numerals, although used infrequently, are included because a few drugs are labeled and a few dosages are ordered using the apothecaries' system of measurement. Knowledge of fractions, decimals, and percentages is needed for most calculations. This section reviews the methods and rules for working with these processes. Exercises provide practice in assessment of knowledge, skill, and accuracy.

It is recognized that pocket calculators and computers are used extensively to solve problems. However, knowing and understanding the basic concepts needed to solve problems involving dosages is mandatory. The health care professional who is able to work problems manually and with proficiency will not be handicapped when an operational calculator is unavailable or manual calculations require rechecking. Whether a hand-held calculator is provided by the agency or carried by the health professional, it must be in working order. Ascertaining that a calculator works correctly should be done prior to each shift. Despite regular checks, calculators may not operate properly. One must be able to solve problems if a calculator is not available. Therefore it is strongly recommended that some or all of the problems in this book be worked manually.

When using a calculator, one must enter the information correctly. Always check to be sure that the numbers and arithmetical operation or function entered are correct. Rechecking manual calculations with a calculator and rechecking answers manually when using a calculator is encouraged.

Whether a problem is worked manually or with the aid of a calculator, always evaluate the answer in terms of the question, "Is this answer reasonable?" If unsure, it is wise to ask another professional to work the problem. When doing this, presenting the problem to the other person, rather then telling or showing them how you have worked the problem, will avoid bias.

Unit One Pretest

EXPLANATION: The following pretest is useful for identifying areas in which arithmetic review is needed. Complete the pretest and check answers. Analyze the reasons for making each error. If more than one problem in a group is answered incorrectly, review the appropriate section in Chapters 1 through 6.

Express in Roman numerals:

1. 5 _____
2. 38 _____
3. 18 _____

4. 56 _____
5. 49 _____
6. 65 _____

7. 115 _____
8. 29 _____
9. 12 _____

Express in Arabic numbers:

10. XXXIII _____
11. XV _____
12. XXIV _____

13. XIV _____
14. XCIV _____
15. CIV _____

16. MC _____
17. CXIII _____
18. LVIII _____

Reduce the following fractions to lowest terms:

19. $\frac{4}{8} =$
20. $\frac{4}{18} =$
21. $\frac{10}{16} =$

22. $\frac{5}{100} =$
23. $\frac{5}{25} =$
24. $\frac{14}{49} =$

Change the following fractions to the higher terms indicated:

25. $\dfrac{3}{4} = \dfrac{}{100}$
26. $\dfrac{4}{5} = \dfrac{}{25}$
27. $\dfrac{5}{7} = \dfrac{}{49}$

28. $\dfrac{1}{3} = \dfrac{}{39}$
29. $\dfrac{3}{8} = \dfrac{}{16}$
30. $\dfrac{5}{6} = \dfrac{}{42}$

Change the following improper fractions to whole or mixed numbers:

31. $\dfrac{32}{8} =$
32. $\dfrac{38}{5} =$
33. $\dfrac{342}{24} =$

34. $\dfrac{56}{3} =$
35. $\dfrac{35}{6} =$
36. $\dfrac{133}{11} =$

37. $\dfrac{18}{5} =$
38. $\dfrac{77}{9} =$
39. $\dfrac{29}{7} =$

Change the following mixed numbers to improper fractions:

40. $3\dfrac{1}{2} =$
41. $4\dfrac{3}{5} =$
42. $4\dfrac{1}{3} =$

43. $13\dfrac{2}{9} =$
44. $6\dfrac{2}{7} =$
45. $43\dfrac{3}{8} =$

Circle the *lesser* fractions:

46. $\dfrac{1}{3}$ or $\dfrac{5}{6}$
47. $\dfrac{2}{3}$ or $\dfrac{2}{9}$

48. $\dfrac{4}{9}$ or $\dfrac{5}{7}$
49. $\dfrac{3}{5}$ or $\dfrac{7}{10}$

Add the following fractions and mixed numbers (reduce answers to lowest terms):

50. $\dfrac{4}{5}$
    $\dfrac{7}{10}$
    $\dfrac{8}{25}$

51. $\dfrac{2}{5}$
    $\dfrac{7}{8}$
    $\dfrac{3}{10}$

52. $5\dfrac{3}{5}$
    $7\dfrac{2}{9}$
    $2\dfrac{4}{45}$

53. $2\dfrac{3}{4}$
    $7\dfrac{4}{7}$
    $8\dfrac{1}{14}$

Subtract the following fractions and mixed numbers (reduce answers to lowest terms):

54. $\dfrac{3}{8} - \dfrac{1}{3} =$

55. $\dfrac{3}{4} - \dfrac{4}{9} =$

56. $2 - 1\dfrac{3}{7} =$

57. $5\dfrac{2}{3} - \dfrac{5}{6} =$

Multiply the following fractions and mixed numbers (reduce answers to lowest terms):

58. $\dfrac{4}{5} \times \dfrac{7}{8} =$

59. $12 \times \dfrac{4}{9} =$

60. $1\dfrac{6}{7} \times \dfrac{3}{8} =$

61. $5\dfrac{3}{4} \times \dfrac{7}{10} =$

Divide the following fractions and mixed numbers:

62. $\dfrac{5}{7} \div \dfrac{6}{10} =$

63. $\dfrac{1}{8} \div 4\dfrac{1}{4} =$

64. $5 \div \dfrac{1}{2} =$

65. $5\dfrac{1}{8} \div 3\dfrac{7}{8} =$

Write the words for the following:

66. 3.25 _____

67. 1.5 _____

68. 201.16 _____

69. 432.868 _____

Change the following fractions to decimals (carry out three decimal places when necessary):

70. $\dfrac{5}{6} =$

71. $\dfrac{7}{8} =$

72. $\dfrac{6}{7} =$

73. $\dfrac{9}{10} =$

Change the following fractions and mixed numbers to decimals:

74. $\dfrac{3}{10} =$

75. $\dfrac{5}{8} =$

76. $5\dfrac{1}{4} =$

77. $3\dfrac{4}{5} =$

Change the following decimals to fractions (reduce answers to lowest terms):

78. 0.4 =

79. 0.06 =

80. 0.05 =

81. 0.015 =

Add the following decimals:

82.   0.4785
            0.428
       +0.8
	83. 0.4
	            0.048
	       +0.33
		84. 0.763
		            0.492
		       +0.6

85.   34.47
            48.62
       +863.52
	86. 74.24
	            0.665
	       +33.8
		87. 62.46
		            794.35
		       +2400.80

Subtract the following decimals:

88.   62.5
         −45.1

89.   44.38
        − 7.92

90.   843.24
         −318.95

91.   239
        −   9.02

Multiply the following decimals:

92.   38.45
         ×   0.3

93.   66.10
         × 0.40

94.   420
         ×0.15

95.   97.7
         ×0.0804

Divide the following numbers, rounding to hundredths when necessary:

96. 54 ÷ 22.7 =

97. 12.4 ÷ 3.4 =

98. 4.7 ÷ 11.3 =

99. 24.93 ÷ 7.2 =

100. 142.5 ÷ 3.8 =

101. 421.2 ÷ 12.75 =

102. 18.08 ÷ 11.27 =

103. 14.27 ÷ 6.032 =

Circle the *greater* of the two decimals:

104. 0.2   or   0.5

105. 0.02   or   0.025

106. 0.750   or   0.075

107. 0.15   or   0.02

108. 0.03   or   0.375

109. 0.07   or   0.4

Solve the following percentage problems:

110. 0.75% of 300 =

111. 0.4% of 200 =

112. 0.5% of 175 =

113. 15% of 500 =

Rewrite the following fractions as ratios, percentages, and decimals:

	Fraction	Ratio	Decimal	Percentage
114.	$\frac{1}{100}$ =	_____ =	_____ =	_____
115.	$\frac{3}{4}$ =	_____ =	_____ =	_____
116.	$\frac{3}{50}$ =	_____ =	_____ =	_____
117.	$\frac{1}{5}$ =	_____ =	_____ =	_____

Solve for x in the following proportions:

118. $1:4 = 6:x$

119. $5:22 = x:66$

120. $0.25:14 = 0.75:x$

121. $\frac{1}{3}:x = \frac{3}{5}:15$

122. $\frac{1}{8}:1 = x:16$

123. $14:x = \frac{7}{8}:10$

1

Roman Numerals and Arabic Numbers

Interpretation of drug orders sometimes requires knowledge of both Roman numerals and Arabic numbers. Roman numerals are used when the dosage of a drug is ordered in the apothecaries' system of measurement. *Roman numerals above thirty are seldom used in prescribing dosage.* When the small letter *i* is used for the Roman numeral *one*, it is usually dotted. On rare occasions the last *i* in a series is written as a *j*. The use of Arabic numbers has largely replaced the use of Roman numerals. This simplifies arithmetical processes. The following list shows the Arabic equivalents for Roman numerals.

Arabic	Roman	Arabic	Roman
1	I	19	XIX
2	II	20	XX
3	III	21	XXI
4	IV	22	XXII
5	V	23	XXIII
6	VI	24	XXIV
7	VII	25	XXV
8	VIII	26	XXVI
9	IX	27	XXVII
10	X	28	XXVIII
11	XI	29	XXIX
12	XII	30	XXX
13	XIII	40	XL
14	XIV	50	L
15	XV	100	C
16	XVI	500	D
17	XVII	1000	M
18	XVIII		

COMBINATION OF BASIC ROMAN NUMERALS

✔ Basic Roman numerals include I, V, X, L, C, D, and M. A combination of Roman numerals may be used to express a numerical value. **To represent a value with combinations of Roman numerals, those numerals with the highest values are used.** For example, X (not VV) would be used to represent 10 and XX (not VVVV or XVV) would be used to represent 20. Acceptable combinations are illustrated in the preceding list.

The numerals, I, X, and C are not repeated more then three times. If that seems necessary, subtraction is used. For example, IV is used rather than IIII; and IX is used rather than VIIII.

✔ ADDITION: *To increase the value of a Roman numeral, place one or more Roman numerals after (to the right of) it.*

Beginning with a numeral having a value of X (10) or more, the same numeral or one of lesser value may be used to add value to the numeral.

EXAMPLES: XI = 11   XVI = 16   XXV = 25

✔ SUBTRACTION: *Placing one Roman numeral of lesser value in front of the basic numeral removes value from it.*

EXAMPLES: IV = 4   IX = 9   XIX = 19   XCI = 91

EXERCISE 1 (answers on page 295)

Fill in the correct Roman numerals:

1. 9 _____
2. 7 _____
3. 26 _____

4. 15 _____
5. 24 _____
6. 19 _____

7. 8 _____
8. 3 _____
9. 16 _____

10. 28 _____
11. 22 _____
12. 1 _____

13. 61 _____
14. 11 _____
15. 20 _____

16. 42 _____
17. 4 _____
18. 13 _____

19. 34 _____
20. 50 _____
21. 1000 _____

22. 90 _____
23. 6 _____
24. 200 _____

25. 12 _____

Fill in the correct Arabic numbers:

26. IV _____   27. VII _____   28. X _____

29. III _____   30. VI _____   31. XIX _____

32. XV _____   33. VIII _____   34. XXX _____

35. XI _____   36. V _____   37. XXIV _____

38. XL _____   39. XIII _____   40. MM _____

41. XXXIX _____   42. XXXV _____   43. II _____

44. XIV _____   45. IX _____   46. XII _____

47. CCCLVIII _____   48. LX _____   49. D _____

50. C _____

2 Fractions

Proficiency in manipulating the addition, subtraction, multiplication, and division of common fractions is necessary if a dose of medication is prescribed using common fractions for an amount less than one. The following review of fractions is designed to aid in recalling basic knowledge of fractions.

A *fraction is part of a whole number or one number divided by another number.* The number above the dividing line is called the *numerator.* It indicates the number of parts of the whole number that are being used. The number below the line is called the *denominator,* and it indicates the number of parts into which the whole is divided.

The number above the dividing line is called the numerator and the number below the line is called the denominator.

$$\frac{1 \text{ (Numerator)}}{2 \text{ (Denominator)}}$$

The numerator indicates the number of parts of a whole number that are being used. The denominator indicates the number of parts into which the whole is being divided.

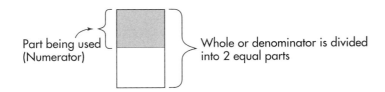

In the fraction ³⁄₈, the whole is divided into 8 equal parts (represented as the denominator) but only 3 parts (the numerator) are being used.

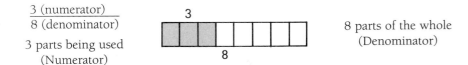

A fraction that has the same numerator and denominator equals the whole number 1. For example, ⁴⁄₄ means that the whole number 1 has been divided into 4 equal parts, and all 4 parts are being used.

✔ *A denominator represents a divisor, a numerator represents a dividend, and, if division is performed, the answer obtained represents a quotient.*

TYPES OF FRACTIONS

Five kinds of fractions are used. These are defined as follows:

Common fractions. The numerator and denominator are both whole numbers.

EXAMPLES: $\dfrac{3}{4} \quad \dfrac{1}{2} \quad \dfrac{5}{2}$

Proper fractions. (sometimes called "true fractions"). The numerator is always less than the denominator.

EXAMPLES: $\dfrac{5}{6} \quad \dfrac{1}{8} \quad \dfrac{1}{4}$

Improper fractions. The numerator is always greater than the denominator.

EXAMPLES: $\dfrac{4}{1} \quad \dfrac{6}{5} \quad \dfrac{16}{9}$

Improper fractions may be changed to mixed numbers and mixed numbers may be changed to improper fractions.

Mixed numbers. A whole number is combined with a fraction.

EXAMPLES: $2\dfrac{3}{4} \quad 3\dfrac{1}{3} \quad 2\dfrac{4}{5}$

Complex fractions. The numerator, the denominator, or both are a proper fraction, an improper fraction, or a mixed number.

EXAMPLES: $\dfrac{2}{1\frac{1}{4}} \quad \dfrac{\frac{1}{2}}{6} \quad \dfrac{\frac{1}{3}}{\frac{1}{4}} \quad \dfrac{\frac{7}{5}}{\frac{19}{20}}$

EXPRESSING FRACTIONS IN HIGHER OR LOWEST TERMS

✔ *If both the numerator and the denominator of a fraction are multiplied by the same number, the value of the fraction remains unchanged.*

EXAMPLES: $\dfrac{3}{4} \times \dfrac{2}{2} = \dfrac{6}{8} \text{ or } \dfrac{3}{4} \qquad \dfrac{5}{10} \times \dfrac{5}{5} = \dfrac{25}{50} = \dfrac{5}{10} \text{ or } \dfrac{1}{2}$

✔ *A fraction may be reduced to lower terms by dividing both the numerator and the denominator by the same number.* A fraction is said to have been reduced to its lowest terms when it is no longer possible to divide the numerator and denominator by the same number. *Reducing a fraction to lowest terms does not change the value of the fraction.*

Because it is easier to work with smaller fractions, it is customary to express fractions in their lowest terms. To reduce fractions, divide both the numerator and denominator by the same number.

EXAMPLES: $\frac{6}{8}\left(\div\frac{2}{2}\right)=\frac{3}{4}$ $\frac{5}{10}\left(\div\frac{5}{5}\right)=\frac{1}{2}$ $\frac{3}{12}\left(\div\frac{3}{3}\right)=\frac{1}{4}$

It is permissible to cancel out or reduce the fraction by dividing both the numerator and the denominator by the same number.

EXAMPLES: $\frac{\cancel{20}^{1}}{\cancel{100}_{5}}=\frac{1}{5}$ $\frac{\cancel{125}^{1}}{\cancel{250}_{2}}=\frac{1}{2}$

If both the numerator and denominator end in zero, the same number of zeros must be cancelled out in each. For each zero cancelled out of the numerator, the same number of zeros must be cancelled out in the denominator.

EXAMPLES: $\frac{1\cancel{0}}{2\cancel{0}}$ $\frac{2\cancel{0}}{40\cancel{0}}$ $\frac{30\cancel{0}}{500\cancel{0}}$

First the zeros are cancelled, which is the same as dividing both the numerator and the denominator by the same number, then the fraction is reduced to its lowest terms. Divide both the numerator and denominator by the largest possible number. One way to find the largest possible number is to determine whether the numerator will divide evenly into the denominator. In the example, $\frac{20}{100}$, the numerator, 20, will divide evenly into the denominator, 100. A cancellation mark is placed through the numerator, 20, and a 1 is placed above it. A cancellation mark is placed through 100, and a 5 (representing the number of times 20 divides evenly into 100) is placed below it. $\frac{\cancel{20}^{1}}{\cancel{100}_{5}}=\frac{1}{5}$ If one zero in the numerator and another in the denominator are cancelled out, the fraction is reduced as follows:

$$\frac{2\cancel{0}}{10\cancel{0}}=\frac{\cancel{2}^{1}}{\cancel{10}_{5}}=\frac{1}{5}$$

EXERCISE 1 *(answers on page 295)*

Express the following fractions in lowest terms:

1. $\frac{6}{10}=$

2. $\frac{6}{12}=$

3. $\frac{4}{20}=$

4. $\frac{48}{98}=$

5. $\frac{15}{24}=$

6. $\frac{18}{72}=$

EXERCISE 1—cont'd

7. $\dfrac{4}{8} =$ 8. $\dfrac{5}{10} =$ 9. $\dfrac{24}{64} =$

10. $\dfrac{9}{12} =$ 11. $\dfrac{5}{40} =$ 12. $\dfrac{10}{45} =$

13. $\dfrac{6}{9} =$ 14. $\dfrac{14}{16} =$ 15. $\dfrac{8}{128} =$

16. $\dfrac{45}{90} =$ 17. $\dfrac{8}{12} =$ 18. $\dfrac{9}{27} =$

19. $\dfrac{12}{20} =$ 20. $\dfrac{8}{10} =$ 21. $\dfrac{4}{32} =$

22. $\dfrac{5}{100} =$ 23. $\dfrac{5}{20} =$ 24. $\dfrac{6}{24} =$ 25. $\dfrac{200}{600} =$

Express the following fractions in the higher terms indicated:

26. $\dfrac{3}{8} = \dfrac{}{16}$ 27. $\dfrac{2}{25} = \dfrac{}{50}$ 28. $\dfrac{7}{10} = \dfrac{}{100}$

29. $\dfrac{4}{5} = \dfrac{}{25}$ 30. $\dfrac{1}{4} = \dfrac{}{12}$ 31. $\dfrac{3}{12} = \dfrac{}{144}$

32. $\dfrac{3}{5} = \dfrac{}{10}$ 33. $\dfrac{2}{3} = \dfrac{}{21}$ 34. $\dfrac{6}{11} = \dfrac{}{121}$

35. $\dfrac{5}{6} = \dfrac{}{150}$ 36. $\dfrac{3}{9} = \dfrac{}{27}$ 37. $\dfrac{1}{2} = \dfrac{}{8}$

38. $\dfrac{3}{8} = \dfrac{}{16}$ 39. $\dfrac{11}{14} = \dfrac{}{28}$ 40. $\dfrac{3}{7} = \dfrac{}{21}$

41. $\dfrac{1}{3} = \dfrac{}{9}$ 42. $\dfrac{3}{4} = \dfrac{}{8}$ 43. $\dfrac{4}{5} = \dfrac{}{25}$

44. $\dfrac{2}{3} = \dfrac{}{9}$ 45. $\dfrac{5}{8} = \dfrac{}{64}$ 46. $\dfrac{2}{5} = \dfrac{}{40}$

47. $\dfrac{2}{19} = \dfrac{}{38}$ 48. $\dfrac{5}{6} = \dfrac{}{18}$ 49. $\dfrac{7}{10} = \dfrac{}{100}$

50. $\dfrac{8}{9} = \dfrac{}{45}$

CHANGING IMPROPER FRACTIONS TO MIXED NUMBERS

✔ *An improper fraction can be changed to a mixed number by dividing the numerator by the denominator.*

EXAMPLE: $\dfrac{6}{5} = 5\overline{)6.0}^{\,1.2}$

or

$$\dfrac{6}{5} = 6 \div 5 = \begin{array}{r} 1.2 \\ 5\overline{)6.0} \\ \underline{5} \\ 10 \\ \underline{10} \end{array}$$

Alternatively, the remainder may be placed over the denominator (the divisor). In the above example the answer could be stated as $1\dfrac{2}{10}$ or $1\dfrac{1}{5}$ instead of 1.2.

EXERCISE 2   (answers on page 295)

Change the following improper fractions to mixed or whole numbers, and reduce the answers to lowest terms:

1. $\dfrac{14}{2} =$ 2. $\dfrac{4}{2} =$ 3. $\dfrac{24}{6} =$

4. $\dfrac{48}{12} =$ 5. $\dfrac{15}{4} =$ 6. $\dfrac{81}{9} =$

7. $\dfrac{10}{5} =$ 8. $\dfrac{45}{15} =$ 9. $\dfrac{15}{10} =$

EXERCISE 2—cont'd

10. $\dfrac{21}{9} =$ 11. $\dfrac{45}{8} =$ 12. $\dfrac{7}{2} =$

13. $\dfrac{38}{7} =$ 14. $\dfrac{54}{7} =$ 15. $\dfrac{19}{3} =$

16. $\dfrac{10}{8} =$ 17. $\dfrac{11}{3} =$ 18. $\dfrac{5}{3} =$

19. $\dfrac{55}{3} =$ 20. $\dfrac{25}{4} =$ 21. $\dfrac{23}{5} =$

22. $\dfrac{42}{8} =$ 23. $\dfrac{40}{3} =$ 24. $\dfrac{75}{11} =$

25. $\dfrac{28}{9} =$

CHANGING MIXED NUMBERS TO IMPROPER FRACTIONS

✔ *A mixed number is changed to an improper fraction by multiplying the whole number by the denominator of the fraction and adding the numerator of the fraction to the result.* Only a mixed number can be changed to an *improper* fraction, and the numerator will always be greater than the denominator.

EXAMPLES: $2\dfrac{1}{2} = \dfrac{(2 \times 2) + 1}{2} = \dfrac{5}{2}$ $3\dfrac{3}{4} = \dfrac{(3 \times 4) + 3}{4} = \dfrac{15}{4}$

EXERCISE 3   (answers on page 295)

Change the following mixed numbers to improper fractions:

1. $2\dfrac{4}{9} =$ 2. $2\dfrac{3}{7} =$ 3. $7\dfrac{1}{2} =$

4. $7\dfrac{2}{3} =$ 5. $6\dfrac{1}{2} =$ 6. $4\dfrac{2}{5} =$

7. $7\dfrac{5}{8} =$ 8. $10\dfrac{3}{5} =$ 9. $7\dfrac{1}{8} =$

10. $10\frac{2}{5} =$ 11. $8\frac{4}{5} =$ 12. $5\frac{2}{3} =$

13. $6\frac{4}{5} =$ 14. $3\frac{7}{8} =$ 15. $9\frac{3}{10} =$

16. $6\frac{1}{4} =$ 17. $5\frac{5}{6} =$ 18. $4\frac{2}{9} =$

19. $9\frac{3}{5} =$ 20. $8\frac{2}{25} =$ 21. $4\frac{7}{100} =$

22. $7\frac{6}{7} =$ 23. $5\frac{1}{2} =$ 24. $4\frac{2}{7} =$

25. $22\frac{3}{4} =$

COMPARING THE SIZE OF FRACTIONS

It is sometimes necessary to determine which of two fractions is the greater, or, if more than two, which is the greatest. Proceed as follows:

To compare the size of fractions, determine if the fractions have the same numerator.

✔ *If two fractions have numerators that are alike, the fraction with the smallest denominator is the greatest.*

For example, the fractions ½ and ¼ have the same numerator (1), but have different denominators (2 or 4). Because there are fewer parts in 2 than in 4, ½ is a larger fraction than ¼. If two rectangles of equal size are divided into 2 or 4 parts, the rectangles look like this:

EXAMPLES:

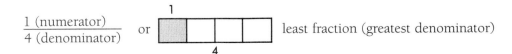

$\frac{1 \text{ (numerator)}}{2 \text{ (denominator)}}$ or greatest fraction (least denominator)

$\frac{1 \text{ (numerator)}}{4 \text{ (denominator)}}$ or least fraction (greatest denominator)

If only one part of each rectangle is used, the fractions would be ½ and ¼, and ½ would be greater than ¼.

Another way to compare the sizes is to find the common denominator of both fractions. For the fractions, ½ and ¼, 4 is the common denominator; therefore ½ is the same as 2/4. The diagrams that follow illustrate that 2/4 or ½ is greater than ¼.

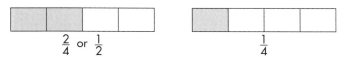

✔ *If two fractions have the same denominators, the fraction with the greater numerator is the greater fraction.*

EXAMPLES:

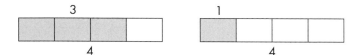

The fractions ¼ and ¾ have the same denominator (4). The fraction having the most parts being used (as shown by the numerator 3) is the greater of the two fractions.

EXERCISE 4

(answers on page 296)

Circle the *greater* fraction in each of the following pairs:

1. $\frac{1}{49}$ or $\frac{3}{49}$
2. $\frac{1}{10}$ or $\frac{9}{10}$
3. $\frac{2}{25}$ or $\frac{3}{25}$
4. $\frac{7}{10}$ or $\frac{3}{10}$
5. $\frac{1}{5}$ or $\frac{2}{5}$
6. $\frac{2}{7}$ or $\frac{1}{7}$
7. $\frac{6}{7}$ or $\frac{5}{7}$
8. $\frac{4}{5}$ or $\frac{3}{5}$
9. $\frac{3}{125}$ or $\frac{1}{125}$
10. $\frac{7}{15}$ or $\frac{9}{15}$
11. $\frac{1}{100}$ or $\frac{1}{150}$
12. $\frac{1}{125}$ or $\frac{1}{150}$

✔ *If fractions have the same denominator but different numerators (for example ⅛, ⅜, ⅞), the fraction with the greatest numerator is the greatest fraction, so ⅞ would be the greatest of these three fractions.*

This is illustrated by the following drawings:

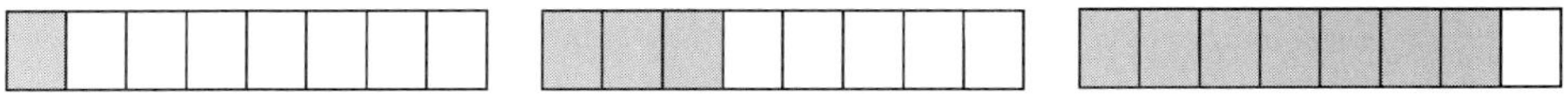

$\frac{1}{8}$ $\frac{3}{8}$ $\frac{7}{8}$

Circle the *lesser* fraction in each of the following pairs:

13. $\frac{2}{5}$ or $\frac{3}{5}$

14. $\frac{3}{50}$ or $\frac{4}{50}$

15. $\frac{1}{6}$ or $\frac{5}{6}$

16. $\frac{4}{5}$ or $\frac{3}{5}$

17. $\frac{7}{24}$ or $\frac{3}{24}$

18. $\frac{3}{75}$ or $\frac{1}{75}$

19. $\frac{4}{150}$ or $\frac{1}{150}$

20. $\frac{3}{10}$ or $\frac{8}{10}$

21. $\frac{9}{70}$ or $\frac{11}{70}$

22. $\frac{1}{125}$ or $\frac{2}{125}$

23. $\frac{4}{150}$ or $\frac{1}{150}$

24. $\frac{1}{200}$ or $\frac{3}{200}$

✔ ***When the numerators and denominators differ, as in $2/3$, $5/6$, $7/9$, it is possible to determine which is greatest and which is least by changing the fractions so that all the denominators are the same.*** This is done by finding a denominator that is common to all the fractions. For the fractions, $2/3$, $5/6$, $7/9$, the number 18 could be the common denominator. Each of these denominators would divide into 18; that is, they could all have 18 as a dividend. Both the *numerator* and the *denominator* of a fraction would have to be multiplied by the same number to keep the fractions balanced.

EXAMPLES: $\frac{2}{3} \times \frac{6}{6} = \frac{12}{18}$ $\frac{5}{6} \times \frac{3}{3} = \frac{15}{18}$ $\frac{7}{9} \times \frac{2}{2} = \frac{14}{18}$

Because $15/18$ is the greatest fraction, $5/6$ is the greatest fraction of the group.

Circle the *greater* fraction in each of the following pairs:

25. $\frac{1}{24}$ or $\frac{1}{12}$

26. $\frac{1}{125}$ or $\frac{3}{150}$

EXERCISE 4—cont'd

27. $\dfrac{5}{6}$ or $\dfrac{8}{9}$ 28. $\dfrac{3}{10}$ or $\dfrac{2}{9}$

29. $\dfrac{7}{30}$ or $\dfrac{4}{5}$ 30. $\dfrac{4}{5}$ or $\dfrac{3}{4}$

31. $\dfrac{12}{25}$ or $\dfrac{5}{9}$ 32. $\dfrac{4}{5}$ or $\dfrac{5}{6}$

33. $\dfrac{1}{25}$ or $\dfrac{1}{75}$ 34. $\dfrac{1}{6}$ or $\dfrac{3}{10}$

35. $\dfrac{5}{8}$ or $\dfrac{7}{9}$ 36. $\dfrac{3}{50}$ or $\dfrac{1}{150}$

ADDING FRACTIONS

✔ *To add two or more fractions, it is necessary to find the common denominator.* Several methods can be used. One method is to find the least denominator that is common to all the fractions to be added. In simple problems, this is likely to be
✔ the greatest denominator in a series of fractions. *Sometimes, it is necessary to multiply denominators to find a common denominator.*

After placing the fractions in a column for addition, find the common denominator. In the following example, the common denominator is represented by 20, the greatest denominator of the fractions:

EXAMPLE: Add $\dfrac{1}{2}$ $\dfrac{1}{5}$ $\dfrac{1}{10}$ $\dfrac{1}{20}$

The fractions are then changed as indicated to obtain fractions of equal value, each with the same denominator. This is done by dividing the new denominator by the original denominator and multiplying the result by the numerator of the original fraction to obtain the new numerator. Next, the numerators of the fractions are added together and placed over the common denominator. Then the fraction obtained as the answer is reduced to lowest terms.

The fractions are placed directly beneath each other. Next, the original fractions are changed to new fractions of equal value, each with the same denominator. The total equivalent fractions are listed. The numerators are added and placed over the common denominator.

EXAMPLE: Add $\dfrac{1}{2}$ $\dfrac{2}{5}$ $\dfrac{3}{10}$ $\dfrac{7}{20}$

First, Place the fractions directly beneath each other.

$$\frac{1}{2}$$
$$\frac{2}{5}$$
$$\frac{3}{10}$$
$$\frac{7}{20}$$

Second, Find the common denominator for all the fractions.

    a. Will all the denominators divide into the greatest denominator of all the fractions?

    b. Is it necessary to multiply some or all of the denominators to find a number into which all the denominators can divide?

In the example given above, all denominators (2, 5, and 10) will divide into the greatest denominator (20).

$$\frac{1}{2} = \frac{}{20}$$
$$\frac{2}{5} = \frac{}{20}$$
$$\frac{3}{10} = \frac{}{20}$$
$$\frac{7}{20} = \frac{}{20}$$

Third, Change all fractions so that they have the same common denominator. To do this, divide the original denominator into the common denominator and multiply the number obtained by the numerator.

    For example, to change ½ to a fraction with the denominator of 20, divide 2 into 20, which equals 10. Multiply the number obtained (10) by the numerator of the original fraction (1), and place the product over the denominator of 20. In the second fraction, ⅖, 5 divides into 20, 4 times. 4 multiplied by the original numerator of 2 equals 8, the new numerator, which is placed over the new denominator, 20.

The problem then appears as:

$$\frac{1}{2} = \frac{10}{20}$$
$$\frac{2}{5} = \frac{8}{20}$$
$$\frac{3}{10} = \frac{6}{20}$$
$$\frac{7}{20} = \frac{7}{20}$$

Fourth, Add the numerators of all fractions (which now have the same common denominator) together and place the number obtained over the common denominator. Finally, reduce the answer to lowest terms. In the example, the answer $^{31}/_{20}$ is reduced to a whole number and a fraction, $1^{11}/_{20}$.

$$\frac{1}{2} = \frac{10}{20}$$
$$\frac{2}{5} = \frac{8}{20}$$
$$\frac{3}{10} = \frac{6}{20}$$
$$\frac{7}{10} = \frac{14}{20}$$
$$\frac{31}{20} = 1\frac{11}{20}$$

✔ *When mixed numbers are added, the whole numbers are placed directly underneath each other, as are the fractions.*

   Example: Add $1\frac{1}{2}$ $2\frac{2}{3}$ $3\frac{3}{4}$

After a common denominator is found for all fractions, the fractions are changed so that all of them share the same denominator. The numerators of the fractions are added together and placed over the common denominator. Next, the whole numbers are added together. If an improper fraction is obtained when the fractions are added together, it is changed to a whole number and a proper fraction. These are then added to the number obtained when the whole numbers are added together.

$$1\frac{1}{2} = 1\frac{6}{12}$$
$$2\frac{2}{3} = 2\frac{8}{12}$$
$$3\frac{3}{4} = 3\frac{9}{12}$$
$$6\boxed{\frac{23}{12}} = 7\frac{11}{12}$$
$$\boxed{\frac{23}{12} = 1\frac{11}{12}}$$

✔ *When mixed numbers are added, the fractions are added first, and then the whole numbers are added.* If addition of the fractions yields an improper fraction, it is changed to a mixed number, and the whole number obtained is added to the other whole numbers.

EXERCISE 5

(answers on page 296)

Add the following fractions and mixed numbers, and reduce the answers to lowest terms:

1. $\dfrac{2}{9}$
   $\dfrac{4}{27}$
   $\dfrac{7}{9}$
   $\dfrac{2}{3}$

2. $\dfrac{5}{32}$
   $\dfrac{1}{48}$
   $\dfrac{1}{24}$
   $\dfrac{1}{16}$

3. $\dfrac{7}{8}$
   $\dfrac{3}{4}$
   $\dfrac{5}{16}$
   $\dfrac{3}{32}$

4. $\dfrac{1}{2}$
   $\dfrac{3}{20}$
   $\dfrac{7}{10}$
   $\dfrac{9}{40}$

5. $\dfrac{3}{4}$
   $\dfrac{11}{32}$
   $\dfrac{7}{8}$
   $\dfrac{5}{16}$

6. $\dfrac{1}{6}$
   $5\dfrac{3}{8}$
   $2\dfrac{1}{2}$
   $\dfrac{7}{9}$

7. $22\dfrac{1}{6}$
   $15\dfrac{4}{9}$
   $36\dfrac{2}{27}$

8. $\dfrac{4}{5}$
   $\dfrac{9}{30}$
   $\dfrac{5}{90}$

9. $\dfrac{2}{3}$
   $5\dfrac{1}{2}$
   $\dfrac{7}{8}$

10. $43\dfrac{1}{2}$
    $78\dfrac{1}{8}$
    $10\dfrac{4}{5}$

11. $3\dfrac{1}{10}$
    $\dfrac{1}{4}$
    $\dfrac{6}{8}$

12. $20\dfrac{3}{4}$
    $14\dfrac{1}{2}$
    $16\dfrac{1}{4}$

13. $\dfrac{4}{21}$
    $\dfrac{1}{84}$
    $6\dfrac{3}{7}$

14. $18\dfrac{2}{3}$
    $12\dfrac{3}{4}$
    $16\dfrac{1}{6}$

15. $9\dfrac{7}{32}$
    $\dfrac{3}{16}$
    $7\dfrac{1}{48}$

EXERCISE 5—cont'd

16. $4\frac{2}{3}$
    $8\frac{5}{6}$
    $3\frac{3}{8}$

17. $\frac{9}{72}$
    $\frac{7}{8}$
    $\frac{4}{9}$

18. $4\frac{1}{8}$
    $\frac{2}{3}$
    $12\frac{3}{4}$

19. $\frac{1}{8}$
    $\frac{1}{16}$
    $\frac{5}{6}$
    $\frac{3}{4}$

20. $\frac{7}{16}$
    $\frac{3}{8}$
    $\frac{5}{32}$
    $\frac{1}{4}$

SUBTRACTING FRACTIONS

✔ *In subtracting fractions, as in adding fractions, it is necessary to find the common denominator.* In the example shown, the equivalent fractions are given.

EXAMPLE: $\frac{3}{4} - \frac{1}{2}$ $\begin{aligned} \frac{3}{4} &= \frac{3}{4} \\ -\frac{1}{2} &= -\frac{2}{4} \\ \hline &\frac{1}{4} \end{aligned}$

✔ *If the fraction to be subtracted is greater than that from which it is to be subtracted, a whole number (1) must be borrowed from the whole number in the mixed number and then added to the fraction.*

EXAMPLE: Subtract $1\frac{1}{2}$ from $2\frac{1}{4}$

First, place the whole number and its accompanying fraction directly beneath the ones from which they are to be subtracted. Find the least common denominator and make the necessary changes in the fractions so that both have the same denominator. In this example, the common denominator for ¼ and ½ is 4 and the fraction ¼ is changed to ²⁄₄.

Next, subtract the numerators of the fractions. Because it is impossible to subtract 2 from 1, the size of the upper fraction (¼) must be increased. This requires borrowing a 1 from the whole number (3) that occurs with the fraction. If 1 is borrowed from 3, it can be added to the fraction ¼ and the whole number changes to 2. 1 and ¼ is the same as 4/4 + ¼ which equals 5/4. The problem is seen as follows:

$$3\tfrac{1}{4} \qquad 3\tfrac{1}{4} \qquad 2\tfrac{5}{4}$$
$$-1\tfrac{1}{2} \;=\; -1\tfrac{2}{4} \;=\; -1\tfrac{2}{4}$$
$$\phantom{-1\tfrac{1}{2} \;=\; -1\tfrac{2}{4} \;=\;} 1\tfrac{3}{4}$$

EXERCISE 6   (answers on page 296)

Subtract the following fractions and mixed numbers, and reduce the answers to lowest terms:

1. $\dfrac{11}{16}$
   $-\dfrac{3}{8}$

2. $\dfrac{9}{16}$
   $-\dfrac{3}{8}$

3. $\dfrac{3}{5}$
   $-\dfrac{4}{10}$

4. $\dfrac{5}{8}$
   $-\dfrac{3}{16}$

5. $\dfrac{8}{9}$
   $-\dfrac{7}{10}$

6. $\dfrac{9}{10}$
   $-\dfrac{3}{5}$

7. $1\dfrac{5}{12}$
   $-\dfrac{3}{24}$

8. $6\dfrac{1}{10}$
   $-\dfrac{3}{20}$

9. $13\dfrac{2}{3}$
   $-8\dfrac{3}{15}$

10. $2\dfrac{7}{12}$
    $-\dfrac{3}{24}$

11. $\dfrac{7}{10}$
    $-\dfrac{5}{8}$

12. $6\dfrac{3}{8}$
    $-2\dfrac{1}{4}$

13. $42\dfrac{2}{3}$
    $-14\dfrac{4}{5}$

14. $16\dfrac{1}{3}$
    $-3\dfrac{2}{3}$

15. $14\dfrac{1}{5}$
    $-3\dfrac{3}{5}$

EXERCISE 6—cont'd

16. $25\frac{1}{2}$
    $-15\frac{1}{4}$

17. $11\frac{2}{5}$
    $-8\frac{7}{30}$

18. $28\frac{3}{4}$
    $-17\frac{5}{9}$

19. $45\frac{1}{4}$
    $-16\frac{3}{4}$

20. $65\frac{1}{6}$
    $-48\frac{1}{12}$

21. $87\frac{3}{5}$
    $-42\frac{7}{10}$

22. $122\frac{3}{25}$
    $-74\frac{3}{50}$

23. $135\frac{4}{5}$
    $-78\frac{5}{12}$

24. $38\frac{4}{5}$
    $-14\frac{1}{10}$

25. $29\frac{3}{10}$
    $-15\frac{4}{5}$

MULTIPLYING FRACTIONS

✔ *To multiply a fraction by a whole number, multiply the numerator by the whole number and place this answer over the denominator, which remains unchanged.*

EXAMPLE: $3 \times \frac{2}{3} = \frac{(3 \times 2)}{3} = \frac{6}{3} = 2$

If desired, the whole number can be changed to an improper fraction by placing the whole number over a denominator of 1. In this case, the numerators are then multiplied together, as are the denominators.

EXAMPLE: $3 \times \frac{2}{3} = \frac{3}{1} \times \frac{2}{3} = \frac{(3 \times 2)}{(1 \times 3)} = \frac{6}{3} = 2$

Reduction or *cancellation* can be carried out by dividing a numerator and a denominator by the same number.

EXAMPLE: $3 \times \frac{2}{3} = \frac{\cancel{3}}{1} \times \frac{2}{\cancel{3}} = 2$

✔ **To multiply fractions, multiply all of the numerators together and place this answer (the product) over the product of all of the denominators.** Again, cancellation may be carried out.

EXAMPLE: $\frac{1}{2} \times \frac{2}{3} = \frac{(1 \times 2)}{(2 \times 3)} = \frac{2}{6} = \frac{1}{3}$ or $\frac{1}{\cancel{2}} \times \frac{\cancel{2}}{3} = \frac{1}{3}$

NOTE: In fractions, the × (multiplication sign) also means "of," so ½ of ⅔ means ½ × ⅔.

✔ **To multiply mixed numbers, change the whole number and fraction to an improper fraction. Then multiply all of the numerators together and place this product over the product of all of the denominators.** Cancellation may be used in solving the problem.

EXAMPLE: $2\frac{1}{2} \times 3\frac{1}{8} = \frac{5}{2} \times \frac{25}{8} = \frac{(5 \times 25)}{(2 \times 8)} = \frac{125}{16} = 7\frac{13}{16}$

EXERCISE 7 *(answers on page 296)*

Multiply the following fractions and mixed numbers, and reduce the answers to lowest terms:

1. $\frac{3}{8} \times \frac{1}{6} =$
2. $\frac{4}{9} \times \frac{7}{10} =$
3. $\frac{5}{8} \times \frac{4}{9} =$

4. $\frac{1}{8} \times \frac{5}{6} =$
5. $\frac{3}{16} \times \frac{2}{5} =$
6. $\frac{2}{5} \times \frac{5}{6} =$

7. $\frac{5}{8} \times \frac{3}{5} =$
8. $\frac{1}{3} \times \frac{6}{12} =$
9. $\frac{8}{9} \times \frac{5}{16} =$

10. $\frac{4}{9} \times \frac{4}{5} =$
11. $\frac{5}{16} \times \frac{3}{5} =$
12. $\frac{2}{25} \times \frac{7}{20} =$

13. $\frac{9}{25} \times \frac{2}{3} =$
14. $6\frac{2}{3} \times 1\frac{7}{12} =$
15. $6\frac{1}{4} \times 4\frac{5}{6} =$

16. $1\frac{7}{8} \times 3\frac{1}{4} =$
17. $7\frac{3}{8} \times 2\frac{1}{4} =$
18. $8\frac{1}{5} \times 8\frac{4}{5} =$

19. $6\frac{2}{3} \times 1\frac{1}{12} =$
20. $8\frac{1}{4} \times 4\frac{4}{5} \times 2\frac{1}{2} =$
21. $3\frac{1}{2} \times 6\frac{1}{4} \times 8\frac{1}{8} =$

EXERCISE 7—cont'd

22. $9\frac{3}{4} \times 8\frac{2}{3} \times 2\frac{1}{12} =$

23. $11\frac{1}{2} \times 8\frac{6}{7} \times \frac{3}{56} =$

24. $10\frac{1}{2} \times 4\frac{1}{4} \times 17\frac{1}{3} =$

25. $20\frac{1}{2} \times 10\frac{1}{3} \times 6\frac{3}{4} =$

DIVIDING FRACTIONS

✔ *To divide a whole number by a fraction, invert the fraction and multiply.*

EXAMPLE: Divide 6 by $\frac{2}{3}$ $6 \div \frac{2}{3} = 6 \times \frac{3}{2} = \frac{18}{2} = 9$

Cancellation may be carried out if the whole number is changed to an improper fraction by placing the whole number over the denominator 1.

EXAMPLE: $6 \div \frac{2}{3} = \frac{\cancel{6}^3}{1} \times \frac{3}{\cancel{2}_1} = 9$

✔ *To divide one fraction by another, invert the fraction that is the divisor, that is, the second fraction, and multiply.* Again, cancellation may be used.

EXAMPLE: Divide $\frac{4}{5}$ by $\frac{1}{5}$

$$\frac{4}{5} \div \frac{1}{5} = \frac{4}{\cancel{5}_1} \times \frac{\cancel{5}^1}{1} = 4$$

✔ *To divide mixed numbers, first change the mixed numbers to improper fractions, invert the divisor (the second fraction) and multiply.*

To divide mixed numbers, it is first necessary to change mixed numbers to improper fractions. Mixed numbers may be found in either the numerator, denominator or both the numerator and denominator. To carry out division, divide the fraction in the numerator by the fraction in the denominator. In this step, invert the fraction found in the denominator and multiply. Cancellation may be used. Reduce the answer obtained to lowest terms.

EXAMPLE: Divide $2\frac{1}{2}$ by $3\frac{1}{8}$

1. Change mixed numbers to improper fractions.

$$\frac{5}{2} \div \frac{25}{8} =$$

2. Invert the divisor and multiply. Reduce the answer to lowest terms, if necessary.

a. The problem solved when cancellation is used.

$$\frac{5}{2} \div \frac{25}{8} = \frac{\cancel{5}^{1}}{\cancel{2}_{1}} \times \frac{\cancel{8}^{4}}{\cancel{25}_{5}} = \frac{4}{5}$$

b. The problem solved when cancellation is not used.

$$\frac{5}{2} \div \frac{25}{8} = \frac{5}{2} \times \frac{8}{25} = \frac{40}{50} \div \frac{10}{10} = \frac{4}{5}$$

EXERCISE 8 *(answers on page 296)*

Divide the following fractions and mixed numbers, and reduce the answers to lowest terms:

1. $\frac{1}{3} \div \frac{3}{9} =$

2. $\frac{3}{8} \div \frac{5}{6} =$

3. $\frac{1}{100} \div \frac{7}{10} =$

4. $\frac{5}{6} \div \frac{7}{12} =$

5. $\frac{1}{12} \div \frac{3}{24} =$

6. $\frac{1}{25} \div \frac{3}{50} =$

7. $\frac{1}{150} \div \frac{1}{2} =$

8. $\frac{3}{4} \div \frac{9}{5} =$

9. $\frac{2}{6} \div \frac{5}{12} =$

10. $1\frac{2}{3} \div 6\frac{1}{5} =$

11. $1\frac{1}{2} \div \frac{3}{4} =$

12. $\frac{1}{10} \div \frac{1}{3} =$

13. $12\frac{3}{5} \div 8\frac{1}{2} =$

14. $\frac{5}{8} \div 1\frac{3}{5} =$

15. $\frac{1}{75} \div \frac{1}{25} =$

16. $\frac{1}{60} \div \frac{1}{2} =$

17. $4\frac{1}{3} \div \frac{1}{2} =$

18. $10\frac{1}{3} \div \frac{7}{10} =$

19. $4\frac{1}{3} \div \frac{6}{7} =$

20. $3\frac{5}{7} \div 10\frac{2}{3} =$

21. $62 \div 3\frac{1}{2} =$

22. $4\frac{1}{8} \div \frac{5}{40} =$

23. $4\frac{3}{4} \div 7\frac{1}{8} =$

24. $14 \div 6\frac{1}{2} =$

25. $7\frac{1}{2} \div 4\frac{2}{3} =$

3
Decimals

Decimal numbers represent fractions that have a denominator of 10, 100, or 1000, or a greater multiple of 10. Decimal numbers are also called decimal fractions. When both a whole number and decimal fraction have the same value, the numbers are called mixed numbers. A decimal point is used to separate a whole number and a decimal fraction. A zero in front of the decimal point of a decimal fraction alerts the person reading the numbers to look for a decimal point. Zeros may be appended to the right of the last number of the decimal fraction without changing its value.

✔ Working with decimals requires an understanding of the decimal system. ***All figures to the left of the decimal point are whole numbers, and those to the right are decimal fractions, representing a part of one whole.*** Decimals are read as follows:

Tenths	Hundredths	Thousandths
.5	6	2

Tenths are located directly to the right of the decimal point; hundredths are two places to the right of the decimal point; thousandths are three places to the right of the decimal point. A fourth figure would be ten thousandths, a fifth would be hundred thousandths, and so on. The above figure would be read five hundred sixty-two thousandths. Since numbers placed in front of the decimal point are read as whole numbers, 2.562 would be read two and five hundred sixty-two thousandths.

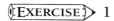 1   (answers on page 297)

Write the words for the following decimals:

1. 0.4 _____

2. 0.3 _____

3. 0.06 _____

4. 0.001 _____

5. 0.01 _____

6. 0.9 _____

7. 7.23 _____

8. 3.05 _____

9. 2.42 _____

10. 1.75 _____

11. 0.015 _____

12. 0.5 _____

ROUNDING DECIMALS

When decimals are to be rounded off, a quantity (usually tenths or hundredths) is either added to or subtracted from the decimal. This is done to make it easier to work with the number and easier to measure the amount of drug or solution.

✔ Rounding is also done when the decimal can be carried out infinitely. **When rounding to tenths, the number in the hundredth position is rounded up if the number is 5 or more (1 is added to the number in the tenth position), and is rounded down if the number is less than 5 (the number in the tenth position is not changed and the number in the hundredth position is dropped).**

EXAMPLE: 1.46 rounded up becomes 1.5
2.73 rounded down becomes 2.7

✔ *To round to hundredths, look at the number in the thousandth position and round up if the number is 5 or more; round down if the number is less than 5. Do not change the number in the hundredths position.*

EXAMPLE: 4.236 becomes 4.24 when rounded up to hundredths
7.542 becomes 7.54 when rounded down to hundredths

EXAMPLE: 5.678 becomes 5.68
5.673 becomes 5.67

EXERCISE 2   (answers on page 297)

Round the following numbers to tenths:

1. 4.46 2. 5.36 3. 6.44 4. 7.23

5. 2.52 6. 10.92 7. 9.81 8. 3.26

9. 7.58 10. 12.13 11. 8.67 12. 5.05

Round the following numbers to hundredths:

13. 7.354 14. 5.125 15. 8.577 16. 4.565

17. 9.3471 18. 11.421 19. 2.542 20. 6.1116

21. 10.2006 22. 3.503 23. 4.441327 24. 1.7527

25. 0.33333 26. 0.6666666

✔ *Fractions may be changed to their decimal forms by dividing the numerator by the denominator.*

EXAMPLE: Change the fraction $\frac{3}{5}$ to a decimal number.

$$\frac{3}{5} = 3 \div 5 = 0.6$$

or

$$\frac{3}{5} = \frac{5\overline{)3.0}}{0.6}$$

EXERCISE 3 *(answers on page 297)*

Change the following fractions to decimals, rounding to thousandths when necessary.

1. $\dfrac{1}{10} =$
2. $\dfrac{1}{200} =$
3. $\dfrac{3}{8} =$
4. $\dfrac{6}{10} =$
5. $\dfrac{7}{25} =$
6. $\dfrac{1}{150} =$
7. $\dfrac{3}{50} =$
8. $\dfrac{3}{100} =$
9. $\dfrac{7}{8} =$
10. $\dfrac{1}{5} =$
11. $\dfrac{6}{7} =$
12. $\dfrac{3}{150} =$
13. $\dfrac{9}{10} =$
14. $\dfrac{3}{5} =$
15. $\dfrac{3}{25} =$
16. $\dfrac{1}{2} =$
17. $\dfrac{4}{5} =$
18. $\dfrac{5}{8} =$
19. $\dfrac{1}{50} =$
20. $\dfrac{3}{4} =$
21. $\dfrac{7}{10} =$
22. $\dfrac{8}{9} =$

23. $\dfrac{5}{6} =$ 24. $\dfrac{4}{25} =$

25. $\dfrac{2}{5} =$

✔ *Decimals may be changed to fractions by dropping the decimal point and using the proper denominator.* For example, 0.5 becomes $\frac{5}{10}$ or $\frac{1}{2}$ (expressing the fraction in lowest terms). Similarly, 0.75 becomes $\frac{75}{100}$ (because the decimal is read seventy-five one hundredths); and 0.005 becomes $\frac{5}{1000}$. The fraction $\frac{75}{100}$ expressed in lowest terms becomes $\frac{3}{4}$, and $\frac{5}{1000}$ becomes $\frac{1}{200}$.

The same principle applies when a decimal containing a whole number is to be changed to a mixed number. Thus 1.5 becomes $1\frac{5}{10}$ or reduced to lowest terms, $1\frac{1}{2}$.

EXERCISE 4   (answers on page 297)

Change the following decimals to fractions, and reduce the answers to lowest terms:

1. 0.1 =   2. 0.25 =

3. 0.12 =   4. 0.35 =

5. 0.65 =   6. 0.8 =

7. 2.5 =   8. 0.04 =

9. 0.4 =   10. 0.75 =

11. 0.15 =   12. 0.88 =

13. 0.06 =   14. 1.5 =

15. 0.2 =   16. 5.928 =

17. 0.72 =   18. 0.9 =

19. 0.24 =   20. 0.375 =

EXERCISE 4—cont'd

21. 0.066 =

22. 0.001 =

23. 0.0002 =

24. 0.0005 =

25. 0.008 =

ADDING DECIMALS

✔ *When adding decimals, align the digits in columns so that the decimal points are placed directly underneath each other.* Aligning the decimal points and digits in columns helps avoid errors in addition.

✔ *Zeros may be added after the decimal number without changing its value.* The empty space following a decimal number is the same as a zero. Placing zeros in empty spaces following the decimal number helps align the columns.

EXAMPLE: Add 0.9, 0.65, 0.225, 0.86

```
  0.900
  0.650
  0.225
  0.860
  -----
  2.635
```

A whole number in a decimal is placed to the left of the decimal point. Zeros preceding a whole number do not change its value. Thus 0002.6 is the same as 2.6.

EXERCISE 5 (answers on page 297)

Add the following decimals:

1. 8.005, 6.25, 18.5

2. 20.3, 18.35, 20.65

3. 10.2, 12.5, 16.8

4. 4.6, 8, 16.8

5. 0.007, 18.1, 4.52

6. 27.1, 0.0001, 0.04

7. 45.4, 7.012, 0.03

8. 0.2, 0.06, 0.05

9. 9.7, 2.063, 14.95

10. 300.6, 5.227, 6.01

11. 9.63, 0.25, 1.395

12. 4.29, 1.001, 0.023

13. 6.007, 0.268, 3.04

14. 0.003, 2.5, 60.8, 4

15. 36.2, 2.064, 72.1

16. 8.25, 6.5, 18.005

17. 6.845, 142.1, 5.75

18. 8.4, 9.15, 4.6

19. 7.24, 84.6, 0.003

20. 0.004, 2.08, 7.34

21. 42.006, 3.7, 2.48

22. 13.2, 0.0003, 0.03

23. 3.276, 4.5, 3.24

24. 2.38, 15.7, 1.431

25. 15.327, 4.05, 2.2

SUBTRACTING DECIMALS

✔ **When subtracting decimals, align the digits in columns so that the decimal points are placed directly underneath each other.** Then, subtract the decimals in the same way as whole numbers. Zeros may be added to the right of the decimal number or to the left of the whole number to help align the columns.

EXAMPLE: Subtract 3.22 from 9.54

$$\begin{array}{r} 9.54 \\ -3.22 \\ \hline 6.32 \end{array}$$

EXERCISE 6   (answers on page 297)

Subtract the following decimals:

1. $54.3 - 7.006 =$

2. $2.7 - 1.2 =$

3. $431.12 - 97.282 =$

4. $4.7 - 1.825 =$

5. $4.5 - 0.9 =$

6. $9.5 - 6.37 =$

7. $18.2 - 15.5 =$

8. $75.3 - 30.2 =$

⟨EXERCISE⟩ 6—cont'd

9. 14.06 − 10.89 =

10. 37.5 − 29.67 =

11. 7.52 − 4.8 =

12. 85.7 − 4.92 =

13. 35.2 − 17.56 =

14. 44.37 − 29.17 =

15. 24.8 − 0.05 =

16. 421.3 − 44.8 =

17. 26.8 − 0.05 =

18. 49.27 − 31.06 =

19. 3.58 − 0.47 =

20. 8.16 − 3.04 =

21. 321.6 − 56.7 =

22. 162.3 − 145.75 =

23. 118.04 − 32.375 =

24. 6.91 − 3.78 =

25. 8.759 − 5.241 =

MULTIPLYING DECIMALS

✔ When multiplying decimals, first align the digits on the far right of the numbers to be multiplied, then multiply. Disregard the decimal points when multiplying. Finally place the decimal point in the product by counting, from the right, the number of places equal to the total number of decimal places in both the multiplier (number by which another is to be multiplied) and the multiplicand (number multiplied).

EXAMPLES:
```
     3562              3.56
   ×  .65            ×  .25
     178 10            1780
    2137 2              712
    2315.30           0.8900
```

In the first example, there are two decimal places in the multiplier, and there is no decimal in the multiplicand; therefore, the decimal point is placed two places from the right in the product. In the second example, there are two decimal places in the multiplicand and two decimal places in the multiplier; therefore, the decimal point is placed four places from the right.

✔ *The number of digits to the right of the decimal point in the product obtained equals the sum of the number of digits to the right of the decimals in the multiplier and multiplicand.*

Zeros may be removed from the end of the decimal number without changing its value. This simplifies multiplication.

EXAMPLE: 7.23Ø × 6.4ØØ

$$\begin{array}{r} 7.23 \\ \times\ 6.4 \\ \hline 2892 \\ 4338 \\ \hline 46.272 \end{array}$$

There is sometimes confusion in multiplying two figures if a zero is contained in one or both of them.

EXAMPLES:

$$\text{(A)}\ \begin{array}{r} 207 \\ \times\ 55 \\ \hline 1035 \\ 1035 \\ \hline 11385 \end{array} \quad \text{(B)}\ \begin{array}{r} 225 \\ \times\ 304 \\ \hline 900 \\ 6750 \\ \hline 68400 \end{array} \quad \text{(C)}\ \begin{array}{r} 360 \\ \times\ 150 \\ \hline 18000 \\ 360 \\ \hline 54000 \end{array}$$

Example A illustrates that multiplication of a zero by another number results in zero. Example B illustrates that multiplication of a number by a zero results in zero. Example C illustrates that multiplication of a zero by a zero results in zero.

✔ *When multiplying by tens, hundreds, or thousands, move the decimal point one, two, or three places, respectively, to the right.*

EXAMPLE: 56 × 10 = 560   (56͜0.)

There is an understood decimal point after any whole number. The number 56 becomes 56. by placing a decimal point after it. To multiply 56 by 10, move the decimal point one place to the right and place a zero in the space to the right of the 56.

When multiplying a figure by 100, move the decimal point two places to the right, which is the position for hundredths.

EXAMPLES: 85 × 100 = 8500   1.7 × 100 = 1͜70.

When multiplying a figure by 1000, move the decimal point three places to the right, the position for thousandths.

EXAMPLES: 76 × 1000 = 76,000   0.75 × 1000 = ͜750.ØØ

EXERCISE 7   *(answers on page 298)*

Move the decimal point the correct direction and number of places to multiply by (a) 10, (b) 100, and (c) 1000:

1. 6.0

2. 0.05

3. 0.8

4. 0.005

EXERCISE 7—cont'd

5. 0.7

6. 0.2

7. 0.001

8. 0.03

9. 1.43

10. 0.01

EXERCISE 8 (answers on page 298)

Multiply the following decimals:

1. 38 × .01 =

2. 7.2 × 40.53 =

3. 0.3 × 4.5 =

4. 1.25 × 6.7 =

5. 2.0 × 60 =

6. 4.3 × 7.24 =

7. 5.75 × 50 =

8. 7.7 × 6.0 =

9. 5 × 0.729 =

10. 9.16 × 7 =

11. 15.4 × 0.06 =

12. 0.8 × 7 =

13. 18.6 × 15 =

14. 0.02 × 0.27 =

15. 0.643 × 0.002 =

16. 0.25 × 110.4 =

17. 7.4 × 82.91 =

18. 9.2 × 0.56 =

19. 8.6 × 9.9 =

20. 0.76 × 73.7 =

21. 49.4 × 3.99 =

22. 74.3 × 2.6 =

23. 0.0074 × 6.2 =   **24.** 0.1 × 60 =

25. 821.4 × 13 =

DIVIDING DECIMALS

✔ *Dividing decimals is more complicated than adding, subtracting, or multiplying decimals. The divisor is the quantity by which a number is divided, the dividend is the quantity that is being divided, and the quotient is the answer that results.*

To divide a whole number by a decimal fraction or mixed number, or to divide a decimal fraction or mixed number by a whole number, decimal fraction, or mixed number, first set up the problem as a standard division problem. Use the following rules for eliminating the decimal point in the divisor and moving the decimal point in the dividend. Finally, divide the numbers.

EXAMPLE:
$$\begin{array}{r} 20.1 \leftarrow \text{quotient} \\ 2\overline{)40.2} \leftarrow \text{dividend} \\ \underline{4} \\ 02 \end{array}$$
divisor

To divide a whole number by a decimal number, move the decimal point in the divisor to the right so that the divisor becomes a whole number. Count the number of places that were added, add that number of zeros to the dividend, and move the decimal point the same number of places. Then carry out the division.

EXAMPLE:
$$\begin{array}{r} 5.97 \\ 6.7\overline{)40.000} \\ \underline{33\;5} \\ 650 \\ \underline{603} \\ 470 \\ \underline{469} \\ 1 \end{array}$$

In the example, the decimal in the divisor, 6.7, is moved one place to the right. Therefore, the decimal point in the dividend (40) is also moved one place to the right. The decimal point in the quotient is placed directly above the decimal point in the dividend. Zeros are added to the right of the decimal point when necessary. Appending zeros to the right of the decimal point does not change the value of a whole number.

Zeros are added to the dividend when dividing a smaller whole number by a larger whole number.

EXAMPLE:
$$\begin{array}{r} 0.5 \\ 7\overline{)4.0} \\ \underline{3.5} \\ 5 \end{array}$$

Similarly, to divide a decimal number by a decimal number, convert the decimal number in the divisor into a whole number; then move the decimal point in the dividend as many places to the right as the decimal point in the divisor is moved. This may require adding zeros. Estimate the quotient and divide as usual.

EXAMPLE:

$$7.682 \overline{)24.500\,0000}$$ 3.1892 or 3.19 or 3.19+

```
         23 046
         1 4540
           7682
          68580
          61456
          71240
          69138
          21020
```

If the numbers do not divide evenly, the answer may be carried out for three decimal places and rounded off. The remainder may be stated as a fraction by placing the remainder over the divisor and reducing it to lowest terms, or a "+" sign may be placed to the right of the whole number to indicate that the division did not end.

✔ *To divide a number by 10, 100, or 1000, move the decimal point one place, two places, or three places, respectively, to the left.*

EXAMPLES: 55 ÷ 10 = 5.5   (5.5ₓ)
            55 ÷ 100 = .55   (.55ₓ)
            55 ÷ 1000 = .055   (.055ₓ)

EXERCISE 9

(answers on page 298)

Divide the following decimals, rounding to thousandths:

1. 4.5 ÷ 6 =   2. 40 ÷ 5.5 =

3. 3 ÷ 0.6 =   4. 15 ÷ 7.5 =

5. 0.6 ÷ 0.03 =   6. 0.042 ÷ 0.013 =

7. 7.2 ÷ 0.9 =   8. 0.9 ÷ 0.6 =

9. 9.6 ÷ 0.7 =   10. 4 ÷ 0.4 =

11. 64.4 ÷ 70 =   12. 5.2 ÷ 2.02 =

13. 0.67 ÷ 7 =   14. 1.4 ÷ 70 =

15. 24.15 ÷ 3.01 =   16. 15.5 ÷ 3.6 =

17. 75 ÷ 0.05 =

18. 25 ÷ 0.5 =

19. 1.5 ÷ 0.3 =

20. 0.004 ÷ 0.05 =

21. 4.01 ÷ 12 =

22. 32.4 ÷ 12.5 =

23. 0.0654 ÷ 0.13 =

24. 0.06 ÷ 0.05 =

25. 0.02 ÷ 12.6 =

COMPARING THE VALUE OF DECIMALS

✔ *The value of a decimal remains unchanged when one or more zeros are appended to it.* For example, 0.5 may be written as 0.50 without changing its value. One method of comparing the size of decimals is to append zeros as necessary to equalize the number of decimal places in each decimal, and then compare the size of the resulting number.

EXAMPLE: Which of the following decimals is larger, 0.5 or 0.085?
0.5 = 0.500 (add zeros to get the same number of decimal places for each fraction)
0.500 is larger than 0.085.

EXERCISE 10

(answers on page 298)

Circle the *greater* decimal in the following pairs of decimals:

1. 0.25 or 0.025

2. 0.7 or 0.75

3. 0.05 or 0.5

4. 0.756 or 0.75

5. 0.73 or 0.85

6. 0.12 or 0.1

7. 0.8 or 0.08

8. 0.06 or 0.6

9. 0.094 or 0.75

10. 0.03 or 0.3

11. 0.57 or 0.75

12. 1.25 or 1.75

EXERCISE 10—cont'd

Circle the *lesser* decimal in the following pairs of decimals:

13. 0.06 or 0.015

14. 0.025 or 0.25

15. 0.01 or 0.10

16. 0.5 or 0.05

17. 0.65 or 0.655

18. 0.12 or 0.012

19. 0.2 or 0.002

20. 0.60 or 0.064

21. 0.33 or 0.325

22. 0.025 or 0.25

23. 0.45 or 0.49

24. 0.125 or 0.025

4

Percentage

Percentage means hundredths. A percent (%) is the same as a fraction in which the denominator is 100; the numerator indicates the part of 100 being considered.

EXAMPLE: $3\% = \dfrac{3}{100}$

In the above example, 3 parts of 100 are being considered.

When one multiplies or divides by a percent, the percent is usually changed ✔ to a decimal. **To change a percent to a decimal, remove the percent sign and divide the number by 100 by moving the decimal point two places to the left.**

EXAMPLE: $3\% = 100\overline{)3.00 \atop 0.03}$ or 0.03

EXERCISE 1 *(answers on page 298)*

Change the following percents to decimal numbers:

1. 45% _____
2. 50% _____
3. 99% _____
4. 2% _____
5. 25% _____
6. 14% _____
7. 82% _____
8. 7% _____
9. 5% _____
10. 32% _____

✔ *To change a decimal to percent, multiply the decimal by 100 by moving the decimal point two places to the right, and appending the percent sign.*

EXAMPLE: $0.03 \times 100 = 0.03.$ or 3%

EXERCISE 2

(answers on page 298)

Change the following decimals to percents:

1. 0.8 _____
2. 0.25 _____
3. 0.125 _____
4. 2.5 _____
5. 0.5 _____
6. 0.459 _____
7. 0.1 _____
8. 0.15 _____
9. 3.45 _____
10. 0.015 _____
11. 0.52 _____
12. 0.28 _____
13. 4.7 _____
14. 0.75 _____
15. 0.19 _____
16. 7.2 _____
17. 0.038 _____
18. 0.12 _____
19. 3.246 _____
20. 0.008 _____
21. 0.30 _____
22. 0.075 _____
23. 0.065 _____
24. 0.006 _____
25. 17.6 _____

To find the percent of a number, change the percent to a decimal and multiply. Review Chapter 3 as necessary.

EXAMPLE: What is 40% of 2000?

a. Change 40% to a decimal.

$$40\% = 0.40$$

b. Multiply together the decimal and the number for which the percentage is sought. Count the total decimal places in both numbers that were multiplied and place the decimal point in the answer by counting the same number of places from the far right.

```
    2000              $480.20
  × 0.40            ×    0.40
  800.00 is equal to  $192.0800 is equal to
      40% of 2000         40% of $480.20
```

EXERCISE 3

(answers on page 298)

Solve the following problems:

1. 3% of 100 = _____

2. 65% of 29 = _____

3. 28% of 250 = _____

4. 92% of 63 = _____

5. 45% of 325 = _____

6. 78% of 300 = _____

7. 80% of 40 = _____

8. 6½% of 2549.86 = _____

9. 15% of 20 = _____

10. 3¼% of 986 = _____

5

Fractions, Decimals, and Percentages

Sometimes it is necessary to solve problems that contain a combination of fractions, decimals, or percentages. Such problems are solved by first converting all numbers in the problem to fractions or to decimal numbers, and then applying the rules for solving the problem. (These rules are found in Chapters 2, 3, and 4.)

Example: $0.4 \times \dfrac{3}{5}$

$0.4 \times 0.6 = 0.24$

or

$\dfrac{\cancel{4}^{\,2}}{\cancel{10}_{\,5}} \times \dfrac{3}{5} = \dfrac{6}{25}$

EXERCISE 1 (answers on page 298)

Solve the following problems by converting the decimals or percents to fractions:

1. $5\% \times \dfrac{2}{5} =$

2. $0.18 \times \dfrac{2}{9} =$

3. $\dfrac{2}{3} \times 0.6 =$

4. $8.52 - 1\dfrac{1}{4} =$

5. $4\dfrac{1}{4} \div 8.5 =$

6. $1.8 - 1\dfrac{3}{10} =$

EXERCISE 1—cont'd

7. $2.8 - 2\frac{4}{5} =$

8. $4\frac{1}{4} \div 3\frac{5}{6} =$

9. $4.8 \div 2\frac{1}{4} =$

10. $\frac{1}{3} \times 0.3 =$

11. $40\% \times \frac{2}{5} =$

12. $5\frac{1}{4} \div 2\frac{1}{5} =$

Solve the following problems by converting the fractions or percents to decimals:

13. $0.35 + \frac{1}{25} =$

14. $0.43 + 8\frac{1}{2} =$

15. $78\frac{5}{8} + 2.1 =$

16. $5\frac{1}{8} - 0.25 =$

17. $4.4 - 2\frac{3}{5} =$

18. $9\frac{2}{5} - 3.7 =$

19. $6\frac{1}{2}\%$ of $180 =$

20. $12 \times 2\frac{1}{2} =$

21. 40% of $75 =$

22. $3\frac{5}{8} \div 4.2 =$

23. $5.6 \div 2\frac{4}{5} =$

24. $2.94 \div \frac{1}{4} =$

EXERCISE 2 *(answers on page 299)*

Change the following percentages to decimals and fractions as indicated by the column headings (reduce fractions to lowest terms):

Percentage	Decimal	Fraction
1. 6%	= _____	= _____

2. 10%   = _____ = _____

3. 75%   = _____ = _____

4. 27%   = _____ = _____

5. 4.5%   = _____ = _____

6. 30%   = _____ = _____

7. 12%   = _____ = _____

8. 15%   = _____ = _____

9. 50%   = _____ = _____

10. 9.6%   = _____ = _____

11. 0.05%   = _____ = _____

12. 20%   = _____ = _____

13. 80%   = _____ = _____

14. 0.005% = _____ = _____

6

Ratio and Proportion

RATIO

A ratio consists of two figures separated by a colon.

EXAMPLES: 1:50   3:100

A ratio indicates that there is a relationship between the two figures. In the above example, the first ratio indicates that 1 is related to 50; in the second, that 3 is related to 100. These examples would be read as 1 is to 50 and 3 is to 100.

✔ ***A ratio is an indicated fraction, and the terms of the ratio are the numerator and denominator.*** A ratio is the relative size of two quantities. The answer obtained by dividing the first part of the ratio by the second is called the quotient.

The value of a ratio is not changed if both terms are multiplied or divided by the same number. Multiplication and division are the only operations that can be performed on a ratio without changing its value.

Any numbers that designate quantities must be expressed in the same units of measure when written as a ratio. Examples of denominate numbers that indicate a quantity of a unit are 3 inches, 4 gallons, and 10 years. In order to establish a ratio of 3 inches to 2 feet, both units of measure must be the same. In this example, the ratio might be established by changing feet to inches, in which case the ratio would be 3:24.

A ratio may be written as a fraction and a fraction may be written as a ratio.

EXAMPLES: $1:50 = \dfrac{1}{50}$ $\dfrac{3}{100} = 3:100$

Ratios are also expressed in their lowest terms. This is done in the same manner as are fractions, that is, by dividing both parts of the ratio by the same number.

EXAMPLE: 2:20 = 1:10

✔ ***To express a percentage as a ratio, first convert it to a fraction with 100 as the denominator.*** For example, $25\% = {}^{25}/_{100} = 25:100$. Expressed in its lowest terms, the ratio 25:100 becomes 1:4.

✔ To change a decimal to a ratio, multiply the decimal by 100, or move the decimal point two places to the right, and use 100 as the denominator of the ratio.

EXAMPLES: $0.87\frac{1}{2} = 87\frac{1}{2}:100$ $0.09 = 9:100$

$0.009 = 0.9:100$ $0.375 = 37.5:100$
or   or
9:1000   375:1000

✔ A fraction with a denominator of 10 or multiple of 10 may be written as a fraction, a decimal, or a ratio.

For example, when the denominator is 10, it may be written as $\frac{1}{10}$, $\frac{3}{10}$, $\frac{5}{10}$; 0.1, 0.3, 0.5; or 1:10, 3:10, 5:10. When the denominator is 100, it may be written $\frac{1}{100}$, $\frac{2}{100}$, $\frac{8}{100}$; 0.01, 0.02, 0.08; or 1:100, 2:100, 8:100. When the denominator is 1000, it may be written as $\frac{3}{1000}$, $\frac{7}{1000}$, $\frac{9}{1000}$; 0.003, 0.007, 0.009; or 3:1000, 7:1000, 9:1000.

EXERCISE 1 (answers on page 299)

Rewrite the following fractions as ratios expressed in lowest terms:

1. $\frac{1}{3}$ 2. $\frac{6}{8}$

3. $\frac{3}{4}$ 4. $\frac{3}{5}$

5. $\frac{5}{10}$ 6. $\frac{4}{10}$

7. $\frac{9}{25}$ 8. $\frac{1}{2}$

9. $\frac{7}{8}$ 10. $\frac{74}{92}$

11. $\frac{5}{9}$ 12. $\frac{4}{6}$

Rewrite the following decimals as ratios expressed in lowest terms:

13. 0.08

14. 0.25

15. 0.75

16. 0.1

17. 0.5

18. 0.07

19. 0.6

20. 0.02

21. 0.45

22. 0.03

23. 0.09

24. 0.04

Rewrite the following percentages as ratios expressed in lowest terms:

25. 9%

26. 40%

27. 0.02%

28. 0.8%

29. $\frac{9}{10}$%

30. $\frac{2}{5}$%

31. 7%

32. 5%

33. 10%

34. 0.06%

35. 0.5%

36. $4\frac{1}{4}$%

PROPORTION

Proportion is a statement showing that two ratios have equivalent value. A proportion is written as follows:

EXAMPLE: 1:50 = 2:100 or 1:50::2:100

✔ The inner terms of the proportion are called *means,* and the outer terms are called *extremes.* **In a true proportion, the product of the means equals the product of the extremes:**

EXAMPLE: 1:50 = 2:100 (inner terms are Means, outer terms are Extremes)

$1 \times 100 = 50 \times 2$ or $100 = 100$
(Extremes)   (Means)

If the value of one term of the proportion is not known, it is commonly represented by an x. The value of the unknown (x) is found by multiplying the means and extremes.

EXAMPLE: $7:x = 4:28$

$4x = 7 \times 28$, or 196

$x = 196 \div 4$, or 49

The computation can be checked or proved by substituting for x the answer obtained and then multiplying to be certain that the product of the means equals the product of the extremes.

$7:49 = 4:28$

$7 \times 28 = 4 \times 49$

$196 = 196$

When the proportion is written to show the relationship of two fractions, cross-multiply either to solve for the value of an unknown or to prove the computation is correct.

EXAMPLE:

$\dfrac{2}{x} = \dfrac{7}{49}$ $\dfrac{2}{14} = \dfrac{7}{49}$

$7x = 2 \times 49$ $7 \times 14 = 2 \times 49$

$7x = 98$ $98 = 98$

$x = 98 \div 7$

$x = 14$

EXERCISE 2 (answers on page 299)

Solve for x in the following proportions; round to the nearest hundredths:

1. $2:1 = x:\frac{1}{2}$
2. $6:1 = x:3$
3. $2:x = 4:22$
4. $8.5:10 = x:200$
5. $15:40 = x:16$
6. $0.6:x = 0.25:2$
7. $25:1 = 45:x$
8. $1.25:1 = 0.625:x$
9. $45:x = 125:1$
10. $1:0.325 = x:0.625$
11. $25:1 = 75:x$
12. $0.625:1 = 2.5:x$
13. $\frac{1}{6}:1 = \frac{1}{4}:x$
14. $0.6:24 = 0.5:x$
15. $25:1 = 50:x$
16. $\frac{1}{2}:\frac{1}{8} = 1:x$
17. $3:1 = 45:x$
18. $\frac{1}{4}:x = 20:80$
19. $\frac{1}{150}:1 = \frac{1}{125}:x$
20. $\frac{1}{8}:20 = x:40$
21. $\frac{1}{4}:6 = x:16$
22. $1:6 = x:9$
23. $1:10 = 0.75:x$
24. $3:2 = 10:x$
25. $0.4:1 = 0.2:x$

Unit One Posttest

EXPLANATION: The following posttest may be used to assess student understanding of arithmetic. If you experience difficulty solving any of the problems accurately, a review of the appropriate chapters may be helpful.

Directions: Work the following problems as indicated.

Express in Roman numerals:

1. 46 _____
2. 132 _____
3. 27 _____
4. 14 _____

Express in Arabic numbers:

5. VIII _____
6. XXIX _____
7. XCI _____
8. XV _____

Change the following fractions to the higher terms indicated:

9. $\dfrac{5}{6} = \dfrac{}{36}$
10. $\dfrac{7}{8} = \dfrac{}{24}$
11. $\dfrac{3}{4} = \dfrac{24}{}$
12. $\dfrac{2}{3} = \dfrac{40}{}$

Change the following improper fractions to whole or mixed numbers (reduce answer to lowest terms):

13. $\dfrac{69}{6} =$
14. $\dfrac{88}{6} =$
15. $\dfrac{24}{6} =$
16. $\dfrac{44}{17} =$

Change the following mixed numbers to improper fractions:

17. $3\frac{3}{8} =$

18. $14\frac{7}{9} =$

Select the *greater* fraction:

19. $\frac{5}{6}$ or $\frac{9}{20}$

20. $\frac{7}{8}$ or $\frac{4}{5}$

21. $\frac{2}{5}$ or $\frac{3}{10}$

Add the following:

22. $\frac{1}{4}, \frac{3}{8}, \frac{2}{3}$

23. $\frac{1}{10}, \frac{3}{5}, \frac{5}{8}$

24. 0.375, 0.7, 0.45

25. 14.03, 1.7523, 0.879

Subtract the following (reduce answers to lowest terms):

26. $\frac{8}{15} - \frac{2}{5} =$

27. $1\frac{3}{10} - \frac{4}{5} =$

28. $45.3 - 19.78 =$

29. $27.6 - 17.6 =$

Multiply the following:

30. $\frac{2}{3} \times \frac{3}{8} =$

31. $4\frac{5}{9} \times 3 =$

Complete the following:

	Fraction	Ratio	Percentage	Decimal
32.	$\frac{3}{4}$ =	_____ =	_____ =	_____
33.	_____ =	_____ =	5%	= _____

Solve the following:

34. 8% of 94 =

35. 0.3% of 20 =

36. 4:7 = x:49

37. $\frac{1}{9}:1 = \frac{7}{8}:x$

38. 4:5 = x:60

39. $\frac{1}{2}:5 = x:2$

40. 7:10 = 14:x

41. $\frac{1}{6}:\frac{1}{4} = 10:x$

42. 0.45:10 = x:20

43. 0.025:1 = 0.01:x

44. 2.5:10 = 1.25:x

45. $0.06:\frac{1}{1000} = 1:x$

46. 12:0.75 = x:3

47. $7\frac{1}{2}:0.5 = 30:x$

48. $\frac{1}{200}:0.0003 = \frac{1}{10}:x$

49. $\frac{1}{20}:3 = x:1$

50. 2.2:1 = 85:x

Unit Two

Systems of Weights and Measures

Computation of dosage from one unit or system of weights and measures to another requires knowledge of three systems of weights and measures—metric/SI, apothecaries', and household. The apothecaries' system is the oldest system, dating from 1617. The metric/SI system was introduced into Europe around 1790, is considered simpler than the apothecaries' system, and is widely used throughout the world.

Although it did not become mandatory in France until 1840, the metric/SI system was developed by the French Academy of Sciences in 1790 to overcome the problems encountered by using a variety of weights and measures. It is considered simpler than the apothecaries' and household systems and is used throughout the world. In 1875 the International Bureau of Weights and Measures, located in Sevres, France, was established to maintain and make revisions in the international standards of measurement.

A major change occurred in 1960 when the International Bureau of Weights and Measures adopted le Système International de'Unités (the SI system). The SI system uses revised standards to define the base units of measurement. Originally, the base units of the metric system including length, volume, and weight were defined in terms of the meter. Currently, the SI system defines the base units of volume and length in terms of physical processes. The kilogram continues to be defined as an object. Revision and additions to the SI system continue to be made. Although the same names for the units of measurement are used, some abbreviations have been modified. These abbreviations are used throughout the text. Other abbreviations continue to be used simply because change occurs slowly for many who learned the previously accepted abbreviations. These will be included in this unit and may be referred to whenever they are encountered.

The Metric Conversion Act of 1975 committed the United States to convert to the metric system/SI but did not specify a date by which this would be completed. Transition to the use of the metric/SI system in the United States is evident in the dual labeling of gauges, road signs, and commercial products. Because the metric/SI system is the only approved system, it is used in the *United States Pharmacopeia (USP)*, and is used on drug labels. Increasingly, the metric/SI system is being used in health care settings. Some use of the apothecaries' and household systems continues in the United States. The household system is the least accurate and is used primarily in the home. Knowledge of these systems is necessary whenever one needs to convert between them or to the metric/SI system.

Basic arithmetic operations are used to convert between systems. The need to convert between systems may be encountered when a physician's order is written in a different system of weights and measures than is found on the drug label. Conversions may be necessary in the home when only household methods of measuring are available. A review of basic arithmetic processes is found in Unit One.

Unit Two Pretest

EXPLANATION: The following pretest is useful for identifying areas in which a review of the systems of weights and measures and temperature is needed. Complete the pretest and check answers. Review the appropriate sections in Chapters 7 through 10 for any questions answered incorrectly.

Convert the following metric/SI measures to the indicated equivalent:

1. 1 g = _____ mg
2. 1 mg = _____ mcg
3. 1 kg = _____ g
4. 1 L = _____ mL
5. 0.001 g = _____ mg
6. 1 mL = _____ cc

Match the following metric/SI units with the correct description:

7. _____ liter   a. unit of weight
8. _____ gram   b. unit of length
9. _____ meter   c. unit of volume

Write out the words for the following metric/SI abbreviations:

10. mg _____
11. cm _____
12. mcg _____
13. kg _____
14. mL _____
15. g _____

Write out the words for the following metric/SI abbreviations:

16. mm _____

17. L _____

18. m _____

Change the following metric/SI units of weight to the indicated equivalents:

19. 4000 mg = _____ g

20. 5.5 kg = _____ g

21. 20 mcg = _____ mg

22. 0.01 g = _____ mg

23. 4500 g = _____ kg

24. 325 mg = _____ g

25. 0.075 g = _____ mg

26. 4 mg = _____ g

Change the following units of volume to the indicated equivalents:

27. 1500 mL = _____ L

28. 2752 L = _____ mL

29. 5 cc = _____ mL

30. 0.8 L = _____ mL

Write the correct symbol and/or abbreviation for each of the following units of measure in the appropriate space:

31. _____ dram

32. _____ gallon

33. _____ grain

34. _____ minim

35. _____ pint

36. _____ pound

37. _____ ounce

38. _____ liter

Change each of the following metric/SI and apothecaries' units to the equivalent indicated:

39. ʒii = _____ mL

40. 3 g = gr _____

41. gr xv = _____ mg

42. 24 mg = gr _____

43. 180 lb = _____ kg

44. 3 mL = fʒ _____

45. fʒ ss = _____ mL

46. 10 mg = gr _____

47. 0 T̊ = _____ mL

48. 2 g = gr _____

49. ʒ̄ iss = _____ mL

50. 80 kg = _____ lb

51. fʒ̄ ii = fʒ _____

52. 60 gr = ʒ̇ _____

53. 3 lb = _____ ounces

54. 60 mg = gr _____

55. gr xxx = _____ mg

56. ℳ xx = _____ gtts

57. 45 kg = _____ lb

58. 3 mL = _____ gtts

59. 250 mg = gr _____

60. 110 lb = _____ kg

Change the following units of linear measure into the indicated equivalents:

61. 40 mm = _____ cm

62. 5 in = _____ cm

63. 200 cm = _____ m

64. 2.3 ft = _____ cm

65. 2200 mm = _____ m

66. 4 yd = _____ m

67. 0.3 m = _____ cm

68. 1 m = _____ in

69. 45 cm = _____ mm

70. 80 cm = _____ in

71. 12 mm = _____ in

72. 5 mi = _____ km

73. 45 cm = _____ in

74. 2 m = _____ in

75. 6 ft = _____ cm

76. 4 in = _____ mm

Convert the following temperatures as indicated:

77. 102.3° F = _____ C

78. 38.2° C = _____ F

79. 99° F = _____ C

80. 36.6° C = _____ F

81. 200° F = _____ C

82. 40° C = _____ F

Change the following household measures to the equivalent indicated:

83. 2 t = _____ T

84. 4 t = _____ mL

85. 1 T = _____ mL

86. 15 mL = ʒ _____

87. ℥ i = ʒ _____

88. 2 cc = ♏ _____

89. 5 mL = gtts _____

90. ℥ ii = _____ mL

Shade the medicine glasses for each of the amounts given:

91. 1 ounce

92. 3 fluidrams

93. 1 tablespoonful

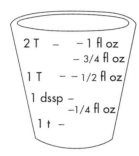
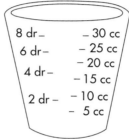

94. 1 teaspoonful

95. 10 milliliters

96. 5 cc

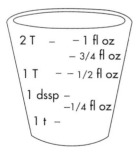
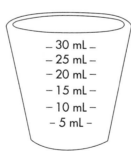
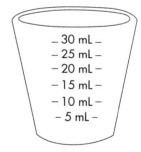

97. 2 tablespoons

98. 2 drams

99. ½ ounce

100. 25 mL

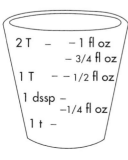
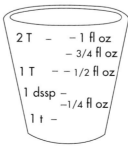
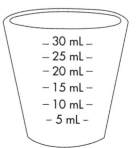

7

Weight and Volume: Metric/SI and Apothecaries' Systems

METRIC SYSTEM

The metric/SI system is the most accurate and flexible system of weights and measures. Calculations within the metric/SI system can be done rapidly and easily.

The metric/SI system is based on the decimal system in which division and multiplication of a unit are in ratios of tens. The units used in the metric/SI system are as follows:

> liter (L)—volume of fluids
> gram (g)—weight of solids
> meter (m)—measure of length

The following prefixes are used to designate the subdivisions of the units of the metric/SI system:

> deci = 0.1 of the unit
> centi = 0.01 of the unit
> milli = 0.001 of the unit

Prefixes used to designate multiples of metric/SI units are as follows:

> deka = 10 times the unit
> hecto = 100 times the unit
> kilo = 1000 times the unit

The following lists illustrate the use of prefixes that show division and multiplication of the metric/SI units. Complete tables of volume and weight are given. As a rule, only the decimal numbers are used to calculate drug dosage. Both whole and decimal numbers are used to calculate weight and length. They are also used for calculating rate of flow for IV solutions.

Metric equivalents

Volume—liter (L)	Weight—gram (g)
	0.001 mg = 1 microgram
0.001 liter = 1 milliliter	0.001 gram = 1 milligram
0.01 liter = 1 centiliter	0.01 gram = 1 centigram
0.1 liter = 1 deciliter	0.1 gram = 1 decigram
10 liters = 1 dekaliter	10 grams = 1 dekagram
100 liters = 1 hectoliter	100 grams = 1 hectogram
1000 liters = 1 kiloliter	1000 grams = 1 kilogram

The following equivalents are used frequently:

Units of weight

1 milligram (mg) = 1000 micrograms (mcg)
1 gram (g) = 1000 milligrams (mg)
0.001 gram (g) = 1 milligram (mg)
1 kilogram (kg) = 1000 grams (g)
0.001 kilogram (kg) = 1 gram (g)

Units of volume

1 liter (L) = 1000 milliliters (mL)
0.001 liter (L) = 1 milliliter (mL)
*1 milliliter (mL) = 1 cubic centimeter (cc)

The following equivalents are needed to change the size of metric units and should be memorized.

Units of weight
1 kg = 1000 g
1 g = 1000 mg
1 mg = 1000 mcg

Units of volume
1 L = 1000 mL
1 mL = 1 cc†

A zero placed to the left of the decimal point helps ensure accuracy by alerting the health care professional to look for a decimal point. Do not place a decimal point and a zero to the right of a whole number. This increases the risk of misreading the number and can lead to serious errors in dosage. For example, write 0.2; do not write 2.0.

Knowing that there are 1000 smaller units in each of the larger units helps in understanding that 0.001 or 1/1000 of the larger units contains only 1 of the smaller units. Understanding this, the above table can be used to derive the following:

1 g = 0.001 kg
1 mg = 0.001 g
1 mcg = 0.001 mg
1 mL = 0.001 L

---

†The term milliliter is preferred. However, cubic centimeter is sometimes used.

Fig. 7-1 illustrates the relationship among metric system/SI units. Table 7.1 shows both the preferred and alternate abbreviations.

Changing greater units to lesser units

To change greater units of measure to lesser units of measure, determine which one is the greater unit. Each of the greater units will always contain more of the lesser units. Therefore when changing a greater unit to a lesser unit, the number of units will increase. The prefix of the lesser unit may indicate the amount of the increase. For example, the prefix *milli* indicates 1000.

✔ *To change grams to milligrams, liters to milliliters, or kilograms to grams, multiply by 1000, moving the decimal point three places to the right.*

EXAMPLE: 3 g = 3$_\times$000. mg

Fig. 7-1 illustrates the relationship among the metric/SI units frequently used in calculations by health care professionals. The solid arrows above the table show the direction for multiplication, and the dotted arrows show the direction for division. The solid arrow above the diagram indicates that there are 1000 grams in 1 kilogram. Kilograms are changed to grams by multiplying kilograms by 1000. The dotted arrow shows that grams are changed to kilograms by dividing by 1000. Grams are changed to milligrams by multiplying by 1000 and milligrams to grams by dividing by 1000. Conversely, micrograms are changed to milligrams by dividing by 1000. The numbers below the table also indicate the relationship between units. For example, there are 1000 grams in 1 kilogram, and 1 milligram equals 0.0001 gram.

The following examples illustrate the use of Fig. 7-1.

EXAMPLE A:

Change 4 L to mL.

L is the base unit and is multiplied by 1000 to find the number of milliliters.

4 (L) × 1000 (number of milliliters in 1 liter) = 4000 mL.

Table 7-1. Commonly used metric/SI abbreviations

Unit of measure	Preferred abbreviations	Other abbreviations
liter	L	l
milliliter	mL	ml
gram	g	Gm, gm
milligram	mg	
microgram	mcg	μg
kilogram	kg	Kg, K
meter	m	M
centimeter	cm	
millimeter	mm	

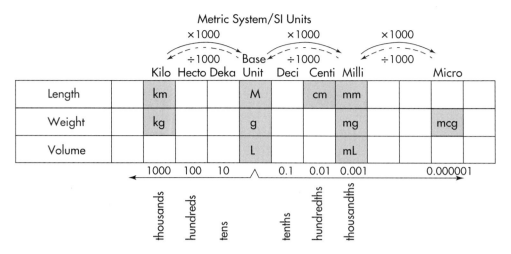

Fig. 7-1. Metric System/SI Units.
(Modified from table by John Martel, St. Clair College, Windsor, Ontario. Reprinted with permission.)

EXAMPLE B:
Change 3500 mg to g.
Divide the number of milligrams by 1000 to find the number of grams.
3500 (mg) ÷ 1000 (mg in 1 g) = 3.5 g.

EXAMPLE C:
Change 2 mg to mcg.
Multiply the number of milligrams × 1000 (the number of micrograms in 1 milligram) to find the total number of micrograms.
2 (mg) × 1000 = 2000 mcg.

EXAMPLE D:
Change 4.6 kg to g.
Multiply the number of kilograms × 1000 (the number of grams in 1 kilogram) to find the number of grams.
4.6 (kg) × 1000 (grams in 1 kilogram) = 4600 g.

Changing lesser units to greater units

When changing lesser units of measure to greater units of measure, determine which is the greater unit of measure. The number of units will decrease because many lesser units are contained in each of the greater units.

✔ *To change milligrams to grams, milliliters to liters, or grams to kilograms, divide by 1000, moving the decimal point three places to the left.*

EXAMPLE: 5000 mL = 5.000ₓL

Health care professionals must be familiar with the various containers available for measuring volume. Fig. 7-2 illustrates two types of graduates marked in milliliters. Fig. 7-3 shows a standard medicine cup.

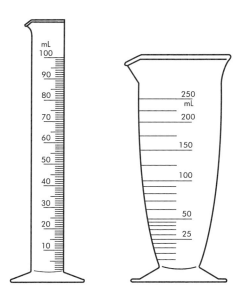

Fig. 7-2. Metric/SI measures suited to measurement of volume. Both containers are marked in milliliters. Cylindrical graduate on left is marked so small amounts can be measured more accurately than with graduate on right.

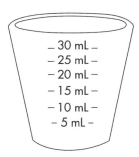

Fig. 7-3. Medicine cup showing volume measures in milliliters.

The same prefixes also apply to the metric/SI unit, the meter. The meter is used for measurements, some of which are related to the size of the area to which a drug is to be applied. It is also used to measure the height of people and to measure distances. Use of the meter and its subdivisions are discussed in Chapter 9, Linear Units of Measure.

The following exercises provide practice in changing one unit of measure to another that is greater or less. This skill is important in clinical practice if the unit of measure printed on the drug label is greater or less than the one given in the physician's order. Some common equivalents will become familiar through frequent use, but calculations should always be rechecked.

EXERCISE 1 (answers on page 301)

Change the following grams to milligrams:

1. 0.32 g = _____ mg
2. 0.0005 g = _____ mg
3. 2 g = _____ mg
4. 0.5 g = _____ mg
5. 0.12 g = _____ mg
6. 1.5 g = _____ mg
7. 0.032 g = _____ mg
8. 10 g = _____ mg
9. 0.1 g = _____ mg
10. 0.016 g = _____ mg
11. 4 g = _____ mg
12. 0.6 g = _____ mg
13. 0.25 g = _____ mg
14. 0.0015 g = _____ mg
15. 0.04 g = _____ mg

EXERCISE 2 (answers on page 301)

Change the following milligrams to grams:

1. 60 mg = _____ g
2. 50 mg = _____ g
3. 640 mg = _____ g
4. 8 mg = _____ g
5. 2200 mg = _____ g
6. 27 mg = _____ g
7. 200 mg = _____ g
8. 6 mg = _____ g
9. 10 mg = _____ g
10. 250 mg = _____ g
11. 16 mg = _____ g
12. 12 mg = _____ g
13. 75 mg = _____ g
14. 335 mg = _____ g
15. 4.8 mg = _____ g

EXERCISE 3 (answers on page 301)

Change the following units of weight in the metric/SI system into the indicated equivalents:

1. 0.2 g = _____ mg
2. 0.5 mg = _____ g

3. 3 g = _____ mg

4. 0.5 g = _____ mg

5. 1 g = _____ mg

6. 40 mg = _____ g

7. 0.005 g = _____ mg

8. 8 mg = _____ g

9. 60 mg = _____ g

10. 5 g = _____ mg

11. 20 mg = _____ g

12. 0.6 g = _____ mg

13. 0.0005 g = _____ mg

14. 30 mg = _____ g

15. 25 mg = _____ g

16. 0.25 g = _____ mg

17. 15 mg = _____ g

18. 1240 g = _____ kg

19. 1.2 g = _____ mg

20. 0.1 mg = _____ g

21. 3000 g = _____ kg

22. 0.08 mg = _____ g

23. 5.7 kg = _____ g

24. 0.0004 g = _____ mg

25. 2500 g = _____ kg

26. 1500 g = _____ kg

27. 2 g = _____ mg

28. 1 mg = _____ g

EXERCISE 4 (answers on page 301)

Change the following units of volume in the metric/SI system into the indicated equivalents*:

1. 15 mL = _____ cc

2. 200 mL = _____ L

3. 0.45 L = _____ mL

4. 5 mL = _____ L

5. 10 cc = _____ mL

6. 0.5 L = _____ mL

7. 1 L = _____ mL

8. 40 mL = _____ L

9. 2000 mL = _____ L

10. 0.001 L = _____ mL

11. 50 cc = _____ mL

12. 30 mL = _____ L

13. 0.02 L = _____ mL

14. 250 mL = _____ L

---

*Find the correct mark on the metric/SI measures after computing the problem.

EXERCISE 4—cont'd

15. 0.75 L = _____ cc
16. 20 mL = _____ L
17. 300 mL = _____ L
18. 4 L = _____ mL
19. 0.9 L = _____ mL
20. 0.1 L = _____ mL
21. 0.25 mL = _____ cc

APOTHECARIES' SYSTEM

Although the apothecaries' system has largely been replaced by the metric/SI system, it continues to be used occasionally.

Health care professionals should know the equivalents and symbols used for the units of measure listed below in the shaded areas.

Volume
60 minims (♏) = 1 fluidram (f℥)
8 fluidrams (f℥) = 1 fluidounce (f℥)
16 fluidounces (f℥) = 1 pint (pt or O)
2 pints (pt or O) = 1 quart (qt)
4 quarts (qt) = 1 gallon (gal or C)

Weight (Troy)*
60 grains (gr) = 1 dram (℥)
480 grains (gr) = 1 ounce (℥)
8 drams (℥) = 1 ounce (℥)
12 ounces (℥) = 1 pound (lb)†

Symbols often are used to indicate the units of measure of the apothecaries' system. The symbol for the unit of measure is followed by the quantity, which is expressed in Roman numerals. However, when a fraction of a unit is expressed, it is placed after the abbreviation or symbol and is written in Arabic numbers. For example, one fourth of a grain is written as gr ¼. A special symbol, ss, is used to represent one half. For example ℥viiss = 7½ drams. Decimal numbers are not used with the apothecaries' system. When the unit of measure is written as a word, the quantity is stated in Arabic numbers and precedes the unit of measure. Note the difference for the symbols for dram and ounce.

EXAMPLES: ℥i = 1 dram
℥ii = 2 ounces
gr xl = 40 grains
♏xl = 40 minims

A greater unit can be changed to a lesser unit by multiplying the greater unit by a fraction or a whole number.

---

*In Troy weight, 11 pennyweight = 24 grains (gr) and 20 pennyweight = 16 ounce (℥).

†16 ounces = 1 pound avoirdupois, which is commonly used as a measure of weight in the United States.

EXAMPLE: Find the number of milliliters in ¼ pint. First, convert pint to milliliters. 1 pint = 500 mL. Then multiply the number of milliliters by the fraction, ¼.

$$¼ \times 500 = 125 \text{ mL in 1 pint}$$
$$(\text{pt}) \quad (\text{mL})$$

A lesser unit can be changed to a greater unit by dividing the lesser unit by a fraction or a whole number.

EXAMPLE: Find the number of milliliters equivalent to 1 pint. There are 2 pints in 1 quart, and there are 1000 mL in 1 liter.

$$1000 \div 2 = 500 \text{ mL in 1 pt}$$
$$(\text{mL/qt}) \quad (\text{pt})$$

The proportion method may also be used to change from one apothecaries' unit to another. To do this, use the same units of measure in the numerator of each ratio. Similarly, the same units of measure are used in the denominators of the ratios. Different units may be used in the numerators than in the denominators. The following example illustrates use of the proportion method.

EXAMPLE: Find the number of milliliters in ½ pt. There are 500 mL in 1 pt. Set up the proportion as follows:

$$\frac{1 \text{ (pt)}}{500 \text{ (mL)}} \times \frac{½ \text{ (pt)}}{x \text{ (mL)}} = 250 \text{ mL in ½ pt}$$

Fig. 7-4 shows two apothecaries' measures.

Because oral doses measured in minims are small and the medicine tends to cling to the measuring glass, the solution is usually diluted and poured into a medicine cup. Then the minim cup is rinsed to be sure that all of the medicine is given. A syringe may be used to measure very small amounts of medicine. The liquid medicine may be placed directly in the patient's mouth with the syringe. If a needle is attached to the syringe when measuring the liquid, the needle must be removed before the syringe is placed into the patient's mouth. A fluidounce measure is used to prepare larger quantities. When a solution is being prepared, the solute (the substance to be dissolved) is placed in the measure and water is added to make the total amount of the solution.

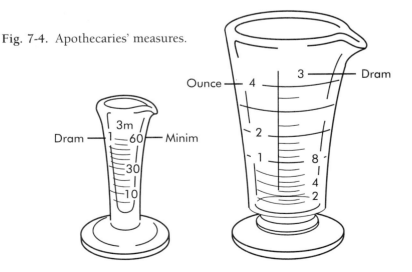

Fig. 7-4. Apothecaries' measures.

EXERCISE 5 *(answers on page 301)*

Change the following units of volume in the apothecaries' system to the indicated equivalents:

1. 1 fluidram = _____ fluidounce
2. 1/8 fluidounce = _____ minims
3. 1/2 fluidounce = _____ fluidrams
4. 1/4 fluidounce = _____ fluidrams
5. 360 minims = _____ fluidrams
6. 4 pints = _____ fluidounces
7. 8 fluidrams = _____ fluidounces
8. 1/2 pint = _____ fluidounces
9. 2 fluidounces = _____ fluidrams
10. 1 pint = _____ fluidounces
11. 4 fluidounces = _____ pints
12. 0.5 quart = _____ pints
13. 8 fluidounces = _____ pints
14. 1 pint = _____ fluidrams
15. 1 quart = _____ gallon
16. 4 pints = _____ gallon
17. 3/4 fluidounce = _____ fluidrams
18. 1 fluidram = _____ minims
19. 30 minims = _____ fluidrams
20. 1/4 fluidounce = _____ minim

EXERCISE 6 *(answers on page 301)*

Change the following units of weight in the apothecaries' system to the indicated equivalents:

1. 1 ounce = _____ drams
2. 1/2 dram = _____ grains
3. 60 grains = _____ dram
4. 2 ounces = _____ drams
5. 4 drams = _____ ounces
6. 1/4 ounce = _____ drams
7. 480 drams = _____ ounces
8. 3 drams = _____ ounce
9. 90 grains = _____ drams
10. 3 pounds = _____ ounces
11. 1/3 pound = _____ ounces
12. 1.5 drams = _____ grains
13. 30 grains = _____ drams
14. 1 1/2 ounces = _____ drams
15. 8 ounces = _____ pound
16. 1/2 ounce = _____ drams
17. 6 drams = _____ ounces
18. 4 ounces = _____ pound
19. 15 grains = _____ dram
20. 3/4 ounce = _____ grains

EXERCISE 7 *(answers on page 301)*

For each of the following units of measure, state the appropriate symbol (questions 1 through 5) or abbreviation (questions 6 through 8):

1. Dram _____
2. Gallon _____
3. Grain _____
4. Minim _____
5. Ounce _____
6. Pint _____
7. Pound _____
8. Quart _____

EXERCISE 8 *(answers on page 301)*

State the units of measure indicated by the following abbreviations or symbols:

1. ℥ _____
2. C _____
3. L _____
4. ♏ _____
5. pt _____
6. lb _____
7. qt _____
8. O _____
9. ʒ _____
10. gr _____
11. f℥ _____
12. fʒ _____

Approximate equivalents: metric/SI and apothecaries' systems

The metric/SI system is more commonly used than the apothecaries' system. Converting from one system to the other is necessary only if an order is written in one system and the available drug is labeled in the other system. To convert from one system to the other requires knowledge of approximate equivalents. Approximate equivalents are not equal, and answers obtained through such conversions may vary as much as 10%. Table 7-2 can be consulted to convert from one system to another. Health care professionals should know the following approximate equivalents:

Volume

Metric/SI system	Apothecaries' equivalents
1 milliliter (mL)*	= 15 minims (♏xv)
4 milliliters (mL)	= 1 fluidram (fʒi)
30 milliliters (mL)	= 1 fluidounce (f℥i)
500 milliliters (mL)	= 1 pint (O i)
1000 milliliters (mL) or 1 liter (L)	= 1 quart (qt)
1 gallon (C)	= 4 quarts (qt)

*Milliliters (mL) and cubic centimeters (cc) are sometimes used interchangeably. However, milliliters refer to liquids and cubic centimeters refer to gases.

Table 7-2. Approximate equivalents: metric/SI and apothecaries' systems. Those in **bold type** are used frequently.

Volume	Weight		
	g	mg	gr
30 mL = 1 fluidounce (f℥)	2	2000	30
15 mL = ½ fluidounce (f℥)	1	1000	15
10 mL = 2½ fluidrams (fℨ)	0.75	750	12
8 mL = 2 fluidrams (fℨ)	0.6	600	10
5 mL = 1¼ fluidrams (fℨ)	**0.5**	**500**	7½
4 mL = 1 fluidram (fℨ)	0.3	300	5
3 mL = 45 minims (♏)	0.25	250	4
2 mL = 30 minims (♏)	0.2	200	3
1 mL = 15 minims (♏)	0.12	120	2
0.75 mL = 12 minims (♏)	**0.1**	**100**	1½
0.6 mL = 10 minims (♏)	0.06	60	1
0.5 mL = 8 minims (♏)	0.05	50	¾
0.3 mL = 5 minims (♏)	0.03	30	½
0.25 mL = 4 minims (♏)	0.02	20	⅓
0.2 mL = 3 minims (♏)	**0.015**	**15**	¼
0.1 mL = 1½ minims (♏)	**0.01**	**10**	⅙
0.06 mL = 1 minim (♏)	**0.008**	**8**	⅛
0.05 mL = ¾ minim (♏)	0.006	6	1/10
0.03 mL = ½ minim (♏)	0.004	4	1/16
	0.003	3	1/20
	0.0015	1.5	1/40
	0.001	1	1/60
	0.0006	0.6	1/100
	0.0005	0.5	1/120
	0.0004	0.4	1/150
	0.0003	0.3	1/200
	0.00012	0.12	1/500
	0.00006	0.06	1/1000

Weight

Metric/SI System	Apothecaries' Equivalents
0.06 gram (g) or 60 milligrams (mg) =	1 grain (gr i)
1 gram (g) or 1000 milligrams (mg) =	15 grains (gr xv)*
4 grams (g) =	1 dram (ℨi)
30 grams (g) =	1 ounce (℥i)
0.45 kilogram (kg) =	1 pound (lb)
1 kilogram (kg) or 1000 grams (g) =	2.2 pounds (lb)

If a dose is ordered in grams and the medication available is in grains, the grams must be converted to grains or the grains to grams.

Remember that metric/SI–apothecaries equivalents will differ depending upon the approach used to convert from one system to another. For example, when con-

---

*15 grains may be changed to milligrams by multiplying 15 by 60 (mg) which would indicate that 15 gr = 900 mg. This is an example of the variation that sometimes occurs when converting from one system to another.

verting 5 grains to the metric/SI system the answer obtained may be either 300 mg or 325 mg, depending upon the approach to the problem.

The proportion method, discussed in Chapter 6, can be used for this purpose.

EXAMPLE: Change 0.25 pint to milliliters.
Known fact: 1 pint = 500 milliliters.
Establish a proportion, using the known fact as one ratio and the problem as the other ratio in the proportion. The order of the parts of each ratio must be the same, such as pints to milliliters.

pints:milliliters = pints:milliliters
1:500 = 0.25:x

$$1x = 0.25 \times 500$$
$$x = 125.00 \text{ milliliters in 0.25 pint}$$

EXAMPLE: Change 15 milligrams to grains.
Known fact: 60 milligrams = 1 grain.
Establish a proportion.

milligrams:grains = milligrams:grains
60:1 = 15:x
60x = 15
$$x = 15 \div 60 \text{ or } \frac{15}{60}$$
$$x = 0.25 \text{ grain or } \frac{1}{4} \text{ grain}$$

When working problems of volume, find the correct measurement on the medicine cups shown in Fig. 8-1.

EXERCISE 9 (answers on page 301)

Change the following apothecaries' units to the metric/SI system*:

1. f℥iv = _____ mL

2. gr x = _____ mg

3. ℨii = _____ mg

4. f℥ss† = _____ mL

5. f℥ii = _____ mL

6. 0.5 lb = _____ kg

7. ♏ lx = _____ mL

8. gr v = _____ mg

---

*Use of various approaches with differing equivalents may, because of the approximation, give correct answers that deviate as much as 10% from the listed answer.

†ss = one half

81

EXERCISE 9—cont'd

9. gr ss = _____ mg
10. gr xv = _____ g
11. 7 lb = _____ g
12. 0.3 gr = _____ g
13. 130 lb = _____ kg
14. ℥ iii = _____ mL
15. 22 lb = _____ kg
16. gr xx = _____ mg
17. ℳxxx = _____ mL
18. 45 f℥ = _____ mL
19. 17.6 lb = _____ kg
20. f℥i = _____ mL

EXERCISE 10 *(answers on page 301)*

Change the following metric/SI units to the apothecaries' equivalent indicated*:

1. 0.06 g = gr _____
2. 1 g = gr _____
3. 61.5 kg = _____ lb
4. 20 g = ℥ _____
5. 2 g = gr _____
6. 500 mg = gr _____
7. 24 mg = gr _____
8. 60 mL = f℥ _____
9. 6 g = gr _____
10. 2 g = gr _____
11. 75 kg = _____ lb
12. 80 kg = _____ lb
13. 1.5 mL = ℳ _____
14. 32 mg = gr _____
15. 2 mL = ℳ _____
16. 5500 g = _____ lb
17. 0.1 g = gr _____
18. 2.5 kg = _____ lb
19. 16 mg = gr _____
20. 6 g = _____ gr

*Use of various approaches with different equivalents may, because of the approximation, give correct answers that deviate as much as 10% from the listed answer.

8

Household Measures

Hospitals provide calibrated medicine cups (Fig. 8-1), calibrated medicine droppers, and other measuring equipment designed to promote accurate measurement of prescribed doses. When such equipment is not available in the home, household utensils may be used to measure dosage. This requires knowledge of household equivalents and the permission of the attending physician. In a few instances, the physician may indicate that the nature of the drug, the condition of the patient, or other factors require greater accuracy of measurement. In such situations, the appropriate calibrated measuring equipment, which is available at drugstores and pharmaceutical supply houses, must be obtained.

Volume

15 drops (gtt xv) = 1 mL or 1 cc
1 teaspoonful (t) = 1 fluidram (fʒi) or 5 (4) mL*
1 tablespoonful (T) = 4 fluidrams (fʒiv)
2 tablespoonfuls (T) = 1 fluidounce (f℥i)
6 fluidounces (f℥vi) = 1 teacupful
8 fluidounces (f℥viii) = 1 glassful

Household, Metric/SI, and Apothecaries' Equivalents

Household	Metric		Apothecaries'
1 drop	= 0.06 mL	=	1 minim
15 drops	= 1 mL	=	15 minims
1 teaspoonful	= 5 (4) mL*	=	1 fluidram
1 tablespoonful	= 15 mL	=	4 fluidrams
2 tablespoonfuls	= 30 mL	=	1 fluidounce
1 teacupful	= 180 mL	=	6 fluidounces
1 glassful	= 240 mL	=	8 fluidounces
1 pint	= 480 mL	=	16 fluidounces (approximately 500 mL)
1 quart	= 960 mL	=	32 ounces (approximately 1 liter)
1 gallon	= 3840 mL	=	128 ounces (approximately 4 liters)

---

*A scant teaspoonful is accepted as 4 mL, whereas a filled teaspoonful is regarded as 5 mL.

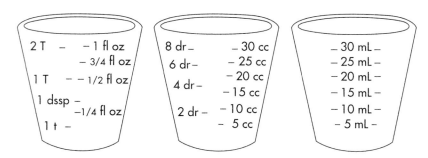

Fig. 8-1. Disposable medicine cups made of plastic material. Household, apothecaries', and metric/SI measures are indicated (dssp indicates dessertspoonful).

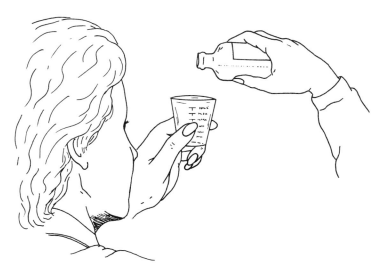

Fig. 8-2. When preparing liquid dose, the health care professional holds measure at eye level, with thumbnail resting on calibration that marks level to which liquid will be poured. Note position of the label. Pouring away from label prevents soiling that can make label difficult or impossible to read.

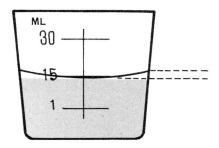

Fig. 8-3. Reading meniscus. The meniscus is caused by the surface tension of the solution against the walls of the container. Surface tension causes the formation of a concave or hollowed curvature on the surface of the solution. Read label at the lowest point of the concaved curve.

(From Clayton BD, Stock YN: *Basic pharmacology for nursing,* ed 10, St Louis, 1993, Mosby.)

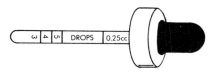

Fig. 8-4. Medicine dropper calibrated for 3, 4, and 5 drops and 0.25 cc.

For the measuring of liquid, the measuring container is held in one hand (usually the left), at eye level, with the thumbnail placed on the exact calibration that coincides with the dose to be measured (Fig. 8-2). The solution may cling to the side of the measure, producing an elliptical curve, called the *meniscus*. The lower curve of the meniscus should rest on the calibration line of the dose being measured (Fig. 8-3).

Some preparations are supplied in bottles fitted with a calibrated dropper (Fig. 8-4). This contributes to accurate measurement. Considerable variation in dosage results when ordinary medicine droppers are used to measure dosage. This can be related to factors such as the size of the opening in the dropper, the angle at which the dropper is held, and the viscosity of the liquid being measured. The dropper should not be tipped during or after measuring the dose of liquid medication. Tipping the dropper causes inaccurate measurement. If the dropper is tipped after the dose is measured, the liquid will enter the bulb and some will cling to it, causing variation in the dose measured. As a rule, medications supplied with calibrated droppers should be measured only in those droppers. The label on the preparation must be read carefully because a dropper may be calibrated to release a specific number of drops per milliliter of solution. The health care provider must be aware that the number of drops per milliliter may differ from the equivalents previously listed.

✔ *To change from household measures to another unit of measure, set up a proportion.* Both ratios of the proportion must be stated in the same order. The same units of measure must be used in both of the numerators and the units of measure used in both of the denominators must be the same. Place the ratio with the unknown quantity on one side of the proportion and the ratio with the known information on the other side.

EXAMPLE: You are asked to give f℥viii (8 fluidrams) of a medicine using a tablespoon measure. One tablespoon is equivalent to f℥iv.

$$\underset{\text{Known}}{\frac{1\ (T)}{4\ (f\mathfrak{Z})}} = \underset{\text{Unknown}}{\frac{x\ (T)}{8\ (f\mathfrak{Z})}}$$

$$4x = 8$$
$$x = 2 \text{ (tablespoon measures needed to give f℥viii)}$$

Another method of establishing the proportion is:

$$1\ (T) : x\ (T) = 4\ (f\mathfrak{Z}) : 8\ (f\mathfrak{Z})$$

$$4x = 8$$
$$x = 2 \text{ tablespoons needed to give f℥viii}$$

✔ *A greater unit may be changed to a lesser unit by multiplying the number of greater units by the number of lesser units contained in it.*

EXAMPLE: Change f℥viii (fluidrams) to f℥. It is known that f℥i (1 fluidounce) contains f℥viii (8 fluidrams).

$$3 \times 8 = 24$$

Therefore f℥iii contains f℥xxiv.

✔ *A lesser unit may be changed to a greater unit by dividing the number of lesser units by the number of greater units.*

EXAMPLE: Change 14 fluidounces to glassfuls. One glassful contains 8 fluidounces. To solve the problem, divide 14 by 8. $^{14}/_{8}$ (f℥) = $1^{3}/_{4}$ (glassfuls). Alternatively, the problem can be solved by setting up a proportion.

$$\frac{8 \text{ (fluidounces)}}{1 \text{ (glassful)}} = \frac{14 \text{ (fluidounces)}}{x \text{ (glassfuls)}}$$
$$8x = 14$$
$$x = 1.75 \text{ glassfuls}$$

Another method of setting up the proportion is:

$$8 \text{ (fluidounces)} : 14 \text{ (fluidounces)} = 1 \text{ (glassful)} : x \text{ (glassfuls)}$$
$$8x = 14$$
$$x = 1.75 \text{ or } 1^{3}/_{4}$$

EXERCISE 1 (answers on page 302)

Change the following units to the indicated equivalents:

1. 3 t = _____ mL

2. 15 mL = _____ T

3. f℥viii = _____ glassful

4. 8 f℥ = _____ mL

5. f℥viii = f℥ _____

6. 2 t = f℥ _____

7. f℥i = _____ t

8. 40 mL = _____ cc

9. 2 T = f℥ _____

10. 3 cc = ♏ _____

11. 60 mL = f℥ _____

12. 1 T = f℥ _____

13. ℥ii = ℥ _____

14. 2 t = _____ mL

15. ♏ lx = _____ t

16. f℥iv = _____ glassful

17. 2 glassfuls = f℥ _____

18. gtt xxx = _____ mL

19. f℥i = f℥ _____

20. 180 cc = _____ glassful

21. 4 mL = _____ t

22. 30 mL = _____ T

23. f℥iv = _____ T

24. f℥i = _____ T

25. 2 T = _____ mL

26. 1 cc = f℥ _____

27. 2 T = f℥ _____

28. $\frac{1}{2}$ t = gtt _____

29. 16 mL = _____ t

30. 4 t = f℥ _____

EXERCISE 2

(answers on page 302)

Shade the medicine cups for each of the following amounts, noting which measurements are equivalent when more than one measurement is provided.

1. a. 1 tablespoon   b. 4 fluidrams   c. 15 cubic centimeters   d. 15 milliliters

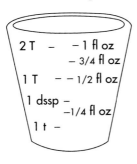 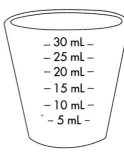 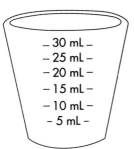

2. a. 1 teaspoonful   b. 5 cubic centimeters   c. 5 milliliters

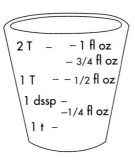 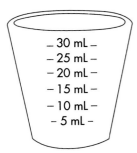 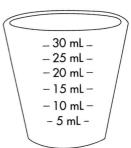

EXERCISE 2—cont'd

3. 2 fluidrams

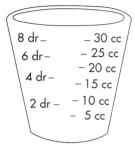

4. 10 milliliters

5. a. 2 tablespoonfuls **b.** 8 fluidrams **c.** 15 milliliters

6. 1 dessertspoonful

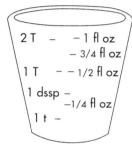

7. a. $\frac{3}{4}$ fluidounce **b.** 6 fluidrams

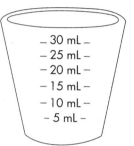

9

Linear Units of Measure

METRIC/SI SYSTEM

Metric/SI units of length may be used to prescribe the size of an area to which medication is to be applied topically, to measure the size of wheals formed by intradermal injection of drugs, and to compare the size of skin reactions to drugs when testing for allergy to selected substances. The tuberculin test is based on this principle. Linear measurements also are used to determine the size of wounds and the size of areas saturated with drainage. Such measurements serve as a baseline with which new measurements can be compared. This information provides guidance in judging whether the size of an area has changed. Measurement of the diameter of a decubitus ulcer provides additional data about it and about the effectiveness of the treatment being used to promote healing. Accurate meausurement in units of length is superior to subjective judgment based on observation alone.

Height, length, and circumference are measured in centimeters, as in measuring the circumference of the head and the length of an infant. The girth of the abdomen may be used to determine whether the amount of distention has changed and how much it has changed within a given period of time. The size of prescribed garments, such as selected abdominal binders and elastic stockings or leotards, is based on multiple measurements that are specified by the manufacturer.

Scientific instruments are calibrated in metric/SI units of length. The sphygmomanometer is calibrated in millimeters of mercury, and the manometer of central venous pressure equipment is calibrated in centimeters of water. Pressure delivered by many mechanical breathing devices and ventilators is measured in centimeters of water. The length of tubes is also calibrated in centimeters.

The distance that a patient ambulates or travels can be recorded in metric/SI units of length. Screening tests for vision and hearing specify the distance between the person being tested and the stimulus—a specified level of sound or a Snellen eye chart—to which he is asked to respond.

The meter is the fundamental unit of linear measure in the metric/SI system. A meter is equivalent to 39.37 inches (39.4 inches), which is about 3½ inches longer than a yard. The prefixes used to indicate subdivisions or multiples of units of metric/SI measures of length are the same as those listed for metric/SI units of weight and volume.

Length—meter (m)

0.001 meter = 1 millimeter (mm)
0.01 meter = 1 centimeter (cm)
0.1 meter = 1 decimeter (dm)
10 meters = 1 dekameter (dm)
100 meters = 1 hectometer (hm)
1000 meters = 1 kilometer (km)

The above table represents a complete table of linear measure. The most commonly used metric/SI measures of length are the kilometer, meter, centimeter, and millimeter. The centimeter and millimeter are used more often in health care practice than are the kilometer and meter. The following list presents commonly used equivalents:

Units of length

1 meter (m) = 1000 millimeters (mm)
0.001 meter (m) = 1 millimeter (mm)
1 meter (m) = 100 centimeters (cm)
1 centimeter (cm) = 10 millimeters (mm)
1 millimeter (mm) = 0.1 centimeter (cm)

✔ *Units of length may be changed by establishing a proportion.*

EXAMPLE: Change 250 millimeters to meters. 1000 millimeters = 1 meter.

$$\frac{1000 \text{ (mm)}}{1 \text{ (m)}} = \frac{250 \text{ (mm)}}{x \text{ (m)}}$$

$$1000x = 250$$

$$x = \frac{250}{1000} \text{ or } \frac{1}{4} \text{ or } 0.25 \text{ m}$$

This problem can also be solved as follows:

$$1000 \text{ (mm)}:1 \text{ (m)} = 250 \text{ (mm)}:x \text{ (m)}$$

$$1000x = 250$$

$$x = \frac{250}{1000} \text{ or } \frac{1}{4} \text{ or } 0.25 \text{ m}$$

Other rules that may be used to change from one unit size to another:

✔ *Multiply to change a greater unit to a lesser unit or to move the decimal point to the right for the correct number of places.*

EXAMPLE: 1 m = 1.000 mm

✔ *Divide to change a lesser unit to a greater unit or to move the decimal point to the left the correct number of places.*

EXAMPLE: 1 mm = 0 001. m

The relationship between sizes of linear units can be illustrated as shown in Fig. 9-1. Note that 1000 meters = 1 kilometer and 1000 milliliters = 1 meter.

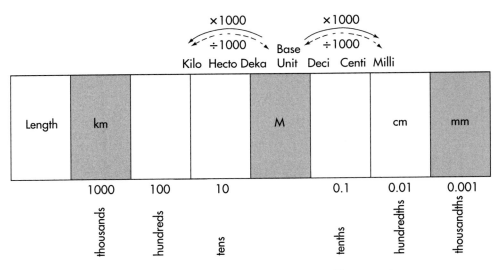

Fig. 9-1. The relationship between sizes of linear units.

EXERCISE 1 *(answers on page 303)*

Change the following units of metric/SI system of linear measure into the indicated equivalents:

1. 0.4 m = _____ cm
2. 1800 cm = _____ m
3. 20 mm = _____ cm
4. 1 m = _____ mm
5. 400 cm = _____ m
6. 40 cm = _____ mm
7. 18 cm = _____ mm
8. 240 mm = _____ m
9. 60 mm = _____ cm
10. 1.5 m = _____ mm
11. 30 mm = _____ cm
12. 5 cm = _____ mm
13. 500 mm = _____ cm
14. 10 cm = _____ mm
15. 42 cm = _____ mm
16. 1327 mm = _____ cm

EXERCISE 1—cont'd

17. 0.55 m = _____ cm   18. 50 mm = _____ cm

19. 300 mm = _____ cm

Solve the following problems:

20. The circumference of the patient's thigh measures 57.25 cm; this is equivalent to _____ mm.

21. The health care provider observes drainage on a wound dressing and charts the following:

    10 PM S: "My incision suddenly stopped hurting so much."
    O: Seropurulent drainage from wound measuring approximately 2.5 cm in diameter.
    A: Early drainage from wound.
    P: Change dressing. Reassess amount of drainage in 1 hour.

    At 11 PM, the area of drainage on the dressing is approximately 5 cm in diameter. The amount of drainage has increased by (a) _____ cm; it is (b) _____ times as large as the area of drainage recorded at 10 PM.

22. The patient complains of abdominal distention. His abdominal girth is measured at 9 AM daily. If his girth is 85 cm today and is 105 cm tomorrow, it can be said that his girth has increased by _____ cm.

23. If the patient's girth is 95 cm today and 870 mm tomorrow, would this represent a(n) _____ (increase or decrease)?

24. If the patient's abdominal girth is 34 cm, this is equivalent to _____ mm.

25. The health care provider is to test a patient's skin reaction to a medication by applying a 0.5 cm circle of ointment containing the medication. This is the same as an area of _____ mm.

26. If the distance from the heel to the popliteal space measures 300 mm, this is equal to _____ cm.

27. If the circumference of the left wrist is 7.5 cm and that of the right is 85 mm, it would be accurate to say that **(a)** the difference between the wrists is _____ cm and **(b)** that the left wrist is _____ (greater or lesser) than the right.

METRIC/SI-ENGLISH CONVERSIONS

The trend is to use metric/SI units to measure length, so persons who have always used the English system will find it necessary to make conversions between the two systems. The common English linear units of measure are:

$$12 \text{ inches (in)} = 1 \text{ foot (ft)}$$
$$3 \text{ feet (ft)} = 1 \text{ yard (yd)}$$

Other units of the English system of length can be reviewed as necessary.

The following charts review common equivalents and conversions from one system to the other.

English system   Metric/SI equivalents
1 inch (in) = 2.5 centimeters (cm)
1 foot (ft) = 30 centimeters (cm)
1 yard (yd) = 0.9 meters (m)
1 mile (mi) = 1.6 kilometers (km)

Metric/SI system   English equivalents
1 kilometer (km) = 0.6 mile (mi)
1 meter (m) = 39.4 inches (in) or 1.1 yard (yd)
1 decimeter (dm) = 4 centimeters (cm)
1 centimeter (cm) = 0.4 inches (in)
1 millimeter (mm) = 0.04 inches (in)

✔ *To convert to the metric/SI system, multiply the English measure by its metric/SI equivalent.* For example, to change the number of inches to centimeters, multiply 2.5, the number of centimeters in each inch, by the total number of inches. Conversely, to change the number of centimeters to inches, divide the total number of centimeters by 2.5, the number of centimeters in an inch. Another method of converting centimeters to inches is to multiply the total number of centimeters
✔ by 0.4, the number of inches in a centimeter. *To convert from the English equivalent to the metric/SI system, multiply the known linear measure in English by the metric/SI unit that is equivalent. To convert to the English system from the metric/SI system, divide the metric/SI unit by its English equivalent.* Proportions may also be used to solve problems of conversion.

EXAMPLE: To find the number of centimeters in 10 in, establish the proportion:

$$\frac{10 \text{ in}}{x \text{ cm}} = \frac{1 \text{ in}}{2.5 \text{ cm}}$$

$$x = 10 \times 2.5 \text{ or } 25 \text{ cm}$$

The proportion can also be established and worked as follows:

10 (inches):x (inch) = 1 (inch):2.5 (centimeters)

$$1x = 10 \times 2.5$$
$$x = 25 \text{ centimeters}$$

EXERCISE 2 *(answers on page 303)*

Change the following units of measure to the indicated equivalents:

1. 10 in = _____ cm
2. 2.5 mi = _____ km
3. 4.5 ft = _____ cm
4. 9 ft = _____ cm
5. 6 m = _____ in
6. 10 cm = _____ in
7. 3 yd = _____ m
8. 2 in = _____ cm
9. 25 mm = _____ in
10. 25 cm = _____ in
11. 1.8 m = _____ yd
12. 6 in = _____ cm
13. 3 mi = _____ km
14. 7 m = _____ in
15. 20 cm = _____ in
16. 35 km = _____ mi
17. 6 m = _____ yd
18. 2 yd = _____ m
19. 14 mm = _____ in
20. 20 in = _____ cm
21. 15 m = _____ cm
22. 55 cm = _____ in
23. 15 in = _____ mm
24. 3 m = _____ in
25. 1.5 yd = _____ m

Solve the following problems:

26. A man who is 6 ft 2 in tall is **(a)** _____ cm, or **(b)** _____ m tall.

27. A lady who is 5 ft 5 in tall is _____ cm tall.

28. An infant who is 21 in long measures _____ cm in length.

29. If you are asked to place an inch of ointment on a particular area, this is equivalent of _____ cm of ointment.

30. If an area of redness is measured as 1.5 in in diameter, this is equivalent to _____ cm in diameter.

31. If the abdominal girth of a person is 75 cm, it is equivalent to _____ in.

32. If the abdominal girth of the person in problem 31 measures 33 in on the following day, the girth can be assessed as (a) _____ (increasing or decreasing) because 33 in is the same as (b) _____ cm.

33. The patient who is ambulated for the first time after surgery may walk a distance of 20 ft, which is the same as _____ m.

34. The following day, the patient may walk 20 m, which is the same as _____ ft.

35. If your friend says that her home is 500 mi away, this is equivalent to _____ km.

36. The highway speed limit that cars are not to exceed is usually 55 mi per hour, or _____ km per hour.

37. If the length of crutches needed is 62 in long, this is the same as _____ cm.

38. If you wish to record the following using the metric/SI system, state the equivalents for each measure:

    a. An area of redness is 1.75 in, or _____ cm, in diameter

    b. Its location is 3 in, or _____ cm, from the shoulder

    c. Its center is elevated and white and measures ⅛ in, or _____ mm.

39. A patient in a cardiac rehabilitation program walked 2.2 mi during an exercise period. This distance is equivalent to _____ km.

40. Another person walked 6 km in 2 hours. This distance is equivalent to _____ mi.

41. A piece of tubing measures ¼ in in diameter. This is equivalent to _____ mm.

42. A length of tubing is 70 cm. This is equivalent to _____ in.

10

Temperature Conversion: Celsius (Centigrade) and Fahrenheit

Countries in which the metric/SI system is used measure temperature in degrees Celsius. The Celsius scale was created by Anders Celsius in 1742 in Sweden. This scale is also referred to as the centigrade scale. The Fahrenheit scale, which is used in the United States, was devised by Gabriel Fahrenheit in 1714 in Germany. The trend to convert to the metric/SI system has increased the use of the Celsius scale in the United States, but continued use of the Fahrenheit scale necessitates conversion from one scale to another. The following table compares some common baselines on these two scales.

	Celsius (centigrade)	Fahrenheit
Water freezes	0°	32°
Water boils	100°	212°
Normal body temperature	37°	98.6°

If a temperature conversion scale such as the one on page 104 is unavailable, conversion from one scale to the other is done with formulas. These formulas use either the decimal 1.8 or the fractions $5/9$ and $9/5$. One of the methods should be chosen and used consistently for converting from one temperature scale to another.

Temperature Conversion Table ($C° = \frac{5}{9}[F° - 32°]$; $F° = \frac{9}{5}[C° + 32°]$)

Celsius	Fahrenheit	Celsius	Fahrenheit	Celsius	Fahrenheit
35.0	95.0	36.9	98.4	38.7	101.8
35.1	.2	37.0	.6	38.8	102.0
35.2	.4	37.1	.8	38.9	.2
35.3	.6	37.2	99.0	39.1	.4
35.4	.8	37.3	.2	39.2	.6
35.5	96.0	37.4	.4	39.3	.8
35.6	.2	37.5	.6	39.4	103.0
35.7	.4	37.6	.8	39.5	.2
35.9	.6	37.7	100.0	39.6	.4
36.0	.8	37.8	.2	39.7	.6
36.1	97.0	37.9	.4	39.8	.8
36.2	.2	38.1	.6	40.0	104.0
36.3	.4	38.2	.8	40.1	.2
36.4	.6	38.3	101.0	40.2	.4
36.5	.8	38.4	.2	40.3	.6
36.6	98.0	38.5	.4	40.4	.8
36.7	.2	38.6	.6	40.5	105.0

FORMULAS USING DECIMALS

The decimal formula for converting the number of degrees Fahrenheit to Celsius is:

$$°C = \frac{°F - 32}{1.8}$$

EXAMPLE: Convert 212 degrees Fahrenheit to Celsius.

$$°C = \frac{212 - 32}{1.8}$$

$$°C = \frac{180}{1.8} \text{ or } 1.8 \overline{)180.0} = 100.0$$

$$°C = 100° F$$

The decimal formula for converting degrees Celsius to Fahrenheit is:

$$°F = 1.8° C + 32$$

EXAMPLE: Convert 37 degrees Celsius to Fahrenheit.

$$°F = (1.8 \times 37) + 32$$

$$°F = 66.6 + 32$$

$$°F = 98.6°$$

Remember: When using the decimal formula, 32 will always be subtracted from the number of degrees Fahrenheit when converting to Celsius because Celsius temperature is lower than Fahrenheit. Conversely, 32 is always added to the number of degrees Celsius when converting to Fahrenheit because Fahrenheit temperature is always higher than Celsius.

FORMULAS USING FRACTIONS

The greater fraction (9/5) is used when converting to Fahrenheit because the Fahrenheit temperature will be more than the Celsius temperature.

Because Celsius is less than Fahrenheit temperature, the lesser fraction (5/9) is used.

In the decimal formula, 32 is subtracted from the number of degrees Fahrenheit when converting to Celsius. Conversely, 32 is added to the number of degrees Celsius when converting to Fahrenheit.

The formula for converting degrees Fahrenheit to degrees Celsius is as follows:

$$°C = \frac{5}{9}(°F - 32)$$

EXAMPLE: Convert 105° F to Celsius.
Substitute into the formula:

$$°C = \frac{5}{9}(°F - 32)$$

$$°C = \frac{5}{9}(105° F - 32)$$

$$\frac{5}{9} \times 73 = \frac{365}{9} \text{ or } 40.56$$

Therefore 105° F is equivalent to 40.56° C or 40.6° C.

The formula for converting degrees Celsius (centigrade) to degrees Fahrenheit is:

$$°F = \frac{9}{5}(°C) + 32$$

EXAMPLE: Convert 37° C to Fahrenheit.
Use the formula:

$$°F = \frac{9}{5}(°C) + 32$$

$$°F = \frac{9}{5}(37° C) + 32$$

$$\frac{9}{5} \times 37 = \frac{333}{5} = 66.6$$

$$66.6 + 32 = 98.6$$

Therefore 37° C is equal to 98.6° F.

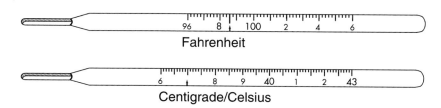

Fig. 10-1. Comparison of Fahrenheit and centigrade Celsius calibrations.
(From Potter PA, Perry AG: *Fundamentals of nursing: concepts, process, and practice,* ed 3, St Louis, 1993, Mosby.)

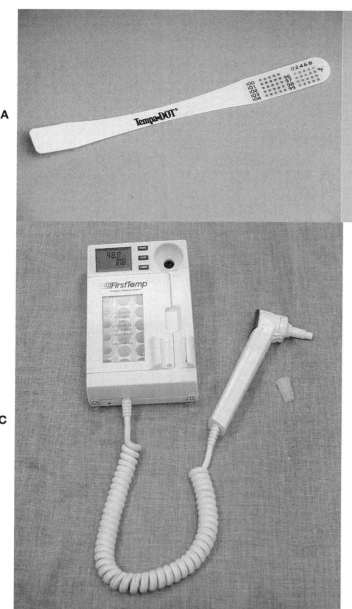
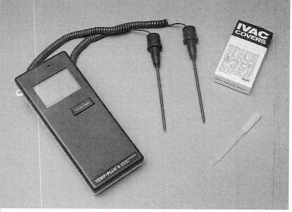

Fig. 10-2. A variety of thermometers are available. A digital readout of temperature appears on the screen of electronic thermometers. **A,** Disposable, single-use thermometer. **B,** Electronic thermometer with disposable plastic sheath. **C,** Tympanic membrane thermometer.
(From Perry AG, Potter PA: *Clinical nursing skills and techniques,* ed 3, St Louis, 1994, Mosby.)

Practice, using the formula preferred, by working the problems in the exercise. For further practice, work all conversions from Fahrenheit to Celsius and then all conversions from Celsius to Fahrenheit.

For each problem, find the calibration on the thermometer in Fig. 10-1 that indicates the temperature given and the temperature to which it was converted.

In addition to the thermometers shown in Fig. 10-1, other types of thermometers are manufactured. A few of these are shown in Fig. 10-2. Electronic thermometers are used by many agencies. These provide quick digital readouts of body temperature.

EXERCISE 1 (answers on page 303)

Work the following problems by converting the temperatures listed to the scale indicated. Round all answers to one decimal place.

1. 37.2 C = _____ F
2. 98.8 F = _____ C
3. 38.2 C = _____ F
4. 101.4 F = _____ C
5. 37.6 C = _____ F
6. 100.2 F = _____ C
7. 36.8 C = _____ F
8. 102 F = _____ C
9. 39.6 C = _____ F
10. 102.5 F = _____ C
11. 39.4 C = _____ F
12. 98 F = _____ C
13. 40 C = _____ F
14. 97.2 F = _____ C
15. 38.4 C = _____ F
16. 103.8 F = _____ C
17. 38 C = _____ F
18. 99.8 F = _____ C
19. 37.4 C = _____ F
20. 100.6 F = _____ C
21. 39.8 C = _____ F
22. 99 F = _____ C
23. 39.2 C = _____ F
24. 103 F = _____ C
25. 36 C = _____ F
26. 100.8 F = _____ C
27. 37.8 C = _____ F
28. 99.6 F = _____ C
29. 38.9 C = _____ F
30. 99.2 F = _____ C

Unit Two Posttest

EXPLANATION: The following posttest may be used to assess understanding of systems of weights and measures. Review the appropriate chapters for any problems answered incorrectly.

Directions: Change the following units of measure to the indicated equivalents:

1. 2 mg = _____ g

2. 2 g = _____ mg

3. 4000 g = _____ kg

4. 10 mg = _____ g

5. 15 cc = _____ mL

6. 0.75 L = _____ mL

7. 0.4 L = _____ cc

8. 600 cc = _____ L

9. 3 mL = _____ L

10. 30 mL = _____ cc

11. ℥iv = ℨ _____

12. 6 lbs = ℨ _____

13. 120 g = ℨ _____

14. O i = ℥ _____

15. ℥viii = ℨ _____

16. ♏lx = ℨ _____

17. ℥iv = ℨ _____

18. O ss = ℥ _____

19. 0.15 g = _____ mg

20. 0.48 g = _____ mg

21. 50 mg = _____ g

22. 340 mg = _____ g

Directions: Change the following units of measure to the indicated equivalents:

23. 120 lb = _____ kg

24. 7.5 lb = _____ kg

25. gr v = _____ mg

26. gr x = _____ mg

27. f₹v = _____ mL

28. ♏xlv = _____ mL

29. gr iss = _____ mg

30. 35 kg = _____ lb

31. 2 g = gr _____

32. 3.5 mL = ♏ _____

33. 12 mL = f₹ _____

34. 0.06 g = gr _____

35. 500 mg = _____ gr

36. f₹ss = f₹ _____

37. 15 mL = _____ T

38. 6 mL = _____ t

39. 20 mL = _____ t

40. 2 cc = ♏ _____

41. 3 g = gr _____

42. 4 m = _____ mm

43. 25 cm = _____ mm

44. 740 mm = _____ m

45. 10 cm = _____ in

46. 50 km = _____ mi

47. 4 m = _____ yd

48. 17 in = _____ cm

49. 102° F = _____ ° C

50. 38.4° C = _____ ° F

51. If Marilyn's oral temperature is 103 degrees Fahrenheit, what is her temperature in degrees centigrade?

52. Mr. Haymand's body temperature is 38.2 degrees centigrade. To how many degrees Fahrenheit is this equivalent?

53. The abdominal girth of a patient at 8 AM measures 56 in. If charted in metric units, how much would this measurement be (a) in centimeters? _____ (b) in millimeters? _____

54. When Mrs. Martin returns to her room after abdominal surgery, there is serosanguineous drainage on her dressing. The diameter of the area of drainage is measured before the dressings are reinforced with additional sterile ones. The area measures 2½ inches in diameter. (a) How would this be accurately recorded in centimeters? _____ Less than a half hour later, her blood pressure falls. Another check of the dressings reveals the area of drainage to be 4 inches or (b) _____ centimeters. The difference between the two measurements in centimeters is (c) _____ .

55. Mr. Lunkel reports that he walked 5 miles today. If he were reporting this distance in kilometers, what would he say?

56. The physician's order reads "Give cascara sagrada ℨ iv hs" This dose is equivalent to (a) _____ mL or (b) _____ t. (c) When is the dose to be given? _____

57. Mrs. Dofinsky telephones Dr. Sznthazke complaining of constipation. She tells her to take 2 T of magnesium hydroxide (Milk of Magnesia). This dose is equivalent to (a) ℨ _____ or (b) _____ mL.

58. When giving his health history to the health care providers, Mr. Everex states that he walks at least 2½ kilometers every day. This is equivalent to how many (a) meters? _____ and (b) miles? _____

59. When oral intake for Miss LeBeth is recorded, she is asked what she has had to drink since midnight. She says that she drank two glasses of water since 9 AM. She also drank a teacup of coffee and a glass of milk for breakfast. She also drank a cup of tea. (a) She has drunk how many milliliters of fluid? _____ (b) To how many pints is this amount equivalent? _____

60. Baby girl K weighed 7½ lb at birth. This is equivalent to (a) _____ g or (b) _____ kg.

Unit Three

Dosages and Solutions

Interpretation of medication orders and administration of medications require extensive knowledge. Not only is it necessary to know and use the systems of weights and measures accurately, but it is also necessary to be able to read, understand, and implement medication orders and to compute dosages correctly. This unit provides explanations and examples of these responsibilities.

In the first chapter of this unit, the many aspects of interpreting and implementing medication orders are presented. These include patient rights, legal concerns, communication of medication orders, various types of orders, storage of medications, computerized medication systems and other systems of drug administration, interpretation of abbreviations, military time, transcription and checking of orders, reading of drug labels, preparation and administration of a dose of medication, documentation, observation and teaching. Pertinent illustrations and exercises are included. These are intended to provide opportunity to practice the various elements involved in interpretation and implementation of orders. Although records, forms, and drug labels may vary in the amount of and location of information, becoming acquainted with some examples provides practice in reading them. This knowledge will help in the interpretation of similar forms when they are encountered.

Computational problems similar to those encountered in clinical practice are discussed in the final chapters of this section. Basic arithmetic and weights and measures should be reviewed as necessary when solving the practice problems. Several methods for solving each type of problem are given. One method should be chosen and used consistently. Because reading labels correctly is essential when preparing dosages, one or more drug labels are included with many of the problems. This gives the opportunity to read labels for different dosages and other information. When appropriate, practice in reading calibrations on syringes and medicine glasses is provided. IV therapy acts very quickly and it is important to be able to read orders for IV therapy correctly. It is also extremely important to work computational problems that occur with IV therapy accurately. Practice in reading the physician's orders and a variety of computations that are encountered with IV therapy are given. Content dealing with drugs and solutions for children's dosages, care of the elderly, and considerations for homecare are also discussed.

Unit Three Pretest

1. State five of the rights of patients receiving drug therapy.

2. What is the best source for learning whether you are allowed to take verbal or telephone orders for a drug?

3. Explain the meaning of the following terms that are used to refer to drug orders.

    a. Standing

    b. prn

    c. Single dose

    d. Stat

    e. Protocol

4. Explain the meaning of the following:

    a. Emergency supply of drugs

    b. Stock medications

    c. Unit doses of medications

5. What is meant by a computerized unit dose system?

6. Compute the total daily dose for the following orders if:

    a. 4 mg of drug is ordered to be given 3 times a day.

    b. One tablet is to be given after breakfast, lunch, and dinner.

    c. 30 mL of solution is to be given every 12 hours

    d. 1000 units are to be given every 8 hours

7. An order has been written for aspirin 0.6 g (orally). You know that aspirin is usually given every four hours prn. What should you do with this order?

8. The following times for drug therapy are used frequently. What are their accepted abbreviations?

    a. Four times a day

    b. Every four hours

    c. Whenever necessary

    d. After meals

    e. Before meals

    f. Twice a day

    g. Immediately

9. Interpret the following physician's orders:

    a. Simvastatin (Zocor), 20 mg orally, qd with evening meal.

b. Calcium carbonate 600 mg, orally, bid, with lunch and dinner.

 c. Thioridazine (Mellaril), 10 mg, orally, daily at hs.

10. Convert the following clock times to military (24-hour) time:

 a. 8 AM

 b. 9:30 PM

 c. 5:15 PM

11. Identify the following information on the drug label shown for Benadryl

 a. Trade name

 b. Generic name

 c. Dosage unit

 d. Dose per unit

 e. Usual dose

 f. Manufacturer

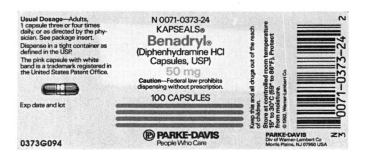

12. You are interrupted while preparing 8 AM medications for your patients. What should you do?

13. Discuss the safety measures that are followed when administering a drug(s) to a patient.

14. What must be documented following the administration of drugs?

15. What is an MAR?

16. Read the charting that follows for the following information:

    a. Patient's name, age, and room number

    b. Name of physician

    c. Known allergies

    d. Names of drugs, dose, method of administration, times and frequency of administration

    e. Initials of person administering last dose and time of last dose

17. What information should the patient know about each medication that is self-administered?

18. If a patient who is to take a drug at equal intervals three times a day usually awakens at 8 AM and goes to bed at 10 PM, when should the drug be taken?

Figure 9-6 A typical MAR for children's medications.

						DATE	2/8			DATE	2/9			DATE	2/10		
DATE	DRUG	DOSE	ROUTE	DATE DC	TIME SCHEDULE	11-7	7-3	3-11		11-7	7-3	3-11		11-7	7-3	3-11	
2/8	Prednisone 30 mg		(PO) IM IV R SC		qd		0900 C.T.				0900 C.T.				0900 C.T.		
2/10	Ery Ped susp 150 mg		(PO) IM IV R SC	2/13	q6h										R.D. 1500	R.D. 2100	

Patient Info:
Foster, Darryl
Age: 16
91-624-35-3
Rm. 501
Dr. Donalds

MEDICATION ADMINISTRATION RECORD

PRN/ONE TIME ONLY ORDERS

2/10	Furosemide 25 mg	(PO) IM IV R SC		stat										0530 M.J.		

Signature	Initials	Signature	Initials	Signature	Initials
Cathy Tag	C.T.	Cathy Tag	C.T.	Mary Jones	M.J.
				Rod Dunn	R.D.

KEY
- **ABD** - ABDOMEN
- **LA** - LT. ARM
- **LT.** - LT. THIGH
- **IVPB** - IV PIGGYBACK
- **LU** - LUQ
- **O** - NOT GIVEN
- **OD** - RT. EYE
- **OS** - LT. EYE
- **SQ** - SUBCUTANEOUS
- **OU** - BOTH EYES
- **RA** - RT. ARM
- **RT** - RT. THIGH
- **RU** - RUQ

ALLERGIES Phenobarbitol

111

19. The physician orders digoxin, 0.125 mg q AM (a) Which strength preparation is most appropriate to use? (b) How many tablets are needed for one dose? (c) How many tablets are needed for 1 week's dosage?

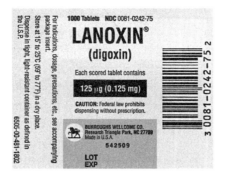
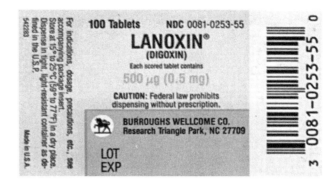

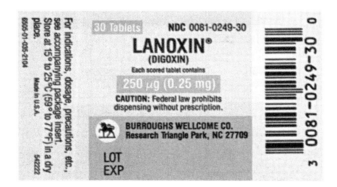

20. Mr. Swurasky is to take aspirin (Ecotrin), 5.2 g/day in divided doses. (a) How many milligrams are in the total daily dose? (b) He is instructed to take this medicine 4 times a day, at mealtime and at bedtime. Tablets containing 325 or 650 mg of drug are available. What amount of drug is required for each dose? (c) If tablets containing 325 mg are used, how many are needed for one dose? (d) If tablets containing 650 mg of drug are used, how many tablets are needed for one dose? (e) If each bottle contains 100 tablets, how many doses are available in 325 mg container? (f) in the 650 mg container? (g) Mrs. Swurasky tells you that she plans to crush the "pills" and put them in applesauce so they will be easier for the mister to swallow. What information does she need about enteric coated tablets?

21. Emery C. has Procardia XL, 60 mg, prescribed q AM. Because he has a large supply of 20 mg Procardia at home, he asks if it will be alright to deplete this supply by taking three 20 mg Procardia tablets every morning? How should you advise him?

22. If the physician orders amoxicillin, 4 g/24 h in divided doses 4 times/day, (a) How much is the total daily dosage in milligrams? (b) how many milligrams of amoxicillin is needed for one dose? (c) Which strength of the following preparations should be used? (d) How many capsules are needed for one dose? (e) How many capsules are needed for the total daily dose?

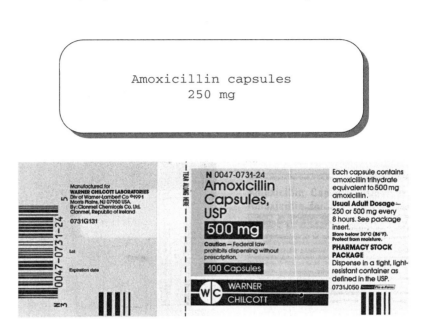

23. If the physician orders lorazepam 1.5 mg at hs, how would you prepare the dose if the following preparations are available?

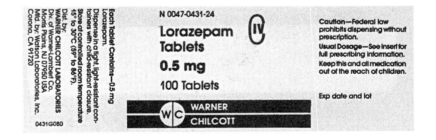

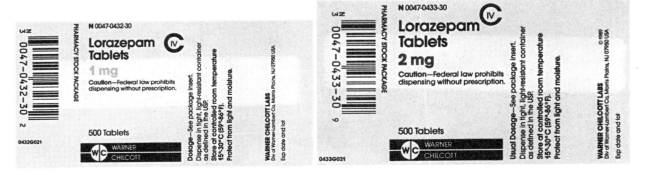

24. If codeine phosphate, gr i is ordered, which of the following preparations will provide this dose in each tablet?

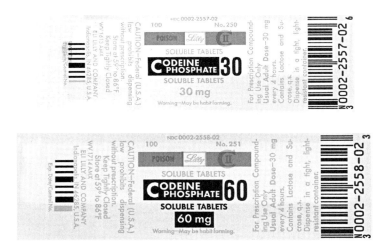

25. If gr iss of a drug is ordered, to how many milligrams is this equal?

26. Saturated solution of potassium iodide [SSKI] 0.3 g is ordered 3-4 times a day, prn. (a) What does this equal in mL? (b) Why should the solution be diluted?

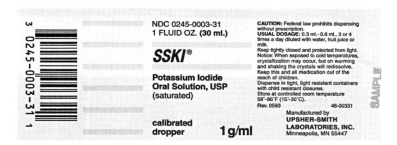

27. If 0.25 g of amoxicillin is ordered, how much of the following oral suspension will provide this dose?

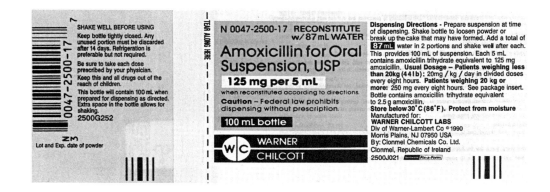

28. The physician orders nafcillin 500 mg IV q 4 h for 24 hours. (a) How many total grams of drug are needed for 24 hours? (b) Which size vial is preferable? (c) How many vials of this size are needed for 24 hours?

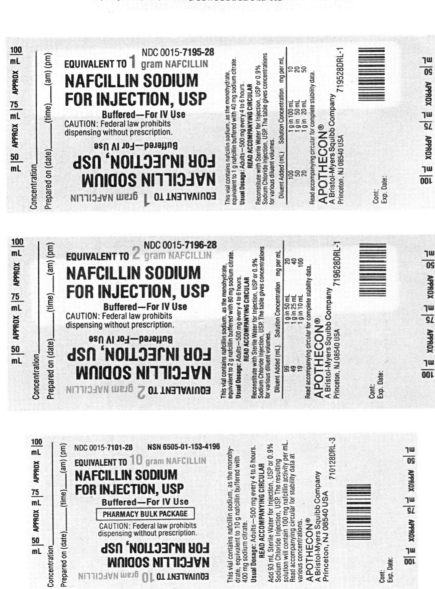

29. Explain exactly how you would prepare a liter of physiologic salt solution.

30. Which insulin is the only one intended for use in external insulin pumps?

31. Which insulin acts most rapidly?

32. Give 26 units of Novo Nordisk Lente pork insulin. (a) Which of the following insulin preparations in problem 33 would you use? (b) Mark the insulin syringe to show the correct dosage (c) Find the label for Lente Iletin II beef insulin. (d) Which of the labels shown represent insulins that have recombinant DNA origin?

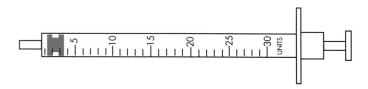

33. Identify the following information on the insulin labeled "i":

   a. Manufacturer

   b. Type of insulin

   c. Brand of insulin

   d. Species of origin

   e. Concentration

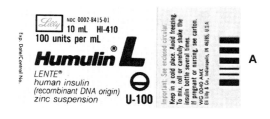

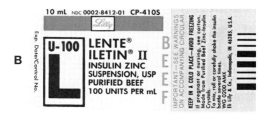

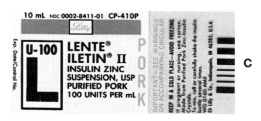

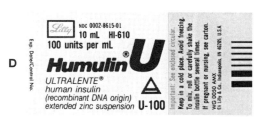

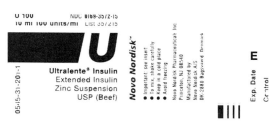

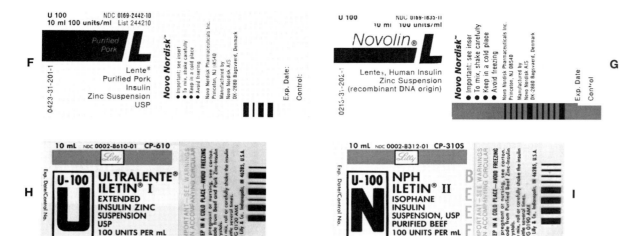

34. Which insulins have (**a**) short action (**b**) intermediate action (**c**) long action?

35. Answer the following questions from an order that reads:

Infuse 3000 mL D5W with 40 mEq KCl in each liter over next 24 hours beginning at 6 AM.

a. Name the kind of solution ordered.

b. State whether this solution is hypotonic, isotonic, or hypertonic.

c. State the total amount of solution ordered.

d. Are any medications to be added to the solution? If so, give the names and amounts.

e. When is the IV infusion to start?

f. Does the order state how long the solution is to run? If yes, how long is it to run?

g. Does the order state the rate of flow to be used? If yes, what is it?

h. How much solution is to be delivered every 8 hours?

i. Calculate the rate of flow in drops per minute if the tubing has a drop factor of 10.

j. Calculate the rate of flow in mL/h.

36. Create a time strip for marking the container of intravenous solution if 1000 mL are to run for 8 hours beginning at 7 PM. Use the mL markings given and use 24-hour time.

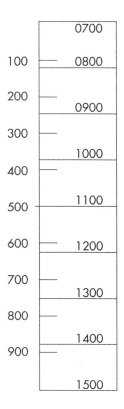

37. When you come to work, you find that Mrs. Divine's IV solution is behind schedule. 1000 mL of solution was scheduled to run 8 h (125 mL/h). Agency policy allows one increase of 25% if there are no contraindications. After assessing Mrs. Devine's condition, you decide to increase the rate of flow by 25% and to observe her closely to be sure that she is tolerating the increased rate of flow. (a) What should the flow rate have been in mL/h? (b) If you increase the rate by 25%, how many additional mL/h will be delivered? (c) What will the new rate of flow be in mL/h?

38. You are instructed to set the IV flow rate at 25 mL/h. (a) If the macrodropper has a factor of 10, what will the rate be in macrodrops/minute? (b) How many milliliters will be delivered in 1 minute? (c) If you use a minidropper that delivers 60 gtts/mL, at what rate will you set the flow in minidrops per minute?

39. Name three abbreviations used to order a "keep open" flow rate.

40. If you are to infuse 2 mEq of potassium chloride hourly using 1000 mL of IV solution that contains 20 mEq of potassium chloride, (a) how many mL of solution is needed to give 2 mEq of potassium chloride? (b) If using a pump, what will the flowrate in mL/h be? (c) Using a macrodrip of 10, how many drops per minute will deliver this amount of potassium chloride hourly?

41. Mrs. K. needs 1000 mL of 5/1 with 40 mEq of potassium chloride added. Because of infiltration, you must discontinue the infusion and chart amount of solution and amount of potassium chloride that she has received. If there are approximately 250 mL of solution remaining, what will you chart for (a) amount of 5/1 taken? (b) amount of potassium chloride taken?

42. You are instructed to flush a heparin lock. Where can you look to learn the amount and kind of solution that is to be used?

43. Where can you find the usual dosage range for a drug?

44. How many units of heparin are in a 4 mL vial that contains 1000 U/mL?

45. If you are to give 1200 units of heparin each hour and the solution you have contains 100 U heparin/mL, how much is needed for one dose?

46. If your patient is receiving 20 mL of solution q1h, and there are 100 U of heparin in each mL of solution, how many units will the patient receive in 24 hours?

47. What kind of syringe will you use to measure heparin that comes in a multi-dose vial?

48. The physician orders 5000 U heparin SC q 12h for Mrs. Hunibrodt. You can choose from preparations that contain 10, 100, 1000, 5000 or 10,000 U/mL. Which strength preparation is most appropriate?

49. Shade the tuberculin syringe shown below to indicate that you are measuring 500 U of heparin using a solution that contains 1000 U/ml.

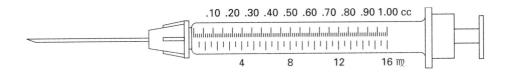

50. If 250 mL of solution contains 50 mg of drug, how much drug is contained in 1 mL of solution?

51. If there are 0.3 mg/mL, how many mcg are there in 1 mL?

52. The physician prescribes a 3 mcg/kg/min dose of a drug to be given intravenously to a patient who weighs 143 lb. (a) What is the patient's weight in kilograms? (b) If there are 25 mg of the drug in 100 mL, how many milligrams of drug are in each mL of solution? (c) How many mcg of drug are there in each mL of solution? (d) How many mcg/min of the prescribed drug is the patient to receive? (e) How many mL/min of solution are needed to deliver this amount of drug? (f) How many mL/h of the prescribed solution will deliver this dose?

53. A child weighs 66 lb. He is to be given an oral suspension of erythromycin (EryPed) 50 mg/kg/day in four divided doses. (a) What will his total daily dosage be? (b) How many mg of drug are needed for each dose? (c) Read the labels that follow and select the one that will provide this dose using the least number of mL of solution. (d) How many mL of solution are needed for one dose?

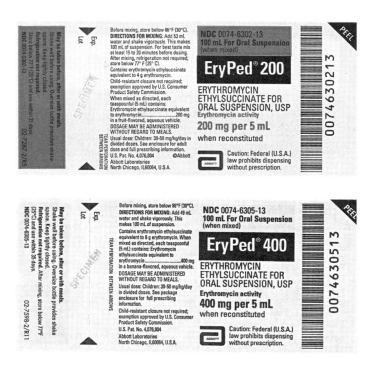

54. Had the physician ordered erythromycin suspension 600 mg/day divided into four doses, (a) how many mg are needed for one dose? (b) How many mL will supply one dose? (c) How many mL are needed for the total daily dose?

55. The physician ordered digoxin (Lanoxin) elixir to digitalize Missy who weighs 56.8 lb. (a) How many kilograms does Missy weigh? (b) Using the usual digitalizing dosage range of 30 to 40 mcg/kg, what is the dosage range for Missy? One-half the total dose is to be given stat and the remainder is to be divided into two doses and given at 8-hour intervals. (c) How much is the dosage range for the stat dose? (d) for each of the two doses that follow the stat dose? (e) Develop a time schedule if the first dose of medicine is given at 6 PM. Use 24-hour time.

56. The physician orders 0.35 mg erythromycin suspension. (a) This is equivalent to how many micrograms? (b) Using the label shown in problem 53, how many mL of suspension are needed for this dose? (c) How can you accurately measure this amount?

57. The adult dose of acetaminophen (Tylenol) is 650 mg. Use body surface area to calculate the dose for Joey who weighs 48.5 lb. **(a)** What is Joey's weight in kilograms? **(b)** What is his body surface area in m^2? **(c)** What is the dosage of acetaminophen for Joey? **(d)** If each tablet of Tylenol contains 350 mg, how many tablets are needed for one dose?

58. Use Clark's formula to obtain a rough estimate of a reasonable dose for a child weighing 50 lb if the adult dose is 650 mg.

59. Use Young's rule to estimate the dose for a child who is 10 years old if the adult dose of the drug is 650 mg.

60. Body surface area provides a fairly accurate method of estimating a child's dose. How do the answers obtained using Clark's and Young's rule compare to the conversion using BSA?

61. What are some reasons that drug dosage may need adjusting for persons who are elderly?

62. Name at least 3 indications of drug interactions.

63. State two common reasons for drug interactions occurring in elderly persons.

64. Health care providers may recommend that patients have all their prescriptions filled at the same pharmacy? Why?

65. What are some reasons that noncompliance with the drug therapy regimen occurs?

66. You are to instruct a hospitalized patient concerning home medication. What are 8 key points that you will include in your teaching plan?

67. On home visits, what would you look for concerning the storage of medicine?

68. What is the meaning of the abbreviation, OTC?

69. Mrs. Linert has had a drug prescribed for rapid heart beat. The prescribing physician instructed her to take it whenever she feels her heart is racing. She has now gone to another physician who told her to follow the instructions on the label "Take 1 a day." She asks you what you think she should do. What will you tell her?

70. Laura has medication for severe hypertension. She tells you that she skips the medicine on the days when she feels fairly good. What does she need to know?

71. Mr. Layton takes procainamide to treat a cardiac arrythmia. After taking the drug for about 5 months, he complains of being extremely fatigued, even when he awakens in the morning. What should you advise him?

72. Maurice stated that he is extremely allergic to aspirin. How can you avoid giving him any medication that contains aspirin?

73. Thelma tells you that the doctor wants to give her a challenge dose of medicine that is thought to be the one most effective against her type of infection. It is similar in chemical structure to another drug to which she is allergic. She asks you to explain what is meant by a challenge dose and why it's necessary.

74. How can people with known allergies protect themselves against receiving specific allergens?

75. It is sometimes recommended that the unpleasant taste of medicine be disguised with milk. Why might you disagree with this thinking?

76. Mrs. Dytace is taking a medication that will lower her serum cholesterol level. She tells you that she is supposed to get blood tests but doesn't understand why she needs them. How might you explain the need for blood tests to her?

11

Interpretation and Implementation of Physician's Order

Interpretation and implementation of medication orders require considerable knowledge of the patient, the patient's age and condition, the plan for therapy, and the drug. The health care provider must know the patient's drug and allergy histories and be aware of any other adverse drug–related reactions which the patient has experienced.

Familiarity with available dosage forms, methods and techniques of administration, expected effects, symptom of adverse effects, and necessary precautions is essential. This knowledge ensures that the "five rights of patients" receiving drug therapy are met. These are:

The right patient
The right drug
The right dosage
The right time
The right route of administration

Additional "rights" include the right to accurate documentation of therapy and knowledge about the prescribed drug therapy, and the right to refuse medication.

✚ THINK CRITICALLY
Is this the right patient?
Is this the right drug?
Is this the right dosage?
Is this the right time?
Is this the right route of administration?

Health care professionals must recognize their own limitations in knowledge or skill and know when to seek appropriate assistance. Whenever a question occurs about the drug or the dose, the health care provider must seek additional information from a reliable source. Many sources of drug information are available. Ideally, official publications of the drugs used in clinical practice should be available on the health care unit. A colleague or a supervisor may be consulted. Pharmacists should be consulted whenever the needed information is not readily available. They have specialized knowledge of drugs and access to many sources of reliable information.

> ### ✚ THINK CRITICALLY
> Is this dose within the usual range?
> Is this the usual method of administration?
> Is this the usual frequency of administration?
> Are these the usual times for taking this medication?
> What are the expected effects of this medicine?
> What symptoms might indicate an adverse reaction to this medicine?

LEGAL ASPECTS OF DRUG THERAPY

State laws and policies established by the employing agency govern the role of health care providers in prescribing, dispensing, and administering medications. Health care professionals may administer only those medications that are legally prescribed. Competency in drug administration must be demonstrated. Laws and agency policies provide guidance in determining who may administer drugs and any restrictions that apply. In many states nurse practitioners, clinical nurse specialists, and physician assistants who have met specified requirements are allowed to prescribe or dispense medications in certain situations.

All health care professionals who administer medications accept responsibility for their own actions even when following a prescription. It is important to know the usual dose, route of administration, frequency of administration, contraindications for the drug, and signs and symptoms of both expected and adverse reactions to the drug. Knowledge and observation of these elements protect the patient from harm and help ensure that needed therapy is received.

MEDICATION ORDERS

Whenever possible medication orders are written by the physician in the physician's order book to decrease misunderstandings and errors. Medication orders are written or given verbally. A written order decreases the potential for misunderstandings and errors. The order should be rechecked and, if it is unclear, assistance with interpretation of the order must be obtained. Examples of a physician's order sheet are shown in Fig. 11-1.

Verbal orders, including telephone orders, are occasionally necessary. Agency policy should always be checked before a verbal order is accepted. Verbal orders are discouraged except in emergencies. Many institutions prohibit students from accepting verbal orders under any circumstances.

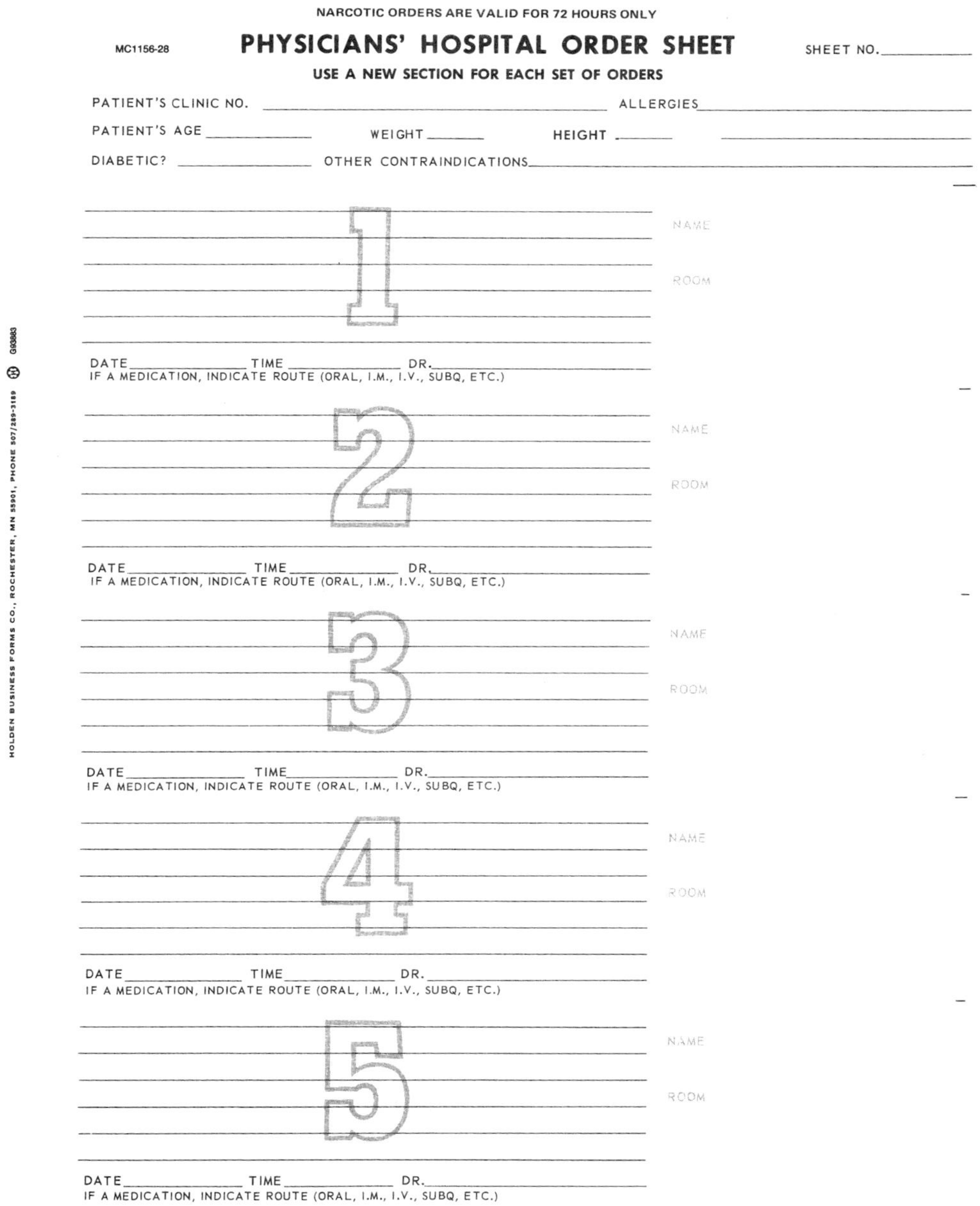
NARCOTIC ORDERS ARE VALID FOR 72 HOURS ONLY

MC1156-28 **PHYSICIANS' HOSPITAL ORDER SHEET** SHEET NO.______

USE A NEW SECTION FOR EACH SET OF ORDERS

PATIENT'S CLINIC NO. ______ ALLERGIES______

PATIENT'S AGE ______ WEIGHT ______ HEIGHT ______

DIABETIC? ______ OTHER CONTRAINDICATIONS______

1 NAME ROOM

DATE______ TIME______ DR.______
IF A MEDICATION, INDICATE ROUTE (ORAL, I.M., I.V., SUBQ, ETC.)

2 NAME ROOM

DATE______ TIME______ DR.______
IF A MEDICATION, INDICATE ROUTE (ORAL, I.M., I.V., SUBQ, ETC.)

3 NAME ROOM

DATE______ TIME______ DR.______
IF A MEDICATION, INDICATE ROUTE (ORAL, I.M., I.V., SUBQ, ETC.)

4 NAME ROOM

DATE______ TIME______ DR.______
IF A MEDICATION, INDICATE ROUTE (ORAL, I.M., I.V., SUBQ, ETC.)

5 NAME ROOM

DATE______ TIME______ DR.______
IF A MEDICATION, INDICATE ROUTE (ORAL, I.M., I.V., SUBQ, ETC.)

HOLDEN BUSINESS FORMS CO., ROCHESTER, MN 55901, PHONE 507/289-3189 G93883

Fig. 11-1. Order sheet with carbon backing. Sections of top sheet containing the order as written and signed by the physician can be removed and given to the pharmacist. The carbon copy of the physician's orders remains on the health care unit. The copy facilitates checking of new orders when the medication is delivered. (Copyright Mayo Foundation for Medical Education and Research. Used with permission.)

The person who accepts a verbal order is responsible for writing the order in the physician's order book. The order, written immediately after it is received, contains the components of an order written by a physician. In addition, the person accepting the order signs the order as follows: "Verbal order by Dr. Shakar to N. Dison, RN" or "V.O. Dr. Shakar/N. Dison, RN." The physician is asked to sign the order at the earliest opportunity, usually within 24 hours. This is specified by agency policy or state and federal laws.

In some settings, the physician's orders are processed with a fax machine. This provides a written record of the order, saves time, and protects both the patient and the health care provider.

Types of medication orders

There are several types of medication orders. A *standing order* is common. It is an order that stands or continues to be in effect until cancelled (Fig. 11-2). Some orders are cancelled automatically when the order has been in effect for a stated period of time. To be considered legally valid, federal laws require the renewal of narcotic orders at stated intervals. The physician may include the length of time for which an order is to stand when writing the order. In most institutions, orders are discontinued and new orders are written when the patient enters an institution or has surgery.

A standing order may indicate that the medicine is to be given at specific times or that it is to be given whenever necessary but no more frequently than specified. The latter is referred to as a prn order. A prn order is a type of standing order. Fig. 11-3 shows an example of a prn order.

Orders for a *single dose order* are carried out one time only—at the time specified in the physician's order or as soon as possible (Fig. 11-4). A *stat order* is a special kind of single dose, one-time order. *Stat* means that the order is to be carried out immediately. Usually, the word *stat* follows the order. An example of such an order is "Give 10 mg morphine sulfate IV stat" (Fig. 11-5).

A *protocol* is a written document that tells the health care provider which actions are permitted without first notifying the attending physician. The order,

Date Ordered	Start Date	Medication and frequency	Dose	Route	Physician Signature
4/1/96	4/2/96	Erythromycin q 6 h	250mg	PO	D. Markes, MD

Fig. 11-2. Example of a standing order, an order that stands until it is discontinued.

Date Ordered	Start Date	Medication and frequency	Dose	Route	Physician Signature
2/4/96	2/4/96	Aspirin q 4 h prn	650mg	PO	B Elemer, MD

Fig. 11-3. Example of a prn order. Medication is given when necessary, but no more often than every 4 hours.

Date Ordered	Start Date	Medication and frequency	Dose	Route	Physician Signature
12/26/96	12/27/96	NPH Insulin tomorrow before breakfast	40U	SC	H Doktor, MD

Fig. 11-4. Example of a single dose order. The dose is not to be repeated.

Date Ordered	Start Date	Medication and frequency	Dose	Route	Physician Signature
11/22/96	11/22/96	Morphine Sulfate stat	10mg	IM	G. Teretta, MD

Fig. 11-5. Example of a stat order. The order is to be carried out immediately and for one time only.

written and signed by a physician, states the circumstances under which the health care provider may implement the order. For example, an order in a protocol for Dr. Sinct's patients might state: "Give aspirin gr. x, q4h prn for relief of headache." This order applies *only* to Dr. Sinct's patients. A protocol allows the health care provider to administer certain medications without first notifying the physician. An existing order specific to the patient *always* supersedes a protocol.

Drug supplies and storage

Emergency supply of drugs. An emergency supply of drugs may be kept on the unit. This supply may contain single or multiple doses of medicines. Some medications may be stored in individually labeled envelopes. Arranging the drugs in alphabetical order facilitates quick finding of needed drugs. Labels must be read very carefully to ensure the correct choice of the strength of a drug and correct number of doses in a vial. If a drug from the emergency supply is used, it must be replaced as soon as possible. Necessary information must be given to the pharmacist by completing a form printed on the drug's packaging envelope or by using a special voucher.

Stock medications. Multiple doses of some drugs may be supplied in a single container. Individual doses are removed when needed. For example, many individual doses may be poured from one large bottle of magnesium hydroxide (Milk of Magnesia), or many doses may be obtained from one container of aspirin tablets. When stocked on the health care unit, these drugs are referred to as *stock medications* (Fig. 11-6). Because the use of stock medications increases the risk of error, use of them has declined.

Individual supplies of medicine. Each patient may have a supply of each of his or her medications stored in a cubicle in the medication cupboard or drawer of the medication cart. Each container may hold multiple doses. Therefore the health care provider must read labels carefully.

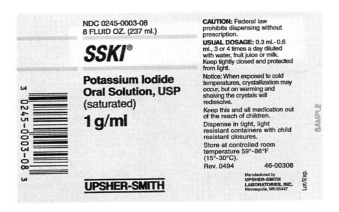

Fig. 11-6. An example of a stock medication that contains multiple doses of medicine.

Single doses or unit doses of medicine. Pharmaceutical companies supply some medications as single doses. The usual dose of the medicine is prepared and labeled by the manufacturer. For example, a small container of magnesium hydroxide (Milk of Magnesia) is available that supplies 1 oz, the usual dose of the drug. Single doses of tablets may be supplied in individual packages, or many single doses may be supplied in one package (Fig. 11-7, 11-8, and 11-9). Unit doses also may be prepared by the pharmacist.

Medication systems. Any of several medication systems, or variations of them, may be used.

COMPUTERIZED UNIT DOSE SYSTEM. The computerized dose system decreases chances for error. When carbonized forms are used, the original copy of the physician's drug order is sent directly to the pharmacy. A carbon copy of the order remains in the physician's order book and is used to check the order on the computerized printout. See Fig. 11-1 on p. 125, which illustrates this type of order sheet. After the pharmacy has received the physician's order, the order is entered into the computer along with pertinent information about the patient. This infor-

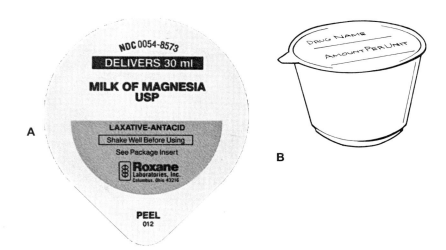

Fig. 11-7. **A**, Label of one-size single-dose container of magnesium hydroxide (Milk of Magnesia). **B**, Unit doses of liquid forms may be packaged in small sealed cups from which the dose is administered. The sealed cover contains identifying information. The physician's order and the labeling information must be compared carefully because many medicines are available in single doses of different strengths. For example, Milk of Magnesia is available in unit dose packages of either 15 mL or 30 mL.

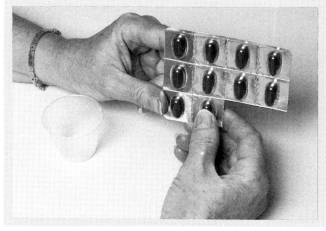

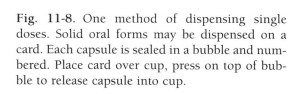

Fig. 11-8. One method of dispensing single doses. Solid oral forms may be dispensed on a card. Each capsule is sealed in a bubble and numbered. Place card over cup, press on top of bubble to release capsule into cup.

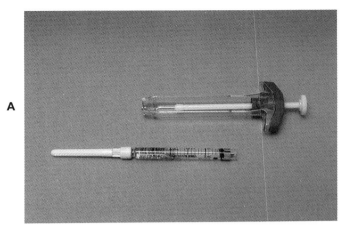

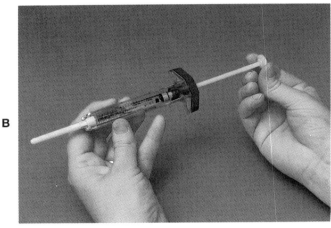

Fig. 11-9. Example of a prefilled cartridge of medication and its assembly. **A,** Carpuject syringe and prefilled sterile cartridge with needle. **B,** The cartridge slides into the syringe barrel, turns and locks at the needle end. The plunger then screws into the cartridge end.

(From Potter PA, Perry AG: *Fundamentals of nursing: concepts, process, and practice,* ed 3, St Louis, 1989, Mosby.)

mation is printed, usually on a printer at the health care provider's station, and checked against the original order. A sample printout is shown in Fig. 11-10.

The unit dose arrives in an envelope on which the information needed by the health care provider for safe administration of the medication has been printed (Fig. 11-11). This information is checked against the information of the drug profile and serves the same purpose as a medication card. If a discrepancy is found, the original physician's order is rechecked and the appropriate personnel are consulted.

The label on each unit dose package states the name of the drug, amount of drug contained in each package, and the amount of drug contained in one tablet or capsule. Unit dose packages of liquid preparations for oral administration state the amount of drug contained in a specified amount of solution. Examples of such labels are: a unit dose label for phenazopyridine hydrochloride (Pyridium) states that one tablet contains 100 mg of drug, a unit dose label for magnesium hydroxide (Milk of Magnesia) states that it contains 30 mL of magnesium hydroxide

```
SCHEDULED DOSES:                                          ADMINISTRATION TIMES
    11 DIGOXIN TAB, 0.25 MG
        DOSE: 0.25 MG     AMT: 1 TAB                                    9
        RT: PO     SCHED: EVERY DAY
        (LANOXIN)         DURATION: OPEN FD:09:00       02/19
NJD_____LD:OPEN_____
    12 SYNTHROID TAB, 0.100 MG (100 MCG) (NF)
        DOSE: 0.1 MG AMT: 1 TAB                                         9
        RT: PO     SCHED: EVERY DAY
        (SYNTHROID)       DURATION: OPEN FD:09:00       02/19
NJD_____LD:OPEN_____
    13 POTASSIUM CL MICROBURST TAB, 10 MEQ
        DOSE: 10 MEQ AMT: 1 TAB                                         8
        RT: PO     SCHED: EVERY DAY WITH MEAL
        (K DUR/TEN-K)     DURATION: OPEN FD:08:00       02/19
NJD_____LD:OPEN_____
    14 CEPHALEXIN CAP, 500 MG
        DOSE: 500 MG AMT: 1 CAP                                  6-10-16-22
        RT: PO     SCHED: QID-6
        NOTE: WHEN UCI/I&O AND ANCEF COMPLETE
        (AKA KEFLEX) DURATION: OPEN FD:OPEN
NJD_____LD:OPEN_____
    23 PNEUMOCOCCAL VACCINE VIAL, 0.5 ML                       ONE DOSE AT 10
 *** DOSE:0.5 ML     AMT: 0.5 ML
        RT: IM     SCHED: ONE DOSE                                      *
        (PNU-IMMUNE/PNEUMOVAX) DURATION: 1 DOSE   FD:10:00   02/20
NJD                                              LD:10:00   02/20
===============================================================
PRN DOSES:
     2 HYDROXYZINE HCL VIAL, 50 MG/ML                          PRN DOSE
        DOSE: 25-50 MG    AMT: 0.5-1 ML
        RT: IM     SCHED: Q3H PRN
        (VISTARIL)        DURATION: OPEN ST:21:32   02/18
NJD_____SP:OPEN_____
     3 ACETAMINOPHEN W/COD 30 MG, *USE STOCK*                  PRN DOSE
        DOSE: 1-2 TAB     AMT: 1-2 TAB
        RT: PO     SCHED: Q3-4H PRN
        (TYLENOL #3) DURATION: OPEN FD:21:32            02/18
NJD_____SP:OPEN_____
     4 PROPOXYPHENE N/ACETAMIN TAB, 100/650MG                  PRN DOSE
        DOSE: 1-2 TAB     AMT: 1-2 TAB
        RT: PO     SCHED: Q4H PRN
        (AKA DARVOCET N 100)  DURATION: OPEN    ST:21:32   02/18
NJD_____SP:OPEN_____
     6 DROPERIDOL VIAL, 5 MG/2 ML                              PRN DOSE
        DOSE: 1.25 MG     AMT: 0.5 ML
        RT: IM     SCHED: Q6-8H PRN
        (INAPSINE) DURATION: OPEN ST:21:33   02/18
NJD_____SP:OPEN_____
     7 TRIMETHOBENZAMIDE CAP, 250 MG                           PRN DOSE
        DOSE: 250 MG AMT: 1 CAP
        RT: PO     SCHED: Q6-8H PRN
        (TIGAN)           DURATION: OPEN ST:21:33   02/18
NJD_____SP:OPEN_____
     8 DIPHENHYDRAMINE CAP, 25 MG                              PRN DOSE
        DOSE: 25-50 MG    AMT: 1-2 CAP
        RT: PO     SCHED: HS PRN
        (AKA BENADRYL)    DURATION: OPEN ST:21:33   02/18
NJD_____SP:OPEN_____
===============================================================
PRN DOSES:
     6 DIPHENHYDRAMINE CAP, 25 MG                              PRN DOSE
 *** DOSE: 25 MG AMT: 1 CAP
        RT: PO     SCHED: HS PRN; MR X 1
        (AKA BENADRYL)    DURATION: OPEN ST:16:29       02/19
NJD_____SP:OPEN_____
     8 **WARNING MESSAGE FOR ACETAMINOPHEN**                   PRN DOSE
 *** DOSE: SEE NOTE  AMT: SEE NOTE
        RT: PO     SCHED: PRN
        NOTE: RECOMMENDED NOT TO EXCEED 4 GRAMS OF APAP / 24 HOURS
                          DURATION: OPEN ST:OPEN
NJD_____SP:OPEN_____
     9 LAXATIVE, ENEMA, OR SUPP. OF CHOICE                     PRN DOSE
 *** DOSE:            AMT:
        RT: PO     SCHED: PRN
                          DURATION: OPEN ST:OPEN
NJD_____SP:OPEN_____
===============================================================
***INDICATES NEW ORDER; **INDICATES CHANGED ORDER; *INDICATES ITEMS CHANGED
PLEASE CHECK AGAINST PHYSICIAN'S ORDER AND CALL PHARMACY IF INCORRECT.
```

Fig. 11-10. Example of a computerized drug profile sheet. Abbreviations are sometimes used to indicate information such as route, start time, and schedule. Note that military time is used on this profile.
(Copyright Mayo Foundation for Medical Education and Research. Used with permission.)

```
CONTINUOUS INFUSIONS:

SERIES: A

A11    5% DEXTROSE IN 0.45% NACL 1,000 ML            START: 10:30 01/20
       20 MEQ KCL                                    STOP:  18:30 01/20
       RUN TIME: 08:00 RATE: 125 ML/HR 2.1 ML/MIN                    MRG

A12    5% DEXTROSE IN 0.45% NACL 1,000 ML            START: 18:30 01/20
       20 MEQ KCL                                    STOP:  02:30 01/21
       RUN TIME: 08:00 RATE: 125 ML/HR 2.1 ML/MIN                    MRG

A13    5% DEXTROSE IN 0.45% NACL 1,000 ML            START: 02:30 01/21
       20 MEQ KCL                                    STOP:  10:30 01/21
       RUN TIME: 08:00 RATE: 125 ML/HR 2.1 ML/MIN                    NKE

A14    5% DEXTROSE IN 0.45% NACL 1,000 ML            START: 10:30 01/21
       20 MEQ KCL                                    STOP:  18:30 01/21
       RUN TIME: 08:00 RATE: 125 ML/HR 2.1 ML/MIN                    NKE

A15    5% DEXTROSE IN 0.45% NACL 1,000 ML            START: 18:30 01/21
       20 MEQ KCL                                    STOP:  02:30 01/22
       RUN TIME: 08:00 RATE: 125 ML/HR 2.1 ML/MIN                    NKE
       END OF CURRENT ORDERS, NEW ORDERS NEEDED

------------------------------------------------------------

SERIES: B

B1     0.9% SODIUM CHLORIDE 1,000 ML                 START: OPEN
                                                     STOP:  OPEN
       RUN TIME: VARIABLE                      ORDER VALID: 20:00 01/19
       NOTE: EMERGENCY FLOOR STOCK                                   SZS

B4     5% NORM. SERUM ALBUMIN 500 ML                *START: 13:00 01/20
**                                                  *STOP:  14:00 01/20
       RUN TIME: 01:00 RATE: 500 ML/HR 8.3 ML/MIN
       NOTE: GIVE IF U0 < 15 ML—INFORM IF NEEDED                     NKE
============================================================

INTERMITTENT INFUSIONS:                         ADMINISTRATION TIMES

INT2   10 MG PROCHLORPERAZINE    IN
       5% DEXTROSE IN WATER 50 ML
       RUN TIME: 00:15 RATE: 200 ML/HR 3.3 ML/MIN
       NOTE: Q4H PRN; INFORM NEEDS (IM OR IV)    FD: OPEN
HRD    SCHED: PRN         DURATION: OPEN         LD: OPEN
------------------------------------------------------------
INT4   500 MG VANCOMYCIN    IN                           11-23
       5% DEXTROSE IN WATER 100 ML
       RUN TIME: 01:00 RATE: 100 ML/HR 1.7 ML/MIN
                                                 FD: 11:00   01/18
HRD    SCHED: Q12H        DURATION: OPEN         LD: OPEN
------------------------------------------------------------
INT5   1 GM AZTREONAM (NF)    IN                         2-10-18
       5% DEXTROSE IN WATER 50 ML
       RUN TIME: 00:20 RATE: 150 ML/HR 2.5 ML/MIN
                                                 FD: 11:00   01/18
HRD    SCHED: Q08H        DURATION: OPEN         LD: OPEN
------------------------------------------------------------
                    ****** CONTINUED ON NEXT PAGE ******
```

Fig. 11-10, cont'd. Example of a computerized drug profile sheet.

```
Dison, Norma                              Room 4-034

Ascription tab, 2 tab                     Dose for: 18:00      9/26/88

Amount: 2 tab

Route: PO                        Schedule: bid with meals
- - - - - - - - - - - - - - - - - - - - - - - - - - - - - - - - - -
 If the dose is not given to the patient, check the reason
 and return the package to the pharmacy.

 _____ It is a prn dose              _____ Patient NPO

 _____ Medication is on nursing unit _____ Patient sleeping

 _____ Replacement dose is needed    _____ Order dc'd by physician

 _____ Patient off the unit          _____ Patient discharged

 _____ Patient refused dose          _____ Other

 _____ Patient vomited dose
```

Fig. 11-11. Sample checklist for computerized unit dose system. The pharmacist places the label on an envelope containing one unit dose. Note that the label contains information similar to that found on medication cards and can be used as a medication card.

(Milk of Magnesia), and a unit dose label for morphine sulfate states that it contains 15 mg in each milliliter of solution for injection. It is important to understand that the amount of drug contained in one tablet or one milliliter can differ even though the drug itself is the same. For example, two strengths of phenazopyridine tablets are available. Unit dose packages of medications intended for injection state the amount of drug contained in each milliliter of solution. The same drug may be available in more than one strength of solution. Calibrations on the syringe containing a unit dose of drug allow the health care provider to expel or add solution accurately when necessary.

Prior to administration of the drug, information on the label of the unit dose must be compared carefully with the physician's order to ascertain that it contains the correct drug and strength. If a discrepancy is found, the original physician's order is rechecked and appropriate personnel are consulted. The need to calculate dosage and time spent in dosage preparation are greatly reduced when a unit dose system is used. This system also decreases the risk of error in calculation.

In some settings, a portable medication cart is used to store and transport drugs to the patient's room. The cart is locked when unattended to protect the drugs contained in it. Medication records, often stored in a notebook, and other items may be placed on the countertop of the cart. Individual drawers in the cart, labeled with the patient's name and room number, contain medicines for that patient only. Stock medications may be stored in the larger drawers. It is customary to keep souffle cups, medicine cups, and a container for used needles on top of the cart. A bag for other waste materials may be taped to the side of the cart. Several models of medication carts are available.

The procedure for medication cart use varies with institutions. In some, the medication cart is a part of the unit dose system and drawers are refilled by the pharmacist. In others, both multiple and single-dose types of containers are placed in the patient's drawer.

Medications are grouped according to their route of administration. This separates the oral medications from those that are to be administered parenterally. Parenteral medications are further grouped so that IV and topical medications are separated. Medicines that are prescribed prn are usually listed separately from those that are to be administered on a regular basis. This helps ensure that the patient receives the right drug by the right route.

Place the medications that are to be given at a particular time, in the same order as listed on the drug profile or kardex. This makes it easier to check the medication against the order. Checks are done (1) when taking the medicine from the drawer, (2) after preparing the dose, and (3) before putting drug container away. Placing a ruler beneath the order makes it easier to follow. Other safeguards may also be followed. The medication administration record will show if the patient has received this drug previously, the time it was last given, the dose given, the route of administration, and scheduled times for doses. Any differences must be assessed carefully. If each dose is individually packaged, the label on the package can be used to identify the drug prior to its administration. Some individual dose packages are labeled with the patient's name. Individual dose packages may be left intact until it is certain that the patient will be able to take the medication at the time intended.

If a dose is not used or needs to be replaced because the patient vomited or the medication was contaminated, this information is communicated to the pharmacist. A checklist on the unit dose package may be used to communicate this information to the pharmacist (Fig. 11-11).

> ✤ **THINK CRITICALLY**
> What is the name of the drug that was ordered?
> Is it to be given orally or by injection?
> Does unit dose package contain the drug that was ordered?
> Is the drug in the correct dosage form?
> Does unit dose package contain the right amount for the dose?

Medication or Identification Cards

Use of medication cards depends on the medication system employed by the particular hospital. Medication cards are not necessary with most unit dose systems. The cards are used primarily when the doses are obtained from multidose containers.

These cards are sometimes referred to as identification cards because they are used to identify the drug, dose, and patient. Although the size, shape, and color of the medication cards used may vary, the information on the cards should always state the date the order was given, name of the patient, location of the patient (room and bed numbers), name of the drug, dosage prescribed, method of administration, frequency or times of administration, and name of the prescribing physician. The name of the transcriber may be written beside the physician's name or on the back of the card. When colored medication cards are used, specific colors may be used to symbolize different times of administration. The color code used is likely to vary from one institution to another; a code is only an aide and does not change the importance of careful reading of the cards by the health care provider.

Medication cards, when used, are completed at the time the order is transcribed. A medication card for an order for James Brown to receive morphine sulfate 15 mg H q4h, might be written as illustrated (Fig. 11-12).

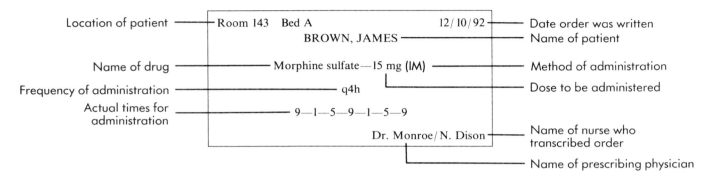

Fig. 11-12. Example of a medication card.

The medication card is used throughout the implementation of the order. The health care provider reads the medication card and compares it with the information on the drug label (1) when taking the medicine from the shelf, (2) again before the dose is removed from the container, and (3) when the container of medication is returned to its place in the medication locker. These comparisons, carried out with diligence, prevent errors.

Interpreting Medication Orders

It is important to interpret medication orders accurately. Abbreviations are translated into words and phrases. Many abbreviations are used; a list of commonly accepted ones appears on the inside back cover of this book. The abbreviations refer to time of day, frequency of administration, dosage form, route of administration, or anatomic parts. For example, if the physician orders colchicine 0.6 mg, 1 tab po qd, the health care provider who reads this would interpret the order to mean "give 1 tablet containing 0.6 mg colchicine orally every day." The meaning of nonapproved abbreviations must be clarified.

The frequency of administration is designed by the physician. The actual time of administration may be dictated by agency policy or procedure. Otherwise, the health care provider schedules these times. The list of abbreviations in Table 11-1 suggests times for administration of drugs along with abbreviations for frequency. Military or 24-hour time is discussed on p. 138.

Orders may be confusing. The health care provider must understand the order perfectly before acting on it. An order can be clarified by consulting appropriate resources. Students should seek assistance from their instructor. Additional information about drugs may be obtained by reading about them and by consulting the pharmacist. An incomplete or illegible order should be clarified with the physician.

EXERCISE 1   *(answers on page 301)*

Compute the total daily dose for the following orders if:

1. 100 mg of drug are ordered to be given four times daily

2. 0.6 g of drug is ordered twice a day

3. 10 mg of drug are ordered three times a day

4. 600 mg are to be given daily in three equal doses

5. 5000 U are to be given twice a day

6. One capsule is to be given with meals and at bedtime

7. Two tablets are to be given every 4 hours

8. One tablet is to be given after breakfast and at bedtime

9. 1000 mL of solution are to be given 3 times over 24 hours

10. 50 mL of solution are to be given every 8 hours

Components of medication orders

A medication order is written in the physician's order book or physician's notes. This order is called a prescription when written for an outpatient. The prescription contains the following parts: name of the patient, date the order was written, name of drug, dose, frequency or times of administration, route of administration, and signature of the person writing the order. The order may also contain additional instructions.

In the hospital setting, the patient's full name, patient identification number, room and bed number, age, address, and other identifying information are stamped on the order sheet. The order forms vary. An example of an order is shown below. Note that the order provides the date and time at which the order was written, the name of the medication (Tylenol), route of administration, PO (by mouth), the amount to be given for each dose (0.6 g), the frequency with which the drug is to be given, q4h prn (every 4 hours when necessary), and the physician's signature.

The health care provider must consider whether an order is reasonable and appropriate for the patient. This requires knowledge of the patient's drug history

DATE AND TIME	M.J. Carry Rm 671
3/10/96 Tylenol 0.6g (O) q 4 h prn	56 1-604-901
Dr. S.J. Tully	

including allergies and adverse reactions, height, weight, age, condition being treated, and general condition of the patient. Assessing whether the dose ordered is within the recommended range of dosages is essential.

Sometimes references give the total daily dose of a drug. The physician decides how to divide the total daily dose into individual doses that will be given throughout the day. The health care provider can compare the total dosage ordered to the recommended total daily dose. To compute the total daily dose that has been ordered, multiply the amount of drug in a single dose by the number of doses ordered for each day. If this amount falls within the recommended total daily dose, it is considered to be within the safe dosage range.

Times of administration

Times at which medications are administered vary from one agency to another and even from one health care unit to another. The schedule used is influenced by many factors. The time interval for a q4h medication might mean that the medication will be given at 8—12—4—8 in one agency but at 9—1—5—9 in another; a schedule of 7—11—3—7 might be preferred by an outpatient. Table 11-1 suggests time patterns that could be used if meals are served at 7:30 AM, 11:30 AM, and 5:30 PM. A q4h order for medication should not be confused with a qid order. The latter is to be given just four times in a 24-hour period; a q4h medication is given at 4-hour intervals through the 24-hour period. In implementation, a q4h order also differs from a q4h prn order. The latter indicates with the abbreviation prn that the drug can be given "if necessary" but not more often than every 4 hours.

Understanding that the prescribed drug exerts its action only when a certain blood level of the drug is maintained helps the health care provider schedule times for administering the drug. Knowledge of the effects of drugs is necessary for establishing and maintaining precise schedules for drug administration. The decision to withhold a drug, even for a short time, must be based on understanding of the drug, the patient, and other influencing factors.

Table 11-1. Suggested times for drug therapy*

Abbreviation	Interpretation	Time of administration
ac	before meals	7—11—5
bid	twice a day	9—7
pc	after meals	9—1—7
prn	whenever necessary	dose may be repeated according to stated time interval
qd	every day	9 AM
qh	every hour	7—8—9—10, and so on
q2h	every 2 hours	7—9—11, and so on
q3h	every 3 hours	6—9—12—3
q4h	every 4 hours	8—12—4—8
q6h	every 6 hours	6—12—6—12
qid	four times a day	9—1—5—9
sos	if necessary	
stat	immediately	

*These are the suggested hours for drug administration if meals are served at 7:30 AM, 11:30 AM, and 5:30 PM.

Knowledge of the effects of a drug is necessary also in order to time its administration for maximum effect. Some drugs must be given with meals, others before meals, and still others are most effective if given after meals. Maintaining a constant blood level of a drug, such as an antibiotic, means that the drug will be administered at equally spaced time intervals. A few drugs, such as those used to treat myasthenia gravis, must be administered at precise times and intervals to maintain the desired effects. Deciding whether to awaken a patient for a medication depends upon a thorough understanding of the drug and of the patient's condition. For example, the amount of time variation between doses of multivitamin preparations may be allowed to vary considerably more than would be reasonable for many other drugs.

EXERCISE 2 *(answers on page 301)*

Interpret in words the meaning of the following physician's orders:

1. Morph. sulf. 10 mg SC q4h prn for abdominal pain

2. Thiamine hydrochloride 100 mg PO qd

3. Digoxin (Lanoxin) 0.125 mg qd PO

4. Codeine sulfate gr 1 per os q4h prn

5. Caffeine sodium benzoate gr ii H

6. Bisacodyl (Ducolax) suppository 10 mg R stat

7. Furosemide (Lasix) 10 mg IV stat

8. Terfenadine (Seldane) 60 mg per os bid

9. Charcocaps caps (activated charcoal) ii O pc repeat in ½ h prn

10. Codeine suspension gr ss IM q4-6h prn

11. Estrogen (Premarin) creme 1 g vaginally 2 × /wk

12. Erythromycin 2% topically to lesion on right cheek bid, after cleansing with hydrogen peroxide

13. KCl 20 mEq PO q AM pc

14. Beclomethasone dipropionate (Vancenase nasal spray) 1 metered dose bid

15. Ferrous sulfate tab 300 mg PO bid with meals

16. Nortriptyline caps 25 mg PO tid

17. Pancrelipase (Viokase) tab i tid with meals

18. Nitroglycerin (Transderm-Nitro 0.2 mg/h) 1 10 mg patch, topically qd for 12 h

19. Acyclovir ung 5% (top) tid to lesion on right lower leg

20. Cyclosporine solution 0.29 mL PO with meals in chocolate milk

21. Homatropine hydrobromide ophthalmic solution 2% ou qid

Twenty-four hour or military time

Use of traditional time can result in misunderstanding because the same numbers are used to indicate both AM and PM time. Therefore *24-hour,* or *military time,* is being used more commonly in patient care situations. In 24-hour time different numbers are used to express each hour of time. This decreases errors related to misunderstanding of time.

Twenty-four hour time is always stated in hundreds of hours. Twenty-four hour time begins with 1 AM, which is written in 24-hour time as 0100, and stated as *zero one hundred hours.* Note that a zero is placed in front of the single digit hours. *A zero is not placed in front of the double digit numbers.* Starting at 10 AM and going through midnight, the hours are written with the double digit followed by two zeros for each hour. Thus 10 AM is written as 1000 and stated as *ten hundred hours,* and midnight is written as 2400 and stated as *twenty-four hundred hours.* Table 11-2 shows the conversion of traditional times to 24-hour time. Fig. 11-13 illustrates a clock that tells both traditional and 24–hour time.

To indicate minutes after the hour in 24-hour time, replace the appended zeros that indicate hundreds by the number of minutes. The traditional time of 9:35 or 25 minutes before 10 becomes 0935; and is stated as *zero nine thirty five hundred hours;* 1945 is stated as *nineteen forty-five hundred hours* and is the same as the traditional time of 7:45 PM.

Table 11-2. Conversion from military time*.

0100 = 1 AM	0900 = 9 AM	1700 = 5 PM
0200 = 2 AM	1000 = 10 AM	1800 = 6 PM
0300 = 3 AM	1100 = 11 AM	1900 = 7 PM
0400 = 4 AM	1200 = 12 Noon	2000 = 8 PM
0500 = 5 AM	1300 = 1 PM	2100 = 9 PM
0600 = 6 AM	1400 = 2 PM	2200 = 10 PM
0700 = 7 AM	1500 = 3 PM	2300 = 11 PM
0800 = 8 AM	1600 = 4 PM	2400 = 12 Midnight

*Colons are sometimes used on computerized labels (01:00, 16:30). This is done to distinguish time from dose.

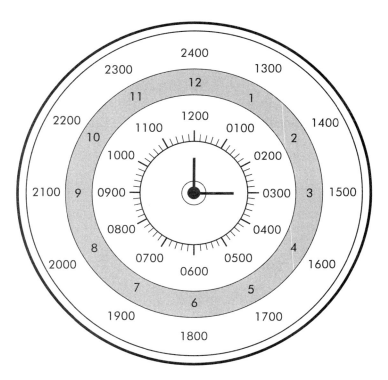

Fig. 11-13. Clock depicting both traditional and 24-hour time. The middle (shaded) circle shows traditional time. The inner circle shows 24-hour time from 1 AM (0100 hours) to 12 noon (1200 hours). The outer circle shows 24-hour time from 1 PM (1300 hours) to 12 midnight (2400 hours).

✚ THINK CRITICALLY

Has one zero been placed in front of each single digit hour of time?
Have two zeros been placed following each hour of traditional time?
Have the zeros for hundreds been replaced with numbers when indicating the correct number of minutes?
Was 12 hours added to traditional time between noon and midnight?

EXERCISE 3 (answers on page 308)

Complete the following table by changing the traditional times to 24-hour times; then write out the way the time would be verbalized. Note that numbers 6 through 10 address times at which medications might be ordered.

	Traditional time	24-hour time	State how the 24-hour is verbalized
1.	9:20 AM		
2.	4:30 PM		
3.	3:15 AM		
4.	6:45 AM		
5.	8:20 PM		
6.	9—7		
7.	6—6		
8.	8—4		
9.	7—1—7		
10.	6—12—6—-12		

EXERCISE 4 (answers on page 308)

Change the following traditional times to 24-hour times.

Traditional time   24-hour time

1. 10 AM

2. 2:10 PM

3. 3 AM

4. 7:45 PM

5. 4 AM

6. 5:15 PM

7. 10:14 PM

8. 8:17 AM

9. 2:42 AM

Transcribing orders

Transcribing an order is usually the first step in order interpretation and implementation. Transcribing an order is often referred to as *signing off* the order. Usually the health care provider in charge or unit secretary transcribes the order. If a secretary transcribes the order, the person in charge must verify that the transcribed order is the same as the original order. When orders are transcribed, they are copied onto the patient's care profile record.

Several methods are used to indicate than an order has been transcribed. A line may be drawn beneath the order followed by the signature of the transcriber. The signature is placed near the end of the line. Alternatively, a check mark is placed at the beginning or end of the order to show that it is in effect. The date of the transcription may be indicated also. A single stat order, which is not to be repeated, may be signed off by placing a check mark beside the order or drawing a line beneath it. The time, date, and signature of the person who implemented the order are written beneath the line.

Some hospitals use an order form that produces carbon copies (Fig. 11-1). When the order has been checked off, the original copy is sent to the pharmacy to obtain a supply of the medication for the patient, and a copy remains in the physician's order book. If the order is written with triplicate copies, the original copy is sent to the pharmacy, a copy is given to the health care provider responsible for administering the medication, and a copy remains in the physician's order book. This alerts the health care provider to the need to initiate a new order.

Checking the transcribed order

The order may also be transcribed to the patient's health plan, or profile, which may be filed in the kardex or in a notebook. Before an order is implemented for the first time, it is important to check the medication card against both the care plan and the physician's order book. If questions about the order arise, it should always be checked against the physician's order. The pharmacist or the physician may be consulted when the order is unclear.

The time at which the health care provider checks the identifying information in the health care plan varies with assigned responsibilities and the particular system of communicating the plan. Some health care providers do this checking when they receive report; others check all medication orders against the health care plans after report is received. Each care provider is responsible for making certain that the health care plan in use agrees with the written orders for the medications. Assembling the medications in the same sequence as listed in the care plan is helpful. One method of verifying that the information on the card agrees

> ### ✚ THINK CRITICALLY
> Is the transcribed order dated and initialed?
> Does it state the following:
>   Name of the drug
>   Dose of the drug
>   Route of administration
>   Schedule for administration
>   Any special instructions

with the information in the care plan is to place the medication card or unit dose package directly beneath the order. When it is ascertained that the information is the same, the card or package is set aside, and the next order is checked.

Students who are given individual reports may check medication orders when they receive report. This permits both the student and the instructor to question information about an order, to seek clarification, and to request other essential information. The student who is not given an individual report is responsible for verifying that the information in the patient's care plan agrees with the physician's order. Clarification must be sought whenever there is a question about interpretation of any part of a medication order. The original order should be checked whenever a discrepancy is found.

READING MEDICATION LABELS

When preparing the dose, the health care provider reads the labels of drugs very carefully. Fig. 11-14 indicates the information found on a drug label. Information contained on all labels includes:

- Trade and generic names for the drug
- Dose per unit
- Dosage form
- Number of dosage units
- Usual dose
- Special cautions or warnings
- Patent number
- Lot number
- Date of expiration

The lot number and date of expiration are stamped on the label at the time of manufacture.

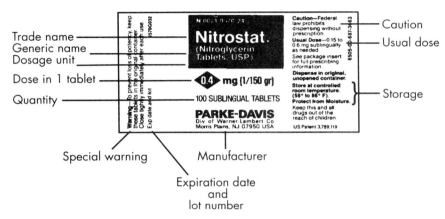

Fig. 11-14. Example of a drug label.

EXERCISE 5

(answers on page 308)

Read the information shown on the labels and complete the following table based on the appropriate label on p. 143.

Label no.	Trade name	Generic name	Dosage unit	Dose per unit	Usual dose	Method of admin.	Amount supplied in container
1							
2							
3							
4							
5							
6							
7							
8							
9							

143

Preparing the Dose Ordered

If stock supply or an individual supply of medicine is used, the health care provider must measure the dose accurately. Accurate reading of the measurement of a liquid dose is facilitated by holding the measure at eye level or placing it on a shelf that is eye level. A suspension must be shaken to suspend particles of the drug in the solution before pouring the dose. This increases the accuracy of measurement. The liquid is poured from the side of the bottle opposite the label; this helps keep the label clean and legible. After pouring the medication, the rim of the bottle may be wiped with a paper towel; this keeps the outside of the bottle clean and prevents the cap from adhering tightly to the bottle. Excess solution, if poured, must be discarded. Changes in the color, consistency, or odor of a medication require that it be returned to the pharmacy for evaluation.

If the drug is supplied in a solid form, such as tablets or capsules, the cap of the bottle can be used to control the number of dosage units removed from the container. Again, if a dose of medication has been removed from its container and cannot be administered, it must be discarded. The manner of disposal used must prevent any person from recovering and using the discarded drugs. Drugs that are controlled by law, such as narcotics, require the use of special disposal procedures.

Solutions intended for injection are available in multiple-dose vials, ampules, and in prefilled syringes. The labels on multiple-dose vials and syringes may state the amount of drug contained in 1 mL of solution. Labels must be read carefully because many drugs are available in different strengths.

Is computation necessary? The health care provider must recognize when computation is necessary. Computation is not necessary if the dosage ordered is the same as the dosage that is available.

Avoiding interruptions while preparing drug dosage. The undivided attention of the health care provider is required during all aspects of drug order implementation. Interruptions should be avoided if at all possible. It is considered good practice to not interrupt the health care provider who is preparing medications, except in an emergency. Waiting quietly and patiently until the provider is finished with preparation helps prevent errors and improves working relationships. If an interruption occurs, the health care provider must recheck the steps in preparing the medication.

ADMINISTERING THE DRUG

The person who administers the drug is legally responsible for giving the drug. Before administering a medication, determine when the patient last received that medication. This can be verified by checking the patient's chart. The medication card, when used, serves to identify the dose until it has been taken by the patient. The card is used to identify the patient and is used for recording administration of the medication. It can also be used to verify that the chart, the number of the room, the bed number, and the patient's name are correct and correspond to the information on the medication card. When the medication cart system is used, the same information is found in the notebook or kardex as on a medication card. In the computerized unit dose system, the labeling information on the envelope containing the unit dose serves the same purpose.

If you do not know the patient, ask him to state his name rather than call him by name or ask, "Are you Mr. Brown?" Patients might misunderstand when called by name and respond to a name other than their own. Identification of the patient is established by checking the information on the identification bracelet worn by the patient. The name on the identification bracelet must match the name on the administration record, medication card, or computerized unit dose envelope. A second bracelet that is color-coded can be used to alert the health care provider to known patient allergies. Although a red identification bracelet is often used to indicate allergies, other schemes for color-coding are sometimes used. It is very important to read the information provided on the bracelets. Some bracelets may have a transparent window that covers an insert on which the patient's allergies can be written. This is a way to protect the patient from receiving potentially harmful drugs. In long-term care facilities, a photograph of the resident may be attached to the medication plan as an additional method of identification.

Knowledge of both the patient and drug enables the health care provider to implement drug orders intelligently. This knowledge equips the health care provider to recognize whether the order is a reasonable one, and to know the pre-

> **✛ THINK CRITICALLY**
> Was the information on the patient's identification bracelet checked against the information found in the records?
> Was the patient asked to state his or her name?
> Does the patient have known allergies to this or a related drug?
> Does this patient have a history of drug dependence or tolerance?
> Does the patient know he or she may refuse medication?

cautions needed, the contraindications, the expected effects, and adverse reactions that may occur. For example, the health care provider who must implement the drug order for Mr. Brown (see Fig. 11-12) should know that it is unusual to give morphine sulfate every 4 hours, and should question whether this order was intended to be a q4h prn order. The drug order may be reasonable for the patient who has intractable pain caused by a terminal disease. The dosage of morphine sulfate, 15 mg, should be questioned if Mr. Brown is a small, frail, elderly man. The health care provider should also question an order to repeat administration of an addicting drug this regularly and frequently. Knowing that morphine causes severe depression of the central nervous system, the health care provider should observe, assess, and record the respiration as well as the level of consciousness of the patient. Drugs that depress respiration are usually withheld if the respirations decrease to 12 or fewer per minute or if the respirations become ineffective. This knowledge should guide the health care provider in a decision to withhold the drug. Consult pharmacology textbooks, drug information resources, and/or the pharmacist when unfamiliar with the drug or unsure about its dose.

Awareness of the need to assess heart action by listening to and counting the apical pulse prior to administering any of the derivatives of digitalis is another example of the importance of knowing the drug. Knowledge that digitalis slows and strengthens the beat of the heart influences the health care provider to take an apical pulse before giving the drug. As a general rule, the drug will be withheld if the heart rate has slowed to 60 or fewer beats per minute. Aware of the expected action of digitalis, the health care provider would consult the physician before repeating the medication if the heart rate increased markedly or became weaker.

Medications should be given at approximately the same time each day. The time at which medication is received is most important to patients who need to know when deviation from the time schedule is permissible. It is suggested that a deviation of no more than 15 minutes before or after the stated time for administration be allowed. Unless extenuating circumstances exist, a total time deviation of ½ hour is reasonable for most drugs that are administered by the health care provider. The importance of administering the drug at the specified time varies with the nature and the purpose of the drug. The health care provider who understands the patient and the action of the medication can exercise discretion about the urgency of administering a drug at a stated time. Some deviation in time of administration is allowed for most drugs, even though the dosage is titrated by the blood levels of the drugs.

Documentation and observation

Immediately after giving the drug, the following must be recorded on the medication administration record (MAR): (1) name of the drug, (2) dose given, (3) time given, (4) route of administration, and (5) the legal name or initials of the person administering the drug. This information should never be recorded before the drug is administered.

> **✚ THINK CRITICALLY**
> Have the drug, dose, time, and route of administration been documented accurately? Has the patient's response to the drug therapy been observed and documented?

Health care providers are permitted to sign their legal name in a designated space on the medication administration record only once for each shift worked. Nicknames are not acceptable. Many different medication administration record forms exist. Health care providers must become familiar with the form used in the setting in which they are administering medications. Examples of various medication administration records are shown in Figs. 11-15, 11-16, and 11-17.

EXERCISE 6 *(answers on page 309)*

Answer the following questions from the information given in Fig. 11-15:

1. What is (a) the patient's name, (b) the patient's age, (c) the patient's room number, and (d) the name of the physician caring for this patient?

2. Two drugs are recorded on the MAR. What are the names of these drugs?

3. By what route of administration was each drug given?

4. How frequently was the drug prednisone ordered?

5. How frequently was the drug furosemide (Lasix) ordered?

6. On which dates were the doses of prednisone given?

7. At what times were the doses of prednisone given?

Foster, Darryl Rm. 501					MEDICATION ADMINISTRATION RECORD								
Age: 16 Dr. Donalds													
91-624-35-3													

DATE	DRUG DOSE ROUTE	DATE DC	TIME SCHEDULE	DATE 2/8			DATE 2/9			DATE 2/10		
				11-7	7-3	3-11	11-7	7-3	3-11	11-7	7-3	3-11
2/8	Prednisone 30 mg (PO) IM IV R SC		qd		0900 C.T.			0900 C.T.			0900 C.T.	
2/10	Ery Ped susp 150 m (PO) IM IV R SC	2/13	q6h								R.D. 1500	R.D. 2100
	IM IV PO R SC											
	IM IV PO R SC											
	IM IV PO R SC											
	IM IV PO R SC											
	IM IV PO R SC											
	IM IV PO R SC											
	IM IV PO R SC											
	IM IV PO R SC											
	IM IV PO R SC											
	IM IV PO R SC											
	IM IV PO R SC											
	IM IV PO R SC											
	IM IV PO R SC											
	IM IV PO R SC											
	IM IV PO R SC											
PRN/ONE TIME ONLY ORDERS												
2/10	Furosemide 25 mg (PO) IM IV R SC		stat								0530 M.J.	

KEY	LU - LUQ	OU - BOTH EYES	Signature	Initials	Signature	Initials	Signature	Initials
ABD - ABDOMEN	**O** - NOT GIVEN	**RA** - RT. ARM	Cathy Tag	C.T.	Cathy Tag	C.T.	Mary Jones	M.J.
LA - LT. ARM	**OD** - RT. EYE	**RT** - RT. THIGH					Rod Dunn	R.D.
LT. - LT. THIGH	**OS** - LT. EYE	**RU** - RUQ						
IVPB - IV PIGGYBACK	**SQ** - SUBCUTANEOUS							
ALLERGIES Phenobarbitol								

Fig. 11-15. An example of a medication administration record (MAR) showing some frequently used abbreviations.

(From Brown M, Mulholland J: *Drug calculations: process and problems for clinical practice,* ed 5, St Louis, 1996, Mosby.)

Fig. 11-16. Medication administration record used at Mayo Foundation for Medical Education and Research, Rochester, Minnesota.

(Copyright Mayo Foundation for Medical Education and Research. Used with permission.)

		ALLERGIES: CODEINE					
		RECOPIED BY INITIALS *L.T.*		R.N. SIGNATURE *B. Wilson, R.N.*			
(Address-o-graph Here)	S I G N A T U R E S	NITES		M. DOERRER, R.N.	M. DOERRER, R.N.	M. DOERRER, R.N.	
		DAYS		P. LITTLE, R.N.	P. LITTLE, R.N.	T. SAX, R.N.	
BARNES HOSPITAL PATIENT ROUTINE MEDICATION RECORD		EVES		D.C. GAIL, R.N.	D.C. GAIL, R.N.		

ORDER DATE / EXP DATE	INIT	ROUTINE MEDICATION Name of drug, strength, and frequency	RTE	SCHEDULE	SHIFT	DATE 6/14/00	DATE 6/15/00	DATE 6/16/00
2/6	PL	LANOXIN 0.25 mg q.d.	PO	10	NITES			
					DAYS	0950 PL	1000 PL	1010 TS
					EVES			
2/7	DG	LASIX 40 mg b.i.d.	PO	10	NITES			
					DAYS			1010 TS
				16	EVES		1545 D.G.	
2/7	DG	ANCEF GM Ī q 6°	IVPB	06	NITES			06 M.D.
				12	DAYS		1215 PL	1200 TS
				18-24	EVES	18 D.G.	2345 D.G.	
2/8	TS	NEOSPORIN OPHTHALMIC OINT. OD	TOP	10	NITES			
					DAYS			1010 TS
				22	EVES			

PERMANENT CHART COPY

Fig. 11-17. An example of a medication administration record (MAR). 24-hour time is used on this MAR. Although the schedule column omits the last two zeros when indicating the hour, the zeros are used when documenting the time of administration.
(From Perry AG, Potter PA: *Clinical skills and techniques*, ed 3, St Louis, 1994, Mosby.)

8. When was the dose of Lasix to be given?

9. At what time was the dose of furosemide actually given?

10. What are the initials of the person who administered the drug **a.** prednisone, **b.** furosemide?

11. What are the names of the person who administered the drug **a.** prednisone, **b.** furosemide?

12. Name the drug to which the patient is allergic.

EXERCISE 7 *(answers on page 309)*

Answer the following questions from the information given in Fig. 11-17 (p. 149):

1. To what drug is the patient allergic?

2. The medication orders were recopied. **(a)** What are the initials of the person who copied them? **(b)** What is the name of the health care provider who checked the orders after they were recopied?

3. Study the information about digoxin (Lanoxin). **(a)** What is the date that digoxin was ordered? **(b)** Who initialed the order? **(c)** How much digoxin is to be given each time? **(d)** How often is the digoxin to be given? **(e)** By what route is the drug to be given? **(f)** On what dates, at what times, and by whom were the doses of digoxin given?

4. Study the information about furosemide (Lasix). **(a)** What is the date that Lasix was ordered? **(b)** Who initiated the order? **(c)** How much Lasix is to be given each time? **(d)** How often is the Lasix to be given? **(e)** By what route is the drug to be given? **(f)** On what dates, at what times and by whom were the doses of Lasix given?

5. Study the information about cefazolin sodium (Ancef). **(a)** What is the date that cefazolin was ordered? **(b)** Who initialed the order? **(c)** How much cefazolin is to be given each time? **(d)** How often is the cefazolin to be given? **(e)** By what route is the drug to be given? **(f)** At what times and by whom were the doses of cefazolin given on February 2? **(g)** At what times and by whom were the doses of cefazolin given on February 8?

6. Study the information about Neosporin ophthalmic ointment. **(a)** On what date was Neosporin ophthalmic ointment ordered? **(b)** Who initialed the order? **(c)** At what times is the Neosporin ophthalmic ointment to be administered? **(d)** By what route is the drug to be administered? **(e)** Where is it to be applied? **(f)** At what time and by whom was the Neosporin ophthalmic ointment applied?

PATIENT EDUCATION

Many opportunities arise for teaching patients about their medications. Information helps patients accept drug therapy. It is customary to provide patients with facts such as the name, purpose, and expected effects of medications. In addition, patients are informed of common side effects, as well as actions that should be taken if such side effects occur. Providing this information in written form is helpful if the medication is to be continued at home.

Discretion is used in determining the amount and kind of information that is conveyed to an individual and the manner in which it is presented. For example, patients who are given drugs that contain a dye that discolors the urine must be told of this effect to avoid alarming them unnecessarily. Patients are also warned of side effects that could jeopardize their safety, such as the dizziness or light-headedness that commonly occurs after the administration of narcotics. Patients who are to continue medication therapy at home must know the signs and symptoms that indicate that the physician should be consulted, the actions to take until the advice of the physician can be obtained, and whether to withhold the drug. Use of investigational drugs requires that patients be fully informed; this is controlled by research protocol and laws.

✢ THINK CRITICALLY

Does the patient know
- The name of the medicine?
- The reason for taking the medicine?
- The expected effects of the medicine?
- Common side effects of the medicine?
- How to contact the physician, if necessary?
- The times or circumstances for taking the medicine?
- The amount of drug to take?
- How to self-administer the drug?
- What to do when drug is not taken because of nausea and vomiting?
- What to do if a dose of medicine is forgotten?

Patients find it helpful to have opportunities to learn to administer the medication under supervision during hospitalization. To do this, the patient needs considerable information, which can be provided in the form of a written plan that includes the name of the drug, its color (when appropriate), the dosage to be taken at specified times, and other helpful information. Some patients find it worthwhile to use a checklist, whereas others devise their own means of remembering the times at which to take medication. Skills in dispensing and administering the drug are practiced until the patient develops the proficiency required for safe administration. Learning to measure and inject insulin usually requires considerable information and multiple opportunities to observe and practice the needed skill. Practice allows the patient to develop skill and confidence in self-administration of medicines and provides the caregiver with opportunities to teach, coach, supervise, and evaluate the competence achieved. With the patient's approval, referrals to community agencies can be made. Assistance with home medication therapy can be obtained through these agencies.

> ### ✛ THINK CRITICALLY
> What does the patient need to know about the drug therapy?
> What does the patient know about the drug therapy?
> How can information best be provided to the patient?
> When can the patient be taught about the drug therapy?

Acquiring the necessary information and skill in medication therapy requires that information and practice be provided as early as possible. Planning and working with patients enables the patients to learn more efficiently and effectively and frees them from being dependent on others to manage medication therapy. Ideally, such teaching begins early in the delivery of health care and is individualized appropriately.

STORAGE AND CONTROL OF DRUGS

Medications should never be accessible to unauthorized people. For this reason, drugs are stored in a locked cupboard, room, or medication cart. Prepared medicines must always be in the sight of and under the control of the person who will administer them. If it is necessary for the health care provider to attend to other duties, the medications should be returned to a safe storage place.

External preparations are stored separately from the medications intended for oral or parenteral administration; this decreases possibilities for error. If refrigerated, drugs must be stored separately from food or beverages.

Drugs that are controlled by federal or state law must be possessed, stored, and used in accordance with the provisions of the law. The Controlled Substances Act of 1970 specifies the requirements that must be met when using controlled substances. These include narcotics, depressants, tranquilizers, and stimulants. Drugs such as narcotics are stored in a locked compartment, and records are kept to document the use of these drugs. The forms used vary, but include the date, time, amount, name of the narcotic, name of the prescribing physician, and name of the health care provider administering the dose. Disposal of a narcotic must be witnessed by two authorized staff members. Although policies differ, the instructor or a registered health care provider is required to witness and co-sign if students sign out narcotics.

EXERCISE 8 *(answers on page 310)*

1. The physician orders meperidine, 75 mg IM. The prepared unit dose is labeled, "Meperidine, 75 mg in 1.5 mL." **(a)** How much solution should be given for the patient to receive 75 mg? **(b)** What does the abbreviation IM mean?

2. The physician orders penicillin V 250 mg PO q8h for 10 days to treat a mild streptococcal infection. The prescription is supplied in 250 mg capsules. **(a)** How many 250 mg capsules are to be given for each dose? **(b)** Establish a schedule using traditional time that assumes a 10 PM bedtime. **(c)** How should the penicillin be administered?

3. The physician orders atropine, 0.4 mg SC. The multidose container is labeled, "Atropine sulfate, 0.4 mg in 1 mL." **(a)** How many milliliters should the health care provider withdraw? **(b)** How is the drug to be given?

4. The physician's order is for phenobarbital, 30 mg O qid. The label on the tablet reads, "Phenobarbital 30 mg." **(a)** How many tablets are needed for each dose? **(b)** How often is this drug to be administered? **(c)** At what times would it be administered in the clinical agency in which you practice?

5. The physician orders propoxyphene hydrochloride (Darvon), plain, 32 mg O q6h. The capsules are labeled, "Darvon, 32 mg." **(a)** How many capsules are needed to give the dose ordered? **(b)** How often is this dose to be repeated?

6. The physician orders Darvon Compound-65, cap i, O q3-4h prn. **(a)** How many capsules of a preparation labeled "Darvon Compound-65" are needed for one dose? **(b)** What is the most frequent time interval at which the dose can be repeated? **(c)** What does the abbreviation prn mean?

7. The physician prescribes heparin, 5000 U IV stat. The drug is labeled, "Heparin, 5000 U/mL." **(a)** What amount of heparin solution should be prepared for the dose ordered? **(b)** What route of administration is to be used? **(c)** When is the dose to be given? **(d)** Is the order to be repeated? **(e)** What does the abbreviation U mean? **(f)** What is the policy of this employer (or school) concerning whether the health care provider can give this drug?

8. The physician prescribes nalidixic acid (NegGram), 1 g orally four times a day for 1 week for Harold B., who has a urinary tract infection resistant to other antibiotics. **(a)** If the prescription is filled with 1 g caplets, how many should be prepared for one dose? **(b)** Develop a time schedule that will maintain a constant level of the drug in the blood.

9. James S., diagnosed with gastritis, has been instructed to take 0.3 g of aluminum hydroxide gel (Amphojel) five times a day, between meals and at bedtime. If needed, he can increase the frequency of the dose to six times a day. He states, "I usually eat my meals at 8, 12, and 6, and I go to bed around 10 PM." (a) Suggest a schedule using traditional time for five times a day. (b) A few days later, he says "My stomach hurts when I first wake up." How can the previous schedule be revised if he usually awakens about 7 AM?

10. The physician orders aminophylline suppositories, gr viiss R stat and non rep. (a) What does the abbreviation R mean? (b) What does the abbreviation non rep indicate to the health care provider? (c) How much drug should each suppository contain?

11. The physician writes an order stating, phenylephrine hydrochloride (NeoSynephrine) ¼%, gtt ii od bid. (a) What does the abbreviation gtt stand for? (b) Which eye is to be treated? (c) How often is the treatment to be done? (d) What abbreviation might be used to indicate that both eyes are to be treated?

12. A woman questions the label on her prescription medication that reads, "Take one capsule 4 times daily for 7 days. Tetracycline 250 mg," and asks when she ought to take the capsules. What is the major principle that she needs to understand to select the times that would allow the medicine to have its maximum effect and that would fit into her time schedule?

13. Susan Z. is to continue taking the drug lithium carbonate at 12-hour intervals when she is discharged from a psychiatric unit. These time intervals are important because the level of drug in the blood affects the quality of control of symptoms. (a) What should Susan be told about lithium levels? (b) How might planning facilitate adherence to a schedule of home medication that requires 12-hour intervals between doses? (c) What method(s) could be used to allow Susan to learn to take her own medication before leaving the institutional setting? (d) Whose responsibility is it to determine that Susan has been given the opportunity to learn acceptable medication administration practices?

14. After Susan has taken lithium for several days, she asks what she should do if she is away from home and finds that she has depleted her drug supply. What are some possible alternatives for consideration in discussion of this problem?

15. Two months after Susan is discharged from the hospital, the level of lithium in her blood indicates that an increase in dosage is needed. The physician increases the dosage by two capsules each day and tells her that she may alter the times at which she takes a particular amount of drug if the increased dosage causes symptoms of nausea or diarrhea. Susan does not understand how the drug amount and schedule are to be altered. If she is now taking six capsules of lithium daily instead of the previous dose of four capsules daily, what should she be told, considering that maintaining the blood levels is essential?

16. The physician writes the following take-home prescription for a patient:

    Nifedipine, 10 mg tid
    Isordil (isosorbide dinitrate), 10 mg qid
    Tenormin (atenolol), 50 mg qd
    Transderm-Nitro (nitroglycerin), (1) qd
    Colace (docusate sodium), 100 mg cap (1) qd

    Make a time schedule for the patient to follow in taking these medications. Assume that the patient will be returning to a job that extends from 8 AM to 4 PM. Plan the schedule so that the medications are evenly distributed without the patient having to take medicine more than three times a day.

17. The physician orders propoxyphene (Darvon N-100), tab i, to be given q3-4h prn for severe muscle pain. (a) How many tablets of the drug are to be administered? (b) What is the name of the prescribed drug? (c) How often may the dose be repeated?

18. You are using prepackaged unit doses of acetaminophen (Tylenol). Each tablet comes individually wrapped and is labeled, "Tylenol, 0.6 g tablets." If the patient refuses to take the drug, under what circumstances can the drug be replaced in the patient's individual supply of medication?

19. Change the following clock time to military time and military time to clock time:

Clock time	Military time	Military time	Clock time
a. 10 AM	_____	e. 0300	_____
b. 4 PM	_____	f. 1400	_____
c. 9:45 PM	_____	g. 2200	_____
d. 12 midnight	_____	h. 1515	_____

Computation of Oral Dosages

Accuracy in computation is essential for the administration of the correct dosage. Inaccurate computation will result in a dose that is too large or too small. Too much drug may produce toxic effects and, in extreme cases, death. Too little drug will not produce the desired effects, allowing the illness or symptoms to continue and progress. In either case, the drug is unlikely to have the desired effects.

Accuracy of computation requires the health care provider to:

1. Convert all units of measure to the same size and system.
2. Use one method of computation consistently and correctly.
3. Determine whether the answer obtained is reasonable.

REVIEW OF RATIO AND PROPORTION

Because ratio and proportion are used in two of the methods presented for solving problems of dosages, they are reviewed briefly in this chapter. For further explanation or practice, refer to Chapter 6, Ratio and Proportion.

A proportion is expressed as two equivalent ratios or fractions. If stated using ratios, *the product of the extremes equals the product of the means.*

EXAMPLE:

$$2:3 = 4:6$$

with means $3, 4$ and extremes $2, 6$

$$2 \times 6 = 3 \times 4$$
$$12 = 12$$

If the product of the means does not equal the product of the extremes, the ratios are not equivalent, and the proportion is not a true proportion.

When the proportion is stated using fractions, *the cross products are equal*. These are obtained through cross-multiplication.

EXAMPLE:

$$\frac{2}{3} = \frac{4}{6} \qquad \begin{array}{c} 2 \times 6 = 3 \times 4 \\ 12 = 12 \end{array}$$

If the cross-products are not equal, the fractions are not equivalent and the proportion is not a true proportion.

Solving for an unknown in a proportion. When computing dosage, one quantity in the proportion is unknown. X is used to represent the unknown. To solve for x, multiply the means and extremes of the proportion when ratios are used.

EXAMPLE:

means
$2:3 = 4:x$
extremes

$$2x = 12$$
$$x = 12 \div 2$$
$$x = 6$$

Substituting 6 for the unknown, the ratio is $2:3 = 4:6$. When fractions are used, cross-multiply to solve for x.

EXAMPLE:

$$\frac{2}{3} = \frac{4}{x} \qquad \begin{array}{c} 2x = 12 \\ x = 12 \div 2 \text{ or } 6 \end{array}$$

The order of the ratios or fractions does not change the proportion. The above proportion could have been stated as $4:x = 2:3$ or $\frac{4}{x} = \frac{2}{3}$. The first ratio is usually complete and the second ratio usually contains the unknown quantity. The same order is used to establish the second ratio as is used in the first or completed ratio.

CHECKING CALCULATIONS

To check calculations, substitute the answer obtained for x, multiply the means, and then multiply the extremes. The two products will equal each other if the computation is correct.

To check calculations when using fractions in the ratio, substitute the answer obtained for x and cross multiply.

$$\frac{2}{3} = \frac{4}{6} \qquad \begin{array}{c} 4 \times 3 = 2 \times 6 \\ 12 = 12 \end{array}$$

If the computation is correct, the two products will be the same. If the products do not equal each other, recheck the computation.

ORAL TABLETS AND CAPSULES

Oral tablets and capsules are available in commonly prescribed strengths. Because common dosages vary, many drugs are available in more than one strength. Read the label carefully to determine the amount of drug available in each tablet or capsule. The following labels show two strengths of the same drug. One contains 325 mg of aspirin in each enteric coated tablet and the other contains 500 mg in each tablet.

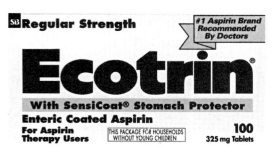 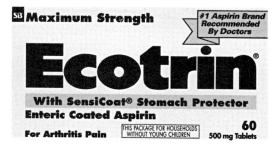

If the tablet or capsule is available in two or more strengths, always select the one that contains the same amount of drug as is ordered for each dose. Ideally, one tablet or capsule will deliver the exact amount of drug prescribed. However, more than one tablet or capsule may be needed for some doses. *As a general guideline, most doses do not require more than one or two tablets or capsules.* Whenever more than one or two tablets or capsules seem necessary for one dose, caution should be used. Recheck the order, reread the label, reassess accuracy, and seek appropriate assistance. Questioning doses of more than two tablets or capsules may prevent serious errors.

Unscored tablets and capsules are not to be divided because this gives an inaccurate amount of drug and may even alter the intended action of the drug. Many solid drug preparations have special coatings to control the amount of drug that is released over time. Some capsules contain several coatings on tiny pellets or granules of the drug. These coatings dissolve at different rates, releasing the drug over a long period of time (Fig. 12-1). When a drug preparation is released over a

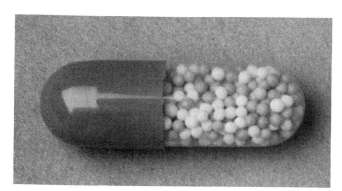

Fig. 12-1. Timed-release capsule. The capsule contains tiny coated pellets or granules of drug. The granules or pellets dissolve at different rates, releasing the drug continuously.

(From Clayton BD, Stock YN: *Basic pharmacology for nurses,* ed 10, St Louis, 1993, Mosby.)

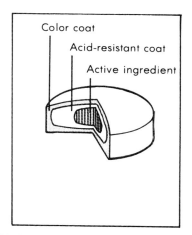

Fig. 12-2. An enteric-coated tablet. Enteric-coated tablets are coated with an acid-resistant substance that does not dissolve in the stomach but dissolves in the intestines.

(From Clayton BD, Stock YN: *Basic pharmacology for nurses,* ed 10, St Louis, 1993, Mosby.)

period of time it is termed a *timed-release, delayed-release,* or *extended release* tablet or capsule. Read the following labels for this information.

A special coating on tablets prevents the drug from being dissolved in the stomach. The drug is not released until it enters the intestines. This is referred to as an enteric coating (Fig. 12-2).

If it seems necessary to divide an unscored or a coated tablet or a capsule, consult the appropriate people. The physician may change the order, or the pharmacist may supply a liquid form of the same drug.

The drug may be available in different strengths, and may be ordered using different units of measure from those found on the label. A drug that is labeled in milligrams may be ordered in milligrams or grams. Sometimes the drug is labeled in grams but is ordered in milligrams. This emphasizes the importance of careful reading of both the order and the drug label. Both types of problems will be presented in this chapter.

DOSAGE CALCULATIONS USING THE SAME UNITS OF MEASURE

Computing dosage when the physician prescribes in the same units of measurement in which the tablets or capsules of drug are available is fairly simple. Make sure the units of strength are the same in both the physician's order and the tablet or capsule. For example, both the drug order and the drug might be labeled in milligrams, grams, or micrograms. Read both the physician's order and the drug label carefully.

> ### ✚ THINK CRITICALLY
> Are the same units of measure used in the physician's order and on the label?
> Is the same order present in both ratios?
> Does the proportion contain true ratios?
> Is the answer obtained reasonable?

METHODS OF CALCULATION

Several methods may be used to solve problems of dosages and solutions. After studying and trying each method, choose the method that is easiest and most comfortable to use. It is important to use one method consistently to avoid confusion. Three methods are presented here. Two methods use ratio and proportion. In method 1, the ratio and proportion are established in terms of amount of drug : unit measure. Method 2 uses a formula. In method 3, the ratio and proportion are established according to size.

Method 1: Using 2 Ratios Established by Drug Label and Prescribed Dose

Method 1 uses true proportion in which two ratios are established. It is logical to establish the first ratio using the information found on the label of the drug preparation. Sometimes the drug preparation is referred to as the drug on hand or the dose available. The label states the amount of drug in one unit of measure. For example, it may state that there are 100 mg in one tablet, 100 mg is the amount of drug. The unit of measure is one tablet. The label may state the amount of drug in a capsule or a tablet.

> EXAMPLE: The physician orders 650 mg of acetaminophen. Information on the label indicates that 325 mg of acetaminophen are contained in each tablet. Information from the label will be used to establish the first ratio of the proportion. The ratio is stated as
>
> Amount of drug:Unit of measure
> 325 (mg):1 (tab)

This ratio is referred to as labeling information or the label side of the proportion.

The other ratio is established from information available in the prescription or physician's order. In the example, the physician ordered 650 mg of drug. To have a true proportion, the second ratio must be stated in the same order and units as the first ratio. Therefore 650 (mg) becomes the first part of the ratio and the unknown (x tablets) becomes the second part of the ratio. This is sometimes referred to as the prescribed dose part of the proportion. In this example, the ratio established from the labeling information is shown on the left side of the proportion and the ratio for the prescribed dose is shown on the right side of the proportion. Although it is mathematically correct to reverse the order, it is less confusing if the ratio from the labeling information is established first.

$$\begin{array}{cc} \text{Labeling} & \text{Prescribed} \\ \text{information} & \text{dose} \\ \text{(Known)} & \text{(Desired)} \end{array}$$

$$325 \text{ (mg)}:1 \text{ (tab)} = 650 \text{ (mg)}:x \text{ (tab)}$$
$$325x = 650$$
$$x = 650 \div 325 \text{ or 2 tabs of acetaminophen, 325 mg per tab}$$

Substituting 2 for x and multiplying the means and extremes verifies that the proportion contains true ratios if both answers are equal.

$$325:1 = 650:2$$
$$650 = 650$$

Always assess whether the answer is reasonable. Because the amount of drug in one tablet is less than the amount of drug prescribed, it is expected that the number of tablets required for the dose will be greater than 1.

The proportion could also be established using fractions as follows:

$$\begin{array}{cc} \text{Labeling} & \text{Prescribed} \\ \text{information} & \text{dose} \end{array}$$

$$\frac{325 \text{ (mg)}}{1 \text{ (tab)}} = \frac{650 \text{ (mg)}}{x \text{ (tab)}}$$
$$325x = 650$$
$$650 \div 325 = 2$$
$$x = 2$$

To check the calculations, substitute the answer obtained for x and cross multiply.

$$\frac{325}{1} = \frac{650}{2}$$
$$325 \times 2 = 650 \times 1$$
$$650 = 650$$

Method 2: Dosage Formula

Method 2 requires substituting information into the following formula:

$$\frac{\text{Desired dose (prescribed dose)}}{\text{Dose that is available (on hand)}} \times \text{Quantity (unit of measure)}$$

$$= x \text{ Unknown (quantity or units of measure to be given)}$$

This formula may be abbreviated as $\frac{D}{H} \times Q(U) = x$. It must be memorized by the person who plans to use it for solving problems.

EXAMPLE: The physician orders 650 mg of acetaminophen and the dose on hand is 325 mg in one tablet. The desired dose is the dose that the physician ordered (650 mg). The dose that is available (on hand) is 350 mg. The quantity of drug is the unit of measure that contains the dose that is available. In this problem, the quantity is one tablet. X is the unknown number of units of measure or tablets needed for the prescribed dose. The substitutions are:

$$\frac{650 \text{ (mg)}}{325 \text{ (mg)}} \times 1 \text{ (tablet)} = x \text{ (number of 325 mg tablets)}$$

$$\frac{\cancel{650}^{2}}{\cancel{325}_{1}} \times 1 = x$$

$$x = 2 \text{ tablets, each containing 325 mg acetaminophen}$$

Method 3: Using 2 Ratios Established According to Size

Method 3 uses the proportion method and the same components as method 1. However, in method 1 one ratio of the proportion was based on information about the drug on hand and the other ratio was based on the desired dosage. In method 3, the ratios of the proportion are established according to size. Usually, the proportion is stated as lesser:greater = lesser:greater.

To establish the first ratio, begin with the known information. What is the dose that is on hand? Is it less or greater than the prescribed dose? If the dose on hand is less than the prescribed dose, the dose on hand would be substituted for lesser and the prescribed dose would be substituted for greater in the first ratio. The second ratio would be established in the same order but would be based on unit of measure. If the dose on hand is substituted for lesser, then the unit of measure for the dose on hand would be substituted for lesser in the second ratio.

EXAMPLE: The prescribed dose is 650 mg of acetaminophen. The available drug contains 325 mg of acetaminophen in one tablet. How many tablets are needed to give 650 mg of acetaminophen, using 325 mg tablets? 325 mg is less than 650 mg.

Therefore 325 mg is substituted into the lesser part of the first ratio and 650 mg is substituted into the greater part of the ratio. Because the 325 mg are contained in one tablet and 650 mg is greater than 325, it is logical that more than one tablet will be needed for the prescribed dose. Therefore one tablet is substituted for lesser and x is substituted for greater.

$$325 \text{ (mg)}:650 \text{ (mg)} = 1 \text{ (tab)}:x \text{ (tab)}$$

Using fractions, the proportion is as follows:

$$\begin{array}{cc} \textbf{Dose} & \textbf{Unit of measure} \\ \dfrac{\text{lesser}}{\text{greater}} & = \dfrac{\text{lesser}}{\text{greater}} \\ \dfrac{325 \text{ (mg)}}{650 \text{ (mg)}} & = \dfrac{1 \text{(tab)}}{x \text{(tab)}} \end{array}$$

$$325x = 650$$
$$650 \div 325 = x$$
$$x = 2 \text{ tablets, each containing 325 mg acetaminophen}$$

To check the calculations, substitute the answer obtained for x and cross multiply.

$$\dfrac{325}{650} = \dfrac{1}{2}$$
$$325 \times 2 = 650 \times 1$$
$$650 = 650$$

If one of the ratios is set up incorrectly, x would equal less than one tablet. Using the information determined before working the problem—that the amount of drug ordered is greater than that contained in one tablet—any errors should be recognized, either in the setting up or working of the problem. Analyze each step for correctness.

ASSESS WHETHER THE ANSWER IS REASONABLE

To assess whether the answer is reasonable or not, compare the dose ordered with the dose available in one unit of measure, such as a tablet or capsule. If the dose ordered is greater than the dose available, the answer will be more than one tablet or capsule. If the dose ordered is less than the dose available, then the answer will be less than one tablet or capsule.

Another way of assessing whether an answer is reasonable is to divide the amount of drug ordered by the amount of drug available to estimate whether the amount needed for the dose will be greater or less. For example, if the physician orders 2 mg of a drug and one tablet available contains 4 mg, 2 would be divided by 4.

$$\dfrac{2}{4} = \dfrac{1}{2} \text{ tablet}$$

$$\dfrac{\text{amount ordered}}{\text{amount available in 1 tablet or capsule}} = \text{number of tablets or capsules needed}$$

The answer, the amount of drug needed for the prescribed dose, is one half of one tablet. If, however, the physician had ordered 8 mg of the drug and the tablet contains 4 mg, 8 divided by 4 indicates that two tablets are needed for the prescribed dose. As a guide, most doses require one or two tablets or capsules.

> ### ✚ THINK CRITICALLY
> How much drug was ordered?
> How much drug is contained in one tablet or capsule?
> Are the same units of measure used in both the drug and the order?
> Is the amount ordered the same, more, or less than the amount in one tablet or capsule?
> How many times greater or less is the dose ordered than the dose available?

EXERCISE 1 (answers on page 310)

Solve the following problems:

1. The physician orders phenytoin, 270 mg/day in three divided doses. **(a)** How many mg of drug are needed for each dose? **(b)** How many tablets are needed for each dose? **(c)** How many tablets are needed for the total daily dose? **(d)** How many tablets are needed for 7 days?

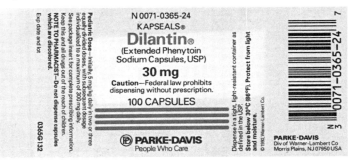

2. The physician orders digoxin, 0.25 mg to strengthen heart action. **(a)** Which strength preparation is most appropriate to use? **(b)** How many tablets are needed for one dose?

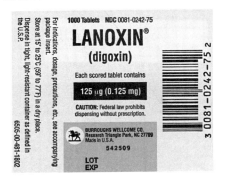 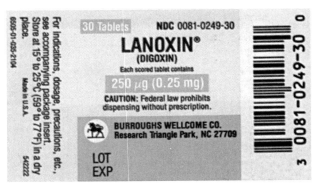

3. The physician orders enteric coated aspirin 650 mg q4h prn to relieve headache. How many tablets are needed for the prescribed dose?

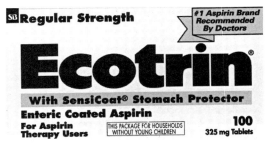

4. The physician orders phenazopyridine, 200 mg, q12h to relieve urinary tract symptoms. (a) Which strength preparation is most appropriate? (b) How many tablets are needed for one dose? (c) What is the total amount of drug that is to be given in one 24-hour period?

5. The physician orders ibuprofen (Motrin), 2400 mg daily in four divided doses to control pain. The tablets available are in strengths of 300, 400, 600 and 800 mg. (a) How much is needed for each dose? (b) Which strength is most appropriate to use? (c) What total number of tablets are needed for the total daily dose? (d) How many tablets are needed for each dose?

6. The physician orders levothyroxine (Synthroid), 0.05 mg as a thyroid replacement drug. There are three strengths of tablets available: 25 mcg (0.025 mg), 50 mcg (0.05 mg), and 75 mcg (0.075 mg). (a) Which strength tablet is most appropriate? (b) How should one dose be prepared?

7. The physician orders warfarin sodium (Coumadin) 10 mg qd. (a) Which strength preparation is most appropriate? (b) How many tablets are needed for this dose?

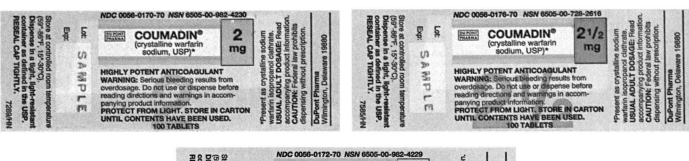

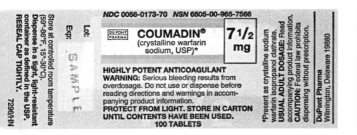
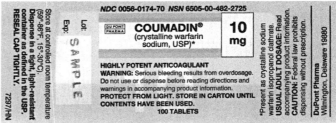

8. The physician orders diphenhydramine HCl, 25 mg qid to relieve itching. **(a)** Which size capsule will provide this dose? **(b)** How many capsules are needed for an entire day? **(c)** If the drug is to be taken for 7 days, how many capsules are needed?

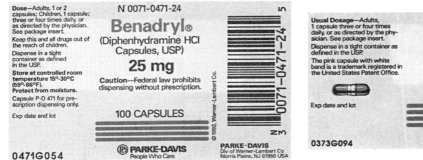
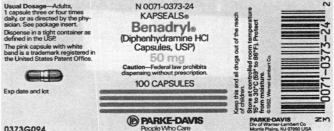

9. The physician orders phenytoin 60 mg q AM. How many capsules are needed for this dose?

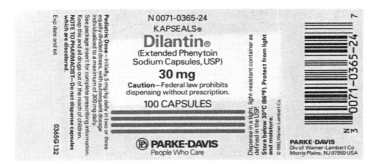

10. If the physician orders 20 mg of chlorpromazine HCl (Thorazine), **(a)** which strength preparation is most appropriate? **(b)** How many tablets are needed for each dose?

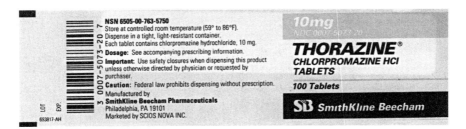

165

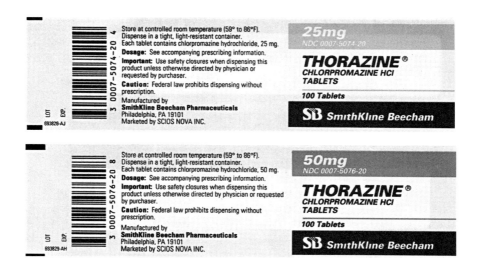

11. Because Mrs. J. has been unable to lower her cholesterol levels adequately with diet and exercise, her physician ordered 20 mg lovastatin (Mevacor) to be taken every evening. The tablets are available in 10, 20, and 40 mg strengths. (a) Which size tablet should be used? (b) How many tablets of the drug will provide this dose?

12. Mr. H. has severe back pain. Diazepam (Valium) 5 mg q6h, prn is ordered to relieve the muscle spasms that are causing the pain. (a) If the tablets containing 2, 5, or 10 mg of Valium are available, which size tablet is most appropriate? (b) How may tablets are needed for each dose?

13. Nifedipine (Procardia), an antianginal drug, is prescribed for Mr. N. in a dose of 20 mg tid. (a) Which of the following capsules is most appropriate for this dose? (b) What will the total daily dosage be? (c) How many capsules are needed for a 30-day supply?

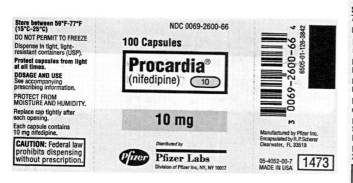
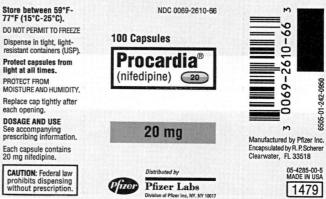

14. Arnold K. has forgotten to refill his prescription for Procardia XL 30 mg q AM. He has on hand some 20 mg capsules of Procardia (shown in previous problem). In this situation, would 1½ capsules of Procardia provide the correct medicine? Please explain.

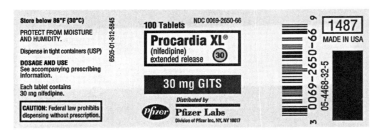

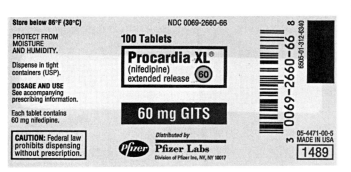

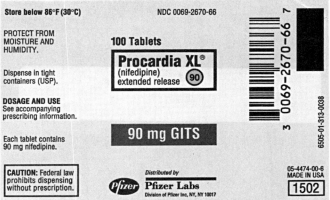

15. Lorazepam (Ativan) 1 mg bid is ordered for Mrs. C. to relieve anxiety associated with depression. (a) Which of the following tablets is most appropriate? (b) How many tablets are needed for each dose? (c) What is the total daily dose?

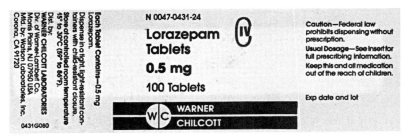

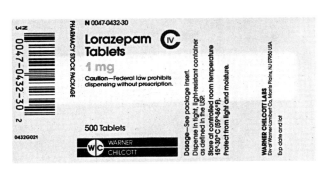

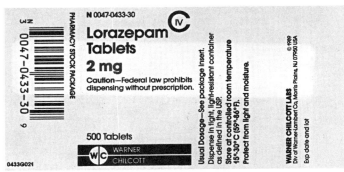

16. Clindamycin hydrochloride (Cleocin HCl) 150 mg q6h is prescribed for the treatment of a severe infection. (a) Which size capsule will provide one dose of this medicine? (b) How many capsules are needed for each 24-hour period of treatment? (c) What is the total daily dose?

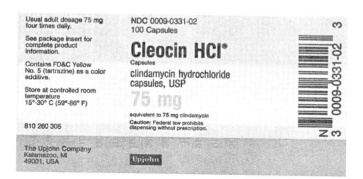

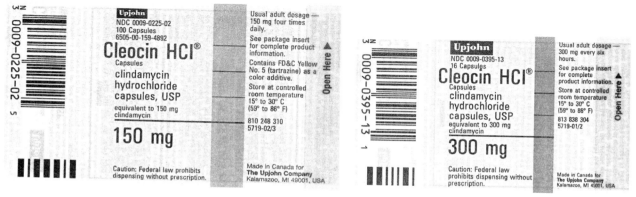

17. The physician orders Mrs. K. to take 325 mg of enteric coated aspirin every morning with her cardiac medications. (a) Which of the following preparations should be used? (b) How many tablets are needed for one dose?

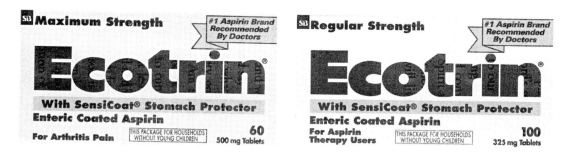

18. Procainamide hydrochloride extended-release tablets (Procan SR) 500 mg q AM is ordered to treat an irregular heart rhythm. (a) Which of the following preparations will provide the correct dose? (b) How many capsules are needed for one dose? (c) How many capsules are needed for a 30-day supply?

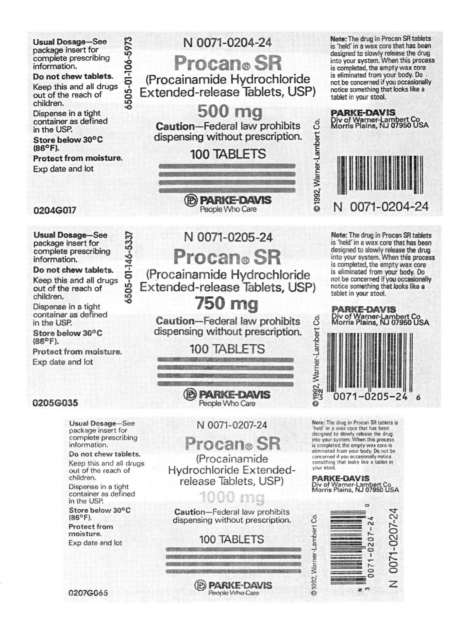

19. Acetaminophen (Tylenol) 650 mg qid for headache is ordered. It is available in regular strength (325 mg) and extra strength (500 mg) caplets and tablets. **(a)** Which size tablet is appropriate? **(b)** How many tablets are needed for one dose?

20. If Extra Strength Tylenol Gelcaps are used and each contains 500 mg of drug, how many milligrams of Tylenol would two gelcaps provide?

USING DIFFERENT SIZE UNITS OF MEASURE IN THE METRIC/SI SYSTEM

Sometimes it is necessary to convert the prescribed units of measure to a greater or lesser unit in the same system. For example, the prescription could be written in milligrams and the drug labeled in grams. Both are metric/SI measures but one is much less than the other. There are several things to consider before deciding how many tablets or capsules are needed for a dose.

Be sure that both the physician's order and the drug label use the same system. If both are stated in the metric/SI system, determine whether both are in the same unit of measure. If each is stated in a different size unit of measure, it is necessary to convert the units named in the order to the same units as those found on the label. If the physician orders 0.5 g of erythromycin and each capsule of erythromycin available contains 250 mg of drug, first change 0.5 g to milligrams.

To change grams to milligrams, multiply by 1000.

$$0.5 \times 1000 = 500$$

It is also correct to move the decimal point 3 places to the right.

$$0.500$$

For more practice in changing one metric/SI unit to another, refer to Chapter 7, Weight and Volume: Metric/SI and Apothecaries' Systems.

After converting grams to milligrams, the problem can be solved in one of the following ways:

METHOD 1: *Using 2 ratios established by drug label and prescribed dose.* State the proportion, using the information on the label as one part of the proportion and the prescribed dose as the other part of the proportion.

Label side of the proportion   Prescribed dose
milligrams:tablets = milligrams:tablets
250 (mg):1 (tab) = 500 (mg):x (tab)

$$250x = 500$$
$$x = 500 \div 250$$
$$x = 2 \text{ tablets of erythromycin, 250 mg per tablet}$$

METHOD 2: *Using the dosage formula.* Substitute into the following formula:

$$\frac{\text{Dose desired}}{\text{Dose available}} \times 1(\text{tab}) = \text{Number of tablets needed to administer prescribed dose}$$

$$\frac{500 \text{ (mg)}}{250 \text{ (mg)}} \times 1 \text{ (tab)} = 2 \text{ tab of erythromycin, 250 mg per tablet}$$

This formula may be abbreviated as:

$$\frac{D}{H} \times U = A$$

D refers to the dose ordered by the physician, H refers to the dose on hand, and U refers to the unit that contains the dose on hand. When working with tablets, one tablet contains the dose on hand.

METHOD 3: *Using 2 ratios established by size.* State the proportion in terms of lesser:greater = lesser:greater.

lesser:greater = lesser:greater
milligrams:milligrams = tablets:tablets

250 (mg):500 (mg) = 1 (tablet):x (tablet)

$250x = 500$
$x = 500 \div 250$
$x = 2$ tablets of erythromycin, 250 mg per tablet

✔ *If the prescribed dose is less than the available dosage form, it is advisable to consult the pharmacist who will, when possible, prepare a liquid form.* Preparation of a liquid form requires considerable knowledge of the drug preparation, for the drug may be insoluble in water or unstable in solution; also the destruction of special coatings may destroy the effectiveness of the drug.

EXERCISE 2 (answers on page 311)

Solve the following problems:

1. The physician orders amoxicillin, 1 g q6h. **(a)** How many milligrams are needed for one dose? **(b)** How many capsules are needed for each dose? **(c)** How many capsules are needed for the total daily dose?

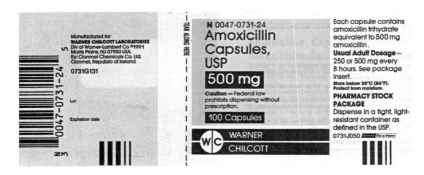

2. The physician orders ampicillin, 0.5 g to be given q12h. **(a)** How many 250 mg capsules are required for one dose? **(b)** How many capsules are needed for the total daily dose?

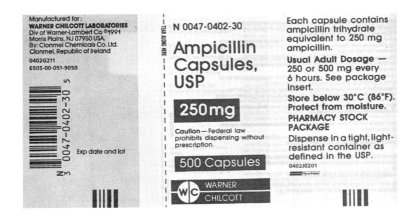

171

3. The physician orders amoxicillin, 0.5 g. Using the previous label, (a) Which strength of preparation is needed? (b) How many capsules are needed for this dose?

4. The physician orders ampicillin, 1 g. Using the previous label, how would one dose be prepared?

5. Respond to an order for a total daily dose of 1.5 g ampicillin in two divided doses if capsules containing 250 and 500 mg are available. (a) How many capsules are needed for one dose? (b) How many capsules are needed for the total daily dose?

6. The physician orders dicloxacillin sodium (Dynapen) 0.5 g q6h. Capsules are available in strengths of 250 mg and 500 mg. (a) Which strength capsule is most appropriate to use? (b) How many capsules are needed for each dose? (c) How many capsules are needed for one 24-hour period? (d) How many capsules are needed for 5 days?

7. The physician orders chlorpromazine hydrochloride, 0.1 g to be given tid. (a) Which strength preparation is most appropriate? (b) How many tablets are needed for each dose? (c) How many tablets are needed for 1 day? (d) How many tablets are needed for 10 days?

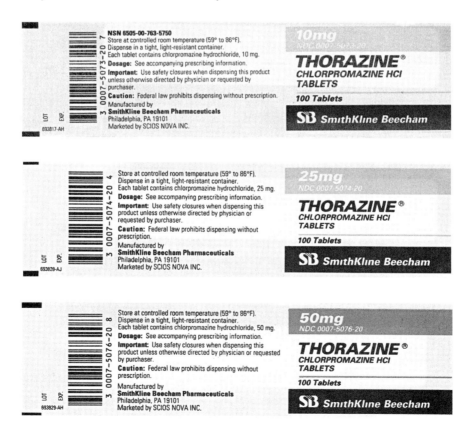

8. The physician orders lexothyroxine sodium (Synthyroid) 0.1 mg. Tablets are labeled as follows: 25 mcg (0.025 mg), 50 mcg (0.05 mg), and 75 mcg (0.075 mg). **(a)** Which strength preparation is most appropriate? **(b)** What would be prepared for the dose?

9. The physician orders cephradine (Anspor), 0.25 g. Capsules available contain 250 milligram or 500 milligram of drug. **(a)** Which strength of preparation is most appropriate? **(b)** How many capsules are needed for the dose?

10. The physician orders sulfisoxazole, 8 g divided into four doses over 24 hours for 4 days. There are two containers of drug that look similar. Each contains 0.5 g tablets. One label reads, "Gantrisin, brand of sulfisoxazole" and the other states "Gantanol, brand of sulfamethoxazole." **(a)** Using the trade name, which preparation is the correct one to use? **(b)** How many grams are needed for each dose? **(c)** How many tablets are needed for one dose? **(d)** How many tablets are needed for 10 days?

USING TWO SIZES OF TABLETS OR CAPSULES

Occasionally a dose will require different sizes of tablets or capsules. For example, if the physician's order is for 10 mg of dexamethasone and the following preparations are available, it is apparent that no one preparation will provide the correct amount of drug for the dose.

Because dexamethasone is not manufactured in 10 mg tablets, how to provide this dose must be determined. To give the least possible number of tablets, look at the various dosages and determine which tablets, when given together, will yield the correct amount of drug for the prescribed dose. *Follow the general rule of administering the fewest possible number of tablets.* Find the size of tablets needed by determining if any two tablets will yield the correct amount of drug for the dose. If this is not immediately obvious, subtract the dose (microgram, milligram, or gram) contained in the largest size tablet available from the dose. *Both numbers must be expressed in the same unit of measure.* The answer tells how many more units of measure are needed in addition to the largest tablet or capsule. Next, look for a tablet or capsule of this size. This problem would be worked as follows:

$$\begin{aligned}&10\ (\text{mg—number of mg of dexamethasone ordered})\\ -\ &6\ (\text{mg—the largest tablet of dexamethasone available})\\ =\ &4\ (\text{mg—the amount that must be added to the 6 mg}\\ &\quad\text{tablet to obtain a 10 mg dose})\end{aligned}$$

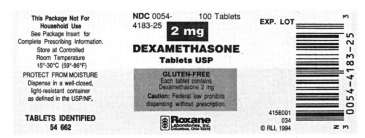

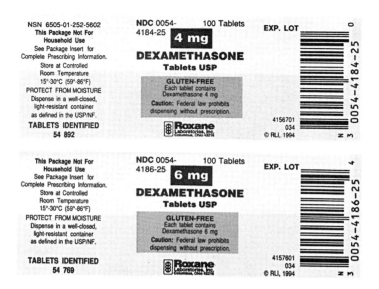

Thus to give 10 mg of dexamethasone one tablet containing 6 mg and another containing 4 mg is the appropriate combination. Twenty tablets of the 0.5 mg size for a 10-mg dose should not be used. Most patients would question taking this many tablets. Counting a large number of tablets introduces potential errors, and many patients would have trouble swallowing this many tablets. Also, additional costs occur each time a prescription is refilled.

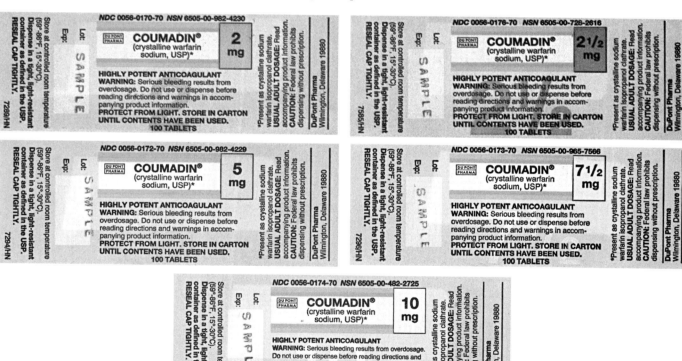

If the prescription is for 4.5 mg of warfarin, first look for a tablet that contains a dose ending in five tenths of a milligram. Subtract this from the prescribed dose to find the amount that must be added to that drug to obtain the prescribed dose.

If for example, the physician orders 4.5 mg of warfarin (Coumadin) and the following preparations are available, first identify the tablet that contains five tenths of a milligram of warfarin and less than 4.5 mg.

0.5 is the same as ½; this easily identifies the tablet that contains 2½ mg of warfarin as the tablet containing the needed five tenths of a milligram. Subtracting this amount from the prescribed dose indicates that an additional 2 mg is needed for the dose.

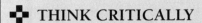

      4.5 (mg in prescribed dose)
    −2.5 (mg in tablet containing fraction)
    =2   (mg additional amount needed for the dose)

One tablet of 2.5 mg plus one tablet of 2 mg equals the prescribed dose of 4.5 mg.

> ✚ **THINK CRITICALLY**
> Is more than one size of tablet needed?
> Can the largest size of tablet available be used?
> Are the same units of measure used for all tablets?
> Is this the least number of tablets needed to supply the dose?

EXERCISE 3 *(answers on page 311)*

Work the following problems, which may require tablets or capsules that contain different amounts of drug:

1. The physician orders dexamethasone, 8 mg to be given as two divided doses daily. **(a)** How many milligrams are in one dose? **(b)** How would the dose be prepared?

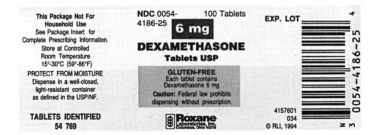

2. If the order is written "Give dexamethasone, 10 mg," how will the dose be prepared?

3. If the physician orders warfarin 7 mg, (a) Which strengths of tablets are appropriate? (b) How would one dose be prepared?

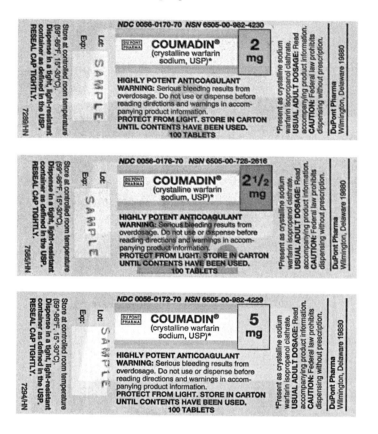

4. If the dose were for 5 mg warfarin (Coumadin), would it be preferable to give (a) two tablets, each containing 2.5 mg or (b) one tablet, 5 mg?

5. If the order were for 4.5 mg warfarin, how would you prepare the dose?

6. If the physician orders 225 mg of clindamycin (Cleocin), (a) which strength tablets would be needed? (b) How many tablets are needed for one dose?

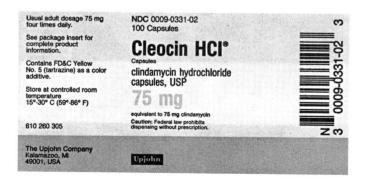

7. The physician orders chlorpromazine hydrochloride (Thorazine) 75 mg. (See labels on p. 172.) (a) Which strengths of preparations are appropriate? (b) How many tablets are needed for one dose?

8. If the order were for 35 mg of chlorpromazine, (a) which strength tablets would be needed? (See labels on p. 172.) (b) How many tablets would be needed for each dose?

9. Had the order been for 60 mg of chlorpromazine (Thorazine), (a) which strengths of preparation would be needed? (See labels on p. 172.) (b) How many tablets would be needed for one dose?

10. The physician orders phenobarbital, 45 milligrams. Tablets are available in strengths of 15 mg and 30 mg. (a) Which strengths of preparation are appropriate? (b) How much of each preparation would be used?

11. The physician orders amoxicillin 1 g. Using this label, how many capsules are needed for this dose?

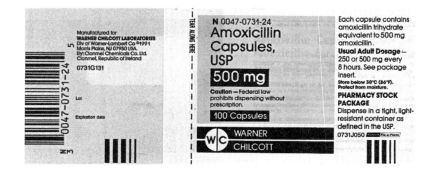

USING DIFFERENT SYSTEMS OF MEASUREMENT

Today, nearly all drug labels and physician's orders use the metric/SI system. Exceptions occur when the dose is ordered in one system and the dose on hand is supplied in another system (such as metric/SI and apothecaries'). *It is necessary to convert the dose ordered into the same system as the dose that is supplied or vice versa.* It is wise to convert the dose ordered into that on hand. The fact that gr i is actually equivalent to 0.0648 g should not be overlooked. However, when converting, it is permissible to use the equivalent 0.06 (some use 0.064 or 0.065) in place of the more exact figure. ✔ *As a rule, 10% greater or less than the exact figure is permissible when converting from one system to another.* When the dose must be measured exactly, the pharmacist computes and prepares the dose.

If, for example, the physician orders atropine sulfate, gr $\frac{1}{200}$, and the dose on hand is 0.0006 g, it is necessary to convert the grains to grams or grams to grains before computing the problem. Both the dose ordered and the dose on hand must be in the same system before the problem can be worked. (See Chapter 7.)

After recalling that 0.06 g is equivalent to gr i, the proportion is set up as follows:

grams:grains = grams: grains

$0.06(g):1 \text{ (gr)} = x(g):\frac{1}{200} \text{ (gr)}$

$x = 0.06 \times \frac{1}{200}$

$x = \frac{0.06}{200} = 200\overline{)0.0600}$

$x = 0.0003$ g, which is equivalent to gr $\frac{1}{200}$

With the knowledge that gr $\frac{1}{200}$ is equivalent to 0.0003 g or that each dose of atropine will be either gr $\frac{1}{200}$ or 0.0003 g, the problem can be solved as follows:

METHOD 1. *Using 2 ratios established by drug label and prescribed dose.* The proportion may be stated, using the labeling information as one part of the proportion.

Label side of the proportion   **Prescribed dose**
gram:tablet = gram:tablet
0.0006 (g):1 (tab) = 0.0003 (g):x (tab)
0.0006x = 0.0003
$x = \frac{0.0003}{0.0006} = \frac{1}{2}$ tab of atropine sulfate, 0.0006 g per tablet

METHOD 2. *Using the dosage formula.* Substitute into the following formula:

$\frac{\text{dose desired}}{\text{dose available}} \times 1$ (tab or unit)

= number of tablets needed to administer the dose prescribed

$\frac{0.0003}{0.0006} \times 1$ (tab) = $\frac{3}{6}$ or $\frac{1}{2}$ tab of atropine sulfate, 0.0006 g per tablet

The formula may be abbreviated as:

$$\frac{D}{H} \times U = A$$

If working with grains instead of grams is preferred, the conversion proportion would be the following:

grams:grains = grams:grains
0.06 (g):1 (gr) = 0.0003 (g):x (gr)
0.06x = 0.0003

$$x = \frac{0.0003}{0.06} = \frac{0.0003}{0.0600} = \frac{1}{200} = \text{gr } \frac{1}{200}$$

or

$$\frac{0.0003}{0.6} \times \frac{10{,}000}{10{,}000} = \frac{3}{600} = \text{gr } \frac{1}{200}$$

Knowing that 0.0006 g is equivalent to gr $\frac{1}{200}$, one can set up the proportion as follows, using grains in place of grams:

grains:grains = tablets:tablets
$\frac{1}{200}$ (gr):$\frac{1}{100}$ (gr) = x (tab):1 (tab)

$\frac{1}{100} x = \frac{1}{200}$

$$x = \frac{1}{200} \times \frac{100}{1} = \frac{1}{2} \text{ tab of atropine sulfate,}$$

0.0006g per tablet

METHOD 3. *Using 2 ratios established by size.* A proportion stating that lesser:greater = lesser:greater may be used.

lesser:greater = lesser:greater
grams:grams = tablets:tablets

0.0003 (g):0.0006 (g) = x (tab):1 (tab)   x = 0.0003 ÷ 0.0006
0.0006x = 0.0003 $x = \frac{3}{6}$ or $\frac{1}{2}$ tab of atropine sulfate, 0.0006 g per tablet

The answer is ½ tab in both instances.

EXERCISE 4 (answers on page 312)

Solve the following problems:

1. The physician orders phenobarbital gr iss. This would be equivalent to how many milligrams?

2. The physician orders 100 mg aminophyilline, which is available in tablets, gr iss. How many tablets will provide this dose?

3. The physician orders nitroglycerine gr $\frac{1}{100}$ sublingually. What would this dose be equivalent to, if stated in milligrams?

4. The physician orders potassium chloride 300 mg PO qd. The dose available is 5 gr tablets. How many tablets will provide the dose ordered?

5. The physician orders sodium salicylate 325 mg. It is available in 5 gr tablets. How many tablets are needed for the dose ordered?

6. The physician orders sodium bicarbonate, gr xv. If the unit dose on hand is 0.3 g tablets, how many tablets are needed for the dose ordered?

7. The physician orders aminophylline 200 mg. It is available in 3 gr tablets. How many tablets are needed for the dose?

8. The physician orders ammonium chloride 1 g. It is available in 7½ gr tablets. How many tablets are needed for the dose?

9. The physician orders thyroid gr ss. It is available in 30 mg tablets. How many tablets are needed for one dose?

10. The physician orders secobarbital (Seconal) gr iss. It is available in 100 mg capsules. How many capsules are needed for one dose?

11. The physician orders aspirin gr x. It is available in 325 mg tablets. How many tablets are needed for one dose?

12. The physician orders digitalis gr iss. It is available in 100 mg tablets. How many tablets are needed for one dose?

13. The physician orders amytal sodium gr i. It is available in 65 mg capsules. How many capsules are needed for one dose?

14. The physician orders thyroid 60 mg. It is available in 1 gr tablets. How many tablets are needed for one dose?

15. The physician orders ammonium chloride viiss gr. It is available in 500 mg tablets. How many tablets are needed for one dose?

16. The physician orders cascara sagrada 650 mg. It is available in 5 gr tablets. How many tablets are needed for one dose?

17. The physician orders ephedrine ¾ gr. It is available in 50 mg tablets. How many tablets are needed for one dose?

18. The physician orders quinidine sulfate gr iii. It is available in tablets of 130 mg, 200 mg, and 325 mg. **(a)** Which size tablet is appropriate and **(b)** how many tablets are needed for the dose?

19. The physician orders amytal sodium gr iii. It is available in 200 mg capsules. How many capsules are needed for the dose?

20. The physician orders calcium carbonate gr x. It is available in 650 mg tablets. How many tablets will provide the dose ordered?

21. The physician orders 10 gr calcium lactate. It is available in 325 mg tablets. How many tablets are needed for the prescribed dose?

13

Computation of Dosage from Solutions: Oral, Injectable, and Diluted

Many drugs are available in solution form from the manufacturer. Extensive knowledge is needed to place some drugs in solution. Unless the solution is prepared correctly, the action of the drug may be altered. The pharmacist should always be consulted if it seems necessary to prepare an oral or injectable solution of a solid drug. Infrequently, the health care professional administering the drug may find it necessary to prepare solutions for external use.

It is important to read the label on solutions very carefully. Information on the label indicates if the solution is intended for oral use only, if it is intended for injection, or if it is to be applied only externally. Labels give other information such as a warning not to use the preparation unless the solution is clear or directions to shake well before pouring.

Solutions used for injection must be sterile. They must be prepared and administered using sterile equipment and aseptic technique. Injectable solutions may be provided as a premeasured dose in a syringe or cartridge, in a single-dose vial, in an ampule, or in a multidose vial. The label on the container states the name of the drug and the amount of drug in a specific amount of solution. This information must be read carefully when selecting the type, strength, and amount of solution, in order to prepare the correct dose. If only part of a dose, premeasured in a syringe, is used, the remainder must be discarded. Any unused solution in an ampule must be discarded also. Multidose vials provide many doses and are used repeatedly unless contamination of the drug occurs. It is necessary to discard any contaminated drug or any multidose vial suspected of contamination.

Not all sterile solutions are intended for injection. The label may indicate that preservatives have been added or that the solution is not intended for injection. A sterile saline solution may be ordered for cleansing body cavities or wounds. Sterile saline may be used to irrigate urinary catheters. Bladder irrigations with sterile solutions are prescribed following surgery and to treat certain bladder conditions.

> ### ✤ THINK CRITICALLY
> Are the units and systems of measurement the same?
> Is the dose ordered in different units than those specified on the label?
> Is this the customary dose?
> Is the dose reasonable?
> If a solid preparation, does the dose exceed 1 to 2 tablets or capsules?
> If an injection, does the dose exceed 1 to 3 mL?

> ### ✤ THINK CRITICALLY
> Is this solution intended for oral administration?
> Should the solution be mixed or shaken before pouring the dose?
> Is it the right solution?
> Is it the right strength of solution?
> What amount will provide the prescribed dose?
> Is this the customary dose?
> How much, if any, additional fluid should be taken with the dose?

Many nonsterile solutions are used externally. The label should state that the solution is for external use only. In large medical centers, the external solutions used are prepared by the pharmacist or by the manufacturer. Some will be provided in the prescribed strength; others will require dilution. In more remote areas and undeveloped countries, the health care provider may find it necessary to prepare external solutions from tablets or powdered forms of the drug. Any solution that has the poison symbol on the label must be used and stored carefully. It is always wise to create and use separate storage areas for oral, injectable, and external solutions. This practice helps prevent errors in the home also.

Calculation of dosage for drugs that are used in solution form is based on ratio and proportion or formula. These will be explained with each type of problem.

ORAL SOLUTIONS OF DRUGS

The physician's order reads that erythromycin 500 mg is to be given orally tid. The label on the bottle states that each 5 mL of oral suspension contains the equivalent of 250 mg erythromycin.

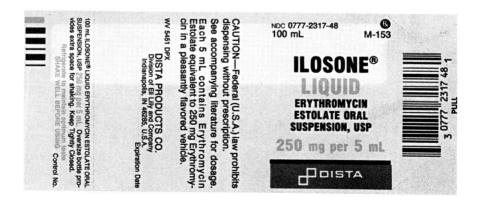

METHOD 1. *Using 2 ratios established by drug label and prescribed dose.* Establish a proportion using the information on the label as one ratio of the proportion and the desired (prescribed) dose as the other.

Label side of proportion   Prescribed dose
milligrams:milliliters = milligrams:milliliters
250 (mg):5 (mL) = 500 (mg):x (mL)

$250x = 5 \times 500$
$250x = 2500$
$x = 2500 \div 250$
$x = 10$ mL of erythromycin solution that contains 250 mg erythromycin in each 5 mL

Thus 500 mg of drug would be contained in 10 mL of solution labeled 250 mg in 5 mL. It is necessary to read the label carefully to learn how much drug is contained in a specific amount of solution. Different strengths of some solutions are available.

METHOD 2. *Using dosage formula.* Substitute into the following formula:

$$\left(\frac{\text{dose desired}}{\text{dose available (in specified amount of solution)}} \right)$$

$\times$ amount of solution containing the stated available dose
= amount of solution needed to give the desired dose

$$\frac{500 \text{ (mg)}}{250 \text{ (mg)}} \times 5 \text{ (mL)} = (500 \div 250) \times 5 = 2 \times 5$$

$= 10$ mL of erythromycin, 250 mg in 5 mL

The formula may be abbreviated as:

$$\frac{D}{H} \times U = A$$

METHOD 3. *Using 2 ratios established by size.* Establish a proportion, using lesser:greater = lesser:greater.

lesser:greater = lesser:greater
milligrams:milligrams = milliliters:milliliters
250 (mg):500 (mg) = 5 (mL):x (mL)
$250x = 2500$
$x = 2500 \div 250$
$x = 10$ mL of erythromycin, 250 mg/5 mL

If a dose is ordered in different system of measurement than the one in which the solution is labeled, before working the problem convert the dose ordered to the system used on the label.

EXERCISE 1 *(answers on page 312)*

Solve the following problems as indicated:

1. The physician orders 400 mg of erythromycin suspension qid. How many milliliters are needed for each dose if there are 250 mg/5 mL?

2. If the physician ordered an oral suspension of erythromycin, gr iii. Using the following preparation, how many milliliters would be needed for this dose?

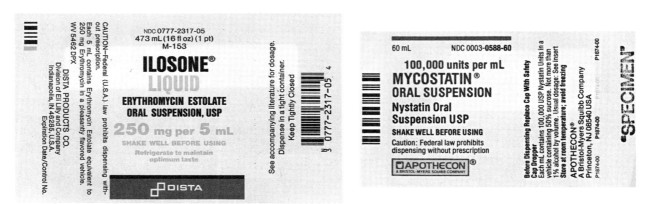

3. Nystatin (Mycostatin) 500,000 U is ordered. Read the above label. How much solution will contain this amount of drug?

4. A daily dose of 500 mg of oral suspension of griseofulvin is ordered to treat a tinea infection. Each 5 mL of solution contains 125 mg of drug. (a) How many milliliters are needed to deliver a dose of 500 mg of griseofulvin? (b) What does this equal in teaspoonfuls? (c) Each bottle contains 4 f℥ or how many 500 mg doses?

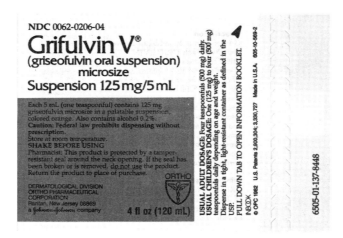

5. Mr. Faresair is to take ranitidine hydrochloride (Zantac Syrup) 150 mg bid to treat symptoms of Zollinger-Ellison syndrome. There are 15 mg of drug in each milliliter of solution. (a) How many milliliters are needed for each dose? (b) By what route is syrup administered? (c) Mark the dose on the medicine cup. (d) How many 10 mg doses are contained in each 16 f℥ bottle?

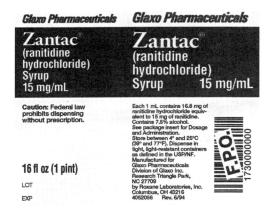
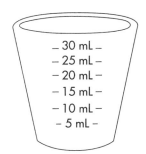

6. A 1 teaspoon dose of iodinated glycerol elixir, a mucolytic expectorant, is to be taken qid by Marney K. (a) If each teaspoonful (5 mL) contains 60 mg of drug, how many milligrams of drug is contained in each dose? (b) How many doses are available from 1 pint of elixir? (c) A pint of elixir would supply doses for how many days, if Marney takes the drug as prescribed?

7. 4 t of Diphenhydramine HCl Elixir qid is ordered. This is equivalent to (a) How many drams, (b) How many tablespoons, and (c) How many ounces?

8. The physician orders an initial dose of 1 mEq/kg sodium bicarbonate to be given to a man who weights 200 pounds. (a) How many milliequivalents of sodium bicarbonate is needed for this dose? (b) If there are 50 mEq in 50 mL, how much solution is needed for the dose?

9. The physician orders penicillin V-potassium (V-Cillin K) 400,000 units. Two solutions are available. One contains 125 mg (200,000 U)/5 mL. The other contains 250 mg (400,000 U)/5 mL. (a) Which solution would you choose? (b) How many milliliters are needed for the dose?

10. If V-Cillin K O is ordered, the solution contains 200,000 U/5 mL, how much solution is needed for the dose of 600,000 units?

11. The physician orders amoxicillin, 0.25 g O. How much of the solution labeled 125 mg/5 mL is needed?

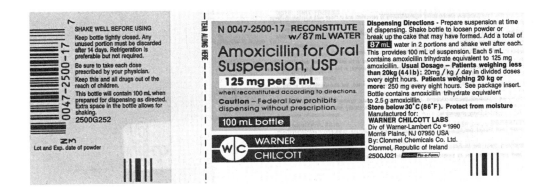

12. Haloperidol (Haldol) 15 mg daily is ordered to maintain control of symptoms of schizophrenia. This drug is available in 0.5, 1, 2, 5, 10, and 20 mg tablets. If this drug is to be given orally in divided doses three times a day, (a) which size tablet is needed for one dose? (b) How many tablets are needed each day? (c) If a liquid preparation is used instead of tablets, how many milliliters are needed for a single dose of 15 mg. Note that there are 2 mg of haloperidol in each 1 mL of solution.

13. Mimi K. is experiencing a major depressive disorder for which the physician has ordered fluoxetine hydrochloride (Prozac) 20 mg q AM. (a) Which of the following capsules is appropriate? (b) When Mimi complains that she feels more depressed in the evening, the prescription is changed to 10 mg bid. Which capsule would provide the correct dose each morning and evening? (c) Has the total daily dose been changed?

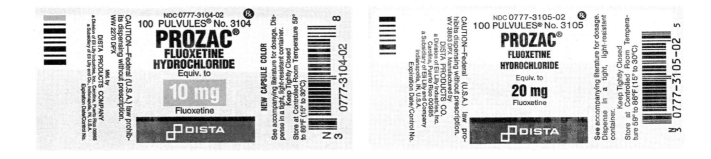

14. Twila S. is to take 300 mg of potassium iodide (SSKI solution), an expectorant, diluted in a glass of juice every 4 to 6 hours. The solution contains 1 g of potassium iodide in each milliliter. (a) How much solution is needed for the 300 mg dose? (b) Mark the calibrated dropper to show how to measure a 0.6 mg dose ordered for another patient.

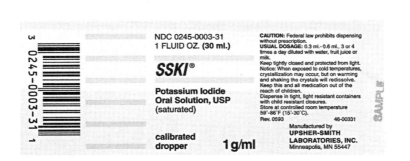 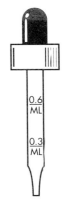

15. A loading dose of 125 mg phenytoin tid is ordered. (a) How much solution is needed for one dose? (b) How many milliliters of solution are in a full bottle of solution? Hint: Read the label carefully.

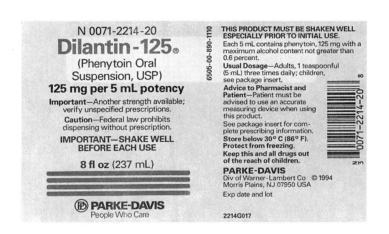 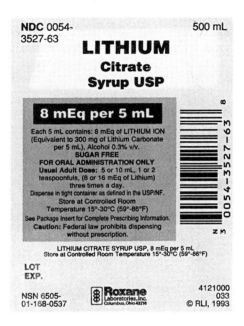

16. The physician orders a total dose of lithium citrate of 24 mEq. How many milliliters of syrup would be needed for this dose? See above label.

17. A daily oral dose of 500 mg of griseofulvin (Grifulvin V) is being used to treat a tinea infection. If each 5 mL of the suspension contains 125 mg of drug, (a) How many milliliters are needed to deliver 500 mg of griseofulvin? (b) To how many teaspoonfuls is this equivalent? (c) How many doses are available in each bottle containing 4 f℥ of suspension?

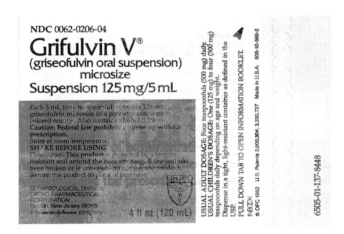

18. Furazolidine (Furoxone), an antimicrobial drug, is ordered for Sergeant Wall, who contracted giardiasis in Haiti. She is to take 2 tablespoonfuls of the liquid drug qid. (a) One dose is equivalent to how many milliliters? (b) To how many teaspoonfuls? (c) How many doses are available from a bottle that contains 60 mL of furazolidine solution?

19. Ira H. has bronchitis accompanied by tenacious mucus. He is to take 600 mg of saturated solution of potassium iodide (SSKI), an expectorant, in a glass of water or juice every 4 hours, to decrease the viscosity of the mucus. The clear solution contains 1 g of potassium iodide in each milliliter. (a) How much SSKI solution is needed for a 600 mg dose? (b) Mark the calibrated dropper to show how to measure this dose.

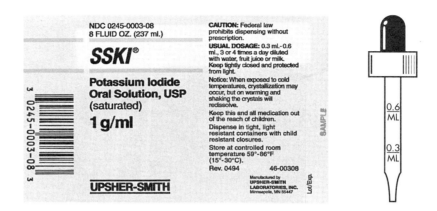

20. Emily T. always takes loperamide hydrochloride with her when she travels. Commonly known as Imodium, it is available as either a liquid or capsules. Emily prefers the liquid form. Each 5 mL (1 t) contains 1 mg of loperamide. (a) If the usual dose is 4 t after the first loose stool, how many milliliters are needed for the dose? (b) She will then take 2 t after each loose stool. This would be measured as how many milliliters?

INTRAMUSCULAR AND SUBCUTANEOUS INJECTIONS: PREPACKAGED STERILE SOLUTIONS

Drugs given by injection are prepared as sterile solutions by the manufacturer. Drugs intended for injection may be supplied in single-dose units, ampules, or multidose vials. Aseptic technique must be used when preparing and administering drugs by injection. Fig. 13-1 shows examples of syringes that may be used to measure solutions to be injected.

Careful reading of drug labels and medication orders is essential. Some sterile solutions are intended for intravenous use only. These are not to be administered by any other route. The same methods are used to calculate dosage for solutions whether they are to be administered subcutaneously or intramuscularly. Small amounts (0.5 to 1 mL) of nonirritating, water-soluble drugs may be administered subcutaneously. Most injections are prescribed and administered intramuscularly. Some irritating drugs are to be given only by deep intramuscular injection. Many solutions are available in more than one strength. A solution may be available in different strengths but packaged in the same-size or a similar-size container. For example, one ampule of hydromorphone hydrochloride (Dilaudid) might contain

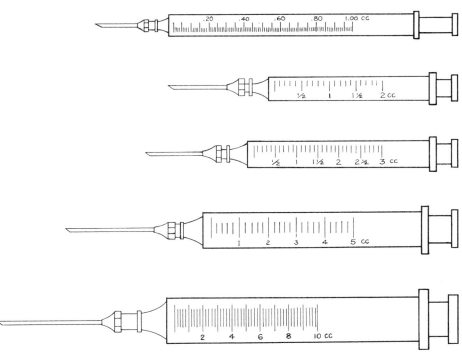

Fig. 13-1. Syringes are used to accurately measure varying amounts of sterile solutions for injection. Uppermost syringe is known as a tuberculin syringe and is graduated in 0.01 mL (cc). It is the syringe of choice for administration of small amounts. A 2 mL (cc) syringe is commonly used to give drug subcutaneously (hypodermically), intramuscularly, or intravenously. It is graduated in 0.1 mL. Larger syringes are used when a larger volume of drug is to be administered. Note that (mL) cc on all except tuberculin syringe contain markings for each one tenth of (mL) cc in addition to ½ and 1 (mL) cc markings.
(From Potter P, Perry A: *Fundamentals of nursing,* ed 3, St Louis, 1993, Mosby.)

> ### ✚ THINK CRITICALLY
> If the solution is to be injected, is it sterile?
> Is it the right kind of solution?
> Is it the right strength of solution?
> Is the amount ordered reasonable for the patient?
> Is the solution considered irritating to tissue?
> Which method is appropriate for administering this drug?

1 mg/mL of drug; another might contain 2 mg/mL of drug; a third might contain 4 mg/mL of drug.

Calculation of dosage for drugs that are to be administered intramuscularly or subcutaneously uses the same methods as described for calculating dosage for oral solutions of drugs. Again, if the order gives a different unit or system of measurement than the label on the drug, convert the ordered dose to the same system of measurement and units as those found on the label.

The physician orders 2 mg of hydromorphone hydrochloride (Dilaudid). The only available strength of hydromorphone that is available on your unit contains 2 mg/mL of drug.

METHOD 1. *Using 2 ratios established by drug label and prescribed dose.* Establish a proportion using the information on the label as one ratio of the proportion and the desired (prescribed) dose as the other.

Label side of proportion	Prescribed dose
milligrams:milliliters	= milligrams:milliliters
4 (mg):1 (mL)	= 2 (mg):x (mL)

$$4x = 2 \times 1$$
$$4x = 2$$
$$x = 2 \div 4$$

$x = \dfrac{1}{2}$ mL of hydromorphone solution containing 4 mg/mL

METHOD 2. *Using dosage formula.* Substitute into the following formula:

$$\frac{\text{dose desired}}{\text{dose available (in specified amount of solution)}} \times \text{amount of solution containing the stated available dose}$$
$$= \text{amount of solution needed to give the desired dose}$$

$$\frac{2 \text{ (mg)}}{4 \text{ (mg)}} \times 1 \text{ (mL)} = \frac{1}{2} \text{ mL of hydromorphone, 4 mg/mL}$$

The formula may be abbreviated as

$$\frac{D}{H} \times U = A$$

METHOD 3. *Using 2 ratios established by size.* Establish a proportion, using lesser:greater = lesser:greater.

lesser:greater = lesser:greater
milligrams:milligrams = milliliters:milliliters
2 (mg):4 (mg) = x (mL):1 (mL)

$$4x = 2$$

$x = 2 \div 4$
$x = \dfrac{1}{2}$ mL of hydromorphone, 4 mg/mL

EXERCISE 2 (answers on page 312)

Solve the following problems as indicated:

1. Francis J. has severe back pain and muscle spasms for which the physician orders orphenadrine citrate (Norflex) 60 mg IM stat. If each 2 mL ampule contains 60 mg of drug, how many milliliters are to be withdrawn for the dose?

2. Pentobarbital (Nembutal), 100 mg IM, is ordered as a hypnotic. Each milliliter contains 50 mg of drug. How many milliliters are required for one dose?

3. Immunizations are needed for a 2-month-old child for diphtheria, tetanus, and pertussis. After shaking the multiple dose vial vigorously, withdraw the dose, which for this child is 0.5 mL of diphtheria and tetanus toxoids and pertussis vaccine adsorbed (DPT). Mark the tuberculin syringe to show how much solution is needed for a single dose.

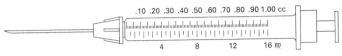

4. The physician orders meperidine, 25 mg IM. If the only solution available contains 50 mg/mL, how much solution is needed for the dose?

5. If the physician orders meperidine hydrochloride, 75 mg IM and the available solution contains 75 mg/mL, (a) how many milliliters of solution is needed for the dose? (b) Shade the syringe to show the correct dose.

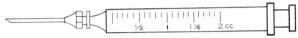

6. Atropine sulfate, gr 1/60 is ordered. Atropine solutions are labeled 0.4 mg/mL, 0.5 mg/mL, and 1 mg/mL. (a) Which solution is appropriate? (b) How much of the solution is needed for the dose? (c) Mark the syringe to show the correct dose.

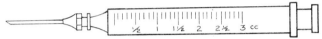

7. If the dose of atropine were for 0.2 mg SC, (a) which strength solution would be most appropriate (see strengths in problem 6)? (b) How much solution would provide this dose? (c) If the order were for 0.3 mg, how much solution would be needed?

8. Codeine gr ss IM is ordered. The solutions available contain either 30 or 60 mg/mL. (a) Which solution is most appropriate? (b) How much of the solution is needed?

9. The physician orders morphine sulfate, gr 1/6. (a) How much of the solution labeled 20 mg/mL is needed for this dose? (b) How much solution is needed for a dose of 10 mg?

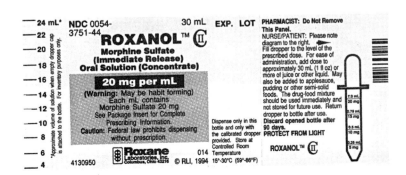

10. Morphine sulfate, gr ¼ is to be given. The strengths of available solutions are 10 mg/mL and 15 mg/mL. (a) Which solution is most appropriate? (b) How much solution is needed?

11. The physician's order for morphine sulfate is for 6 mg SC. (a) Which solution is most appropriate if the two strengths available contain 10 mg/mL or 15 mg/mL? and (b) How much is needed for the dose?

12. The physician orders morphine sulfate, gr ¼. You have the choice of the two solutions given in problem 11. (a) Which solution is appropriate? (b) How much of the solution is needed for the dose?

13. Mr. H. Z. is experiencing an acute psychiatric episode. To alleviate this, trifluoperazine (Stelazine) 1.5 mg deep IM is ordered. (a) If there are 2 mg of drug in each milliliter, how much solution is needed for the prescribed dose? (b) Mark the syringe to show the amount of solution required.

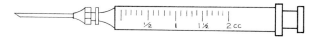

14. Hydromorphone hydrochloride (Dilaudid), 1 mg SC q4-6h is ordered to alleviate postsurgical pain. It is available in 3 sizes of ampules and a multidose vial. The ampules contain 1 mg/mL, 2 mg/mL, or 4 mg/mL. (a) Which size ampule is most appropriate to use? (b) How much solution will provide the dose ordered? (c) If the multidose vial which contains 2 mg/mL of hydromorphone hydrochloride is to be used, how much solution is needed for the dose?

15. Mr. O. has pernicious anemia. Once a month he receives cyanocobalamin (vitamin B_{12}) 200 mcg IM for this condition. How much solution is needed for this dose (a) if it contains 100 mcg/mL, (b) if it contains 1 mg/mL?

16. Pentazocine lactate (Talwin) 30 mg is ordered q3-4h prn for pain. Which of the following preparations is most appropriate for this dose? Unit dose ampules containing 1 mL (30 mg), 1.5 mL (45 mg), and 2 mL (60 mg) are available.

17. If the dose were for 45 mcg of pentazocine, which of the ampules in the previous problem would provide the correct dose?

18. Epinephrine 0.2 mg SC is ordered to treat an asthma attack. If the available solution contains 400 mcg/mL (a) How much solution is needed for this dose? (b) How much of the same solution will provide a dose of gr 1/150?

19. Oxymorphone hydrochloride (Numorphan) 1.5 mg SC is ordered for the relief of severe pain. (a) Which preparation is appropriate? (b) How much solution is needed for this dose?

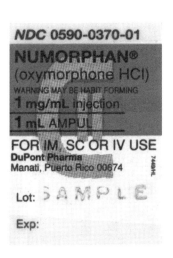
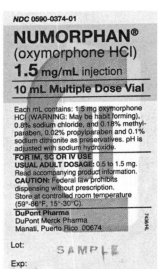

RECONSTITUTION AND DOSAGE OF CRYSTALLINE AND POWDERED DRUGS: ORAL AND INJECTABLE

Some drugs deteriorate relatively quickly when placed in a solution. These drugs are supplied in crystal or powder form and are diluted just before administration. The diluted drugs must be stored and used according to the manufacturer's instructions. Some drug preparations must be used within 24 hours after reconstitution; after this they become unstable and no longer have the desired effects.

Injectable Solutions

Drugs intended for injection are supplied as a sterile powder in a sterile vial and must be dissolved in the diluent recommended by the manufacturer. The commonly used diluents are 0.9% normal saline, sterile water for injection, or bacteriostatic water for injection. These diluents are not to be confused with solutions containing preservatives. Sterile technique must be followed when reconstituting a powdered drug that is to be injected.

It is necessary to read the manufacturer's directions found on the package insert carefully, because the amount of diluent, and sometimes the diluent itself, will vary with the drug preparation. The amount and kind of solution that is to be added to the powdered drug, the total volume of finished solution that will result, and the amount of drug in each milliliter of solution is stated in the directions provided by the manufacturer. The volume of the finished solution may vary from the amount of diluent added. For example, adding 1 mL of sterile water may produce a greater volume than 1 mL of solution, such as 1.2 mL.

Finally, the amount of drug contained in each milliliter of solution will vary with the particular drug and the amount of a powder in the vial. The correct amount of the drug will be given to the patient only if the correct volume of correctly reconstituted solution is used. ***It is important to know that the same drug is often available in different amounts per vial.*** For example, the drug cefazolin (Kefzol) could be available in vials of 250 mg, 500 mg, and 1 g quantities. The amount of diluent to be used to dissolve the drug in each of the vials differs, as does the volume of solution obtained and the average concentration of the drug (Table 13-1). After the solution is prepared, the vial must be labeled accurately to show the amount and kind of diluent added, the approximate average concentration, and the date and time of reconstitution.

If the prescribed dose is 500 mg of cefazolin and the vial contains 500 mg of powdered drug, 2 mL of diluent would be added and 2.2 mL of the reconstituted drug would be administered. However, if the 250 mg vial were used, it would be necessary to reconstitute two vials and to give a total of 4 mL of solution. If a vial containing 1 g of drugs were used, 2.5 mL of diluent would be used and the volume needed to give 500 mg of drug would be about 1.5 mL. In this case it would be easiest to use one vial containing the amount of drug that was prescribed.

In addition to information about reconstituting the drug, the package insert will contain extensive information about the drug. Some package inserts will provide the information about diluting the drug in a table form (Table 13-1), whereas others will give this information in narrative form. Usually, information about dilution follows the description of the drug, its uses, actions, adverse effects, warnings, precautions, and contraindications. Customarily, a statement about the stability of the solution follows the dilution information. This indicates how long the solution of the drug will remain stable under specified circumstances. **After reconstituting the drug, the volume of drug needed can be computed by setting up a proportion, or by dividing the concentration of the drug into the vial size and multiplying the number obtained by the available volume.** Using Table 13-1, 225 mg of drug can be given by using the 500 mg vial. Divide 225 by 500 and multiply the answer obtained by the volume in the vial.

EXAMPLE: Give 250 mg from a 500 mg vial.

First add the correct amount of diluent (2 mL)

$$250 \text{ (mg per dose)} \div 500 \text{ (mg in one vial)} = \frac{1}{2} \text{ the contents of one vial}$$

$$\frac{1}{2} \text{ (the contents of 1 vial)} \times 2.2 \text{ (mL per vial)} = 1.1 \text{ (mL per dose)}$$

Table 13-1. Dilution table for sterile cefazolin sodium (Kefzol).

Vial size	Diluent to be added	Approximate available volume	Approximate average concentration
250 mg	2 mL	2 mL	115 mg/mL
500 mg	2 mL	2.2 mL	225 mg/mL
1 g	2.5 mL	3 mL	330 mg/mL

Using the proportion method, dissolve the drug as instructed and set up the following proportion:

$$250 \text{ (mg per dose)}:x \text{ (mL of drug)} = 500 \text{ (mg of drug)}:2.2 \text{ (mL of solution)}$$
$$500x = 250 \times 2.2$$
$$500x = 550$$
$$x = 550 \div 500$$
$$x = 1.1 \text{ mL of reconstituted solution}$$

Some powdered drugs intended for injection are supplied with the premeasured amount of sterile diluent that is to be used to obtain the correct concentration of drug per milliliter. The directions for mixing the powder and the diluent are also provided.

Oral Solutions

Preparation of powdered drugs that are to be given orally requires reconstitution with the recommended volume and type of diluent, usually water, and given to the patient to drink or through a nasogastric or gastrostomy tube. Clean technique rather than sterile technique is usually permissible when reconstituting drugs that are to be administered orally. The same methods are used for calculation as for injectable drugs.

> ### ✚ THINK CRITICALLY
> How much drug does the unmixed, premeasured powder contain?
> Is sterile technique required for mixing the drug with diluent?
> What diluents are recommended for this drug?
> How much diluent is needed?
> How much drug will be in the finished solution?
> Is the finished solution labeled completely?
> What conditions are necessary for storing the finished solution?
> How long can the finished solution be stored?
> Is the finished solution intended for ingestion, injection, or external use?

EXERCISE 3 (answers on page 313)

Solve the following problems:

1. The physician orders 250 mg cefazolin q8h IM. **(a)** How many grams are needed for the total daily dose? **(b)** How much total diluent is to be added to the vial? **(c)** How much reconstituted drug is needed for each dose? Please consult Table 13-1 on p. 194.

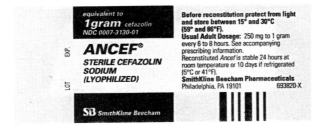

2. The physician orders cephoperazone, sodium 500 mg to be given intravenously q12h. (a) How many milligrams are needed for each 24-hour period? (b) Which vial contains the total amount needed for each 24-hour period?

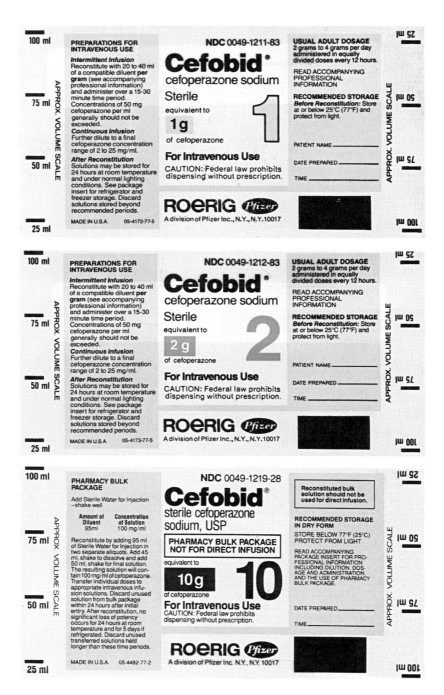

3. The physician orders cefoperazone sodium 4 g/day to be given intravenously in two divided doses. (a) How many grams of drug are needed for each dose? (b) If the available vial contains 10 g of drug, how much diluent is added for its reconstitution? (c) What is the concentration of the solution in a 10 g vial that has been mixed correctly? (d) State the name of the diluent that is used to reconstitute this drug. (e) How long can the reconstituted drug be stored?

4. The physician orders amoxicillin 250 mg q8h O for 10 days. Directions on the package insert state:

Product	Bottle size	Amount of water required for reconstitution
125 mg/5 mL	80 mL	62 mL
	100 mL	78 mL
	150 mL	116 mL
250 mg/5 mL	80 mL	59 mL
	100 mL	74 mL
	150 mL	111 mL

(a) How much of each of the products would be needed for this dose? (b) Which product provides the prescribed dose using the least amount of solution? (c) Which bottle size will provide the exact amount of medication needed for 10 days? (d) How much water is needed to reconstitute a 150 mL bottle to obtain a solution that contains 125 mg of drug in 5 mL of solution?

5. The physician orders nafcillin 500 mg IV q4h for 48 hours. (a) How many total grams of drug are needed for the total prescription? (b) To procure the exact amount of drug needed, select the 2 g vial. How many vials of this size are needed for the 48 hours? (c) To reconstitute a 10 g vial of nafcillin, which diluent is needed? (d) How much diluent will be added to the vial containing 10 g?

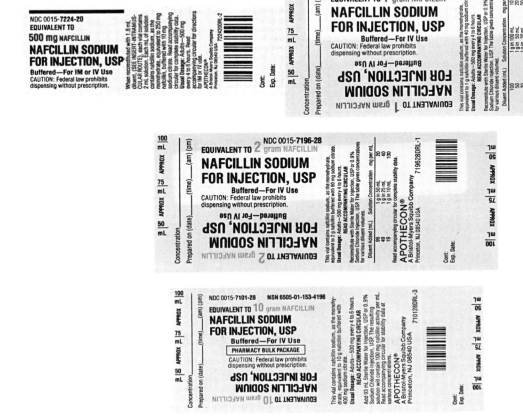

6. A dose of methicillin sodium (Staphicillin), 1 g q6h IM is ordered. There are different vials of methicillin available. Each must be mixed. (a) Which size vial will provide the exact amount needed for 24 hours? (b) How much diluent should be added to the vial to reconstitute the solution? (c) What diluent is to be used? (d) How much reconstituted drug is needed for each dose?

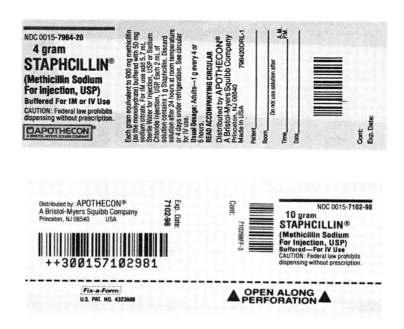

7. The physician orders 500 mg cephalothin sodium (Keflin) q6h IV. (a) How many grams are needed for the total daily dose? (b) Name the diluent that is to be added to the powdered drug. (c) How much diluent is to be added to the vial?

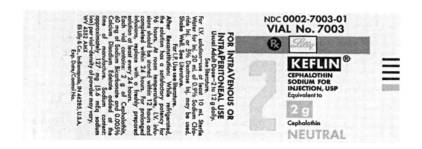

8. Piperacillin sodium (Pipracil), 2 g IM stat and non rep is ordered for the treatment of uncomplicated gonorrhea. Vials in 2, 3, and 4 gram sizes are available. Directions for reconstitution include: Reconstitute each gram of piperacillin with 2 mL of a suitable diluent to achieve a concentration of 1 g per 2.5 mL. Shake well until dissolved. **(a)** Which size vial is most appropriate for this dose? **(b)** How much sterile diluent is to be added to a vial containing 2 g of drug? **(c)** After dilution, how much solution will the vial contain? **(d)** How much solution contains 1 g of drug?

PREPARATION OF EXTERNAL SOLUTIONS FROM STRONGER DRUGS

Most solutions are supplied in the required strength by the pharmacist or pharmaceutical supply houses. Occasionally it may be necessary to make solutions for irrigations or soaks from tablets, crystals, or powders, or by diluting stronger solutions. This practice is necessary most often in community health or home care and in remote areas and undeveloped countries. The physician may prescribe soaks, irrigations, or rinses using specific solutions. A variety of wet dressings, baths, or soaks are used to treat skin conditions. Irrigations are used to cleanse wounds, indwelling catheters and tubes, and body cavities such as the stomach. Although sterility is required when the solution contacts areas that are normally sterile, many solutions such as those that are applied topically or introduced into the gastrointestinal tract rarely need to be sterile. However, nonsterile solutions are prepared using clean technique.

Teaching the patient, family members, and other care providers to make solutions from solid drugs (tablets, crystals, or powders) or to dilute stronger solutions to a weaker strength means that the health care provider must be able to perform the necessary computations. The patient and family members or other care givers must be taught how to prepare the solution. When the solid form of the drug (tablets, crystals, or powders) is used to make the solution, the drug must be dissolved completely. Even tiny particles of some drugs are capable of producing damage to the skin and mucus membranes.

When doing calculations, solid forms of drugs (tablets, crystals, powders) are always 100% strength. Sometimes, these are referred to as pure drugs. Most full strength solutions are 100% also. In a ratio, 100% becomes 1:1. A notable exception is boric acid, which is only 5% when it is full strength. Stock solutions may be of any strength. Careful reading of labels will identify the name of the drug and its strength, if it is already in solution. The amount of drug that is to be placed into solution or diluted is always less than the total volume of solution that is being prepared. The amount of the weakest solution (the diluted drug) will always be greater than the amount of the stronger drug. The finished volume of solution is stated as a liquid measurement such as milliliters.

The amount of drug being used to make the diluted solution is stated in the same units of liquid measurement as the stronger solution. When a solid drug is being used, the diluted solution is stated in units of liquid measurement, which are the equivalent of the units of weight for the solid drug. If the liquid measure is in milliliters, its equivalent measure in weight is grams.

The correct amount of solid drug or stronger strength used to prepare the weaker strength of solution is placed into a measuring container. Enough diluent (often water) is added to a solid drug or a stronger solution to make the total amount of the diluted or weaker solution.

Making 400 mL of 5% solution using a pure drug (100%) or a pure solution (100%), can be sketched as follows:

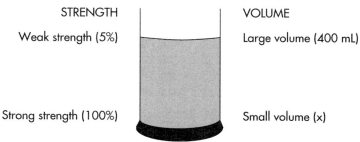

When making a solution, the amount (by weight or volume) of the strong solution or drug is placed into the container, then enough diluent is added to obtain the total amount of the dilute solution.

Some powdered drugs will displace more solution than others. Placing the correct amount of the drug in the container and adding the amount of diluent needed to make the total volume of finished solution will provide the correct strength of solution. This procedure is also used when diluting a strong solution. For example, if 10 mL of 90% solution is to be diluted to a total of 500 mL, one would measure 10 mL into a container and add enough solution to make a total of 500 mL. The amount that would be added would be 490 mL (500 − 10 = 490). It is less efficient and less accurate to measure each solution in separate containers because some solution may adhere to the sides of the container. When the strength of the drug that is being diluted is not given, the pure drug (100%) is used regardless of whether it is in solid or liquid form.

The following formula may be used to solve problems of dilution:

Strength   Volume/weight
weak:strong = lesser:greater

EXAMPLE: Make 400 mL of 5% solution. The final (weak) solution will have a strength of 5%. The strong solution or solid drug that will be diluted has a strength of 100%. The total volume of solution that will be made is 400 mL. It is unknown how much drug should be diluted to make this solution. Substitute into the formula as follows:

Strength   Volume/weight
weak:strong = lesser:greater $100x = 400 \times 5$ or 2000
$5(\%):100(\%) = x(g):400$ (mL) $x = 20$ g solid drug

The same formula is used to make a dilute solution from a stronger solution.

EXAMPLE: Make a 20% solution using 10 mL of 80% solution.

The weak solution will have a strength of 20%. The strong solution that will be diluted has a strength of 80%. The small amount of drug that will be diluted is 10 mL. Substitute into the formula as follows:

Strength   Volume/weight
weak:strong = lesser:greater $20x = 800$
$20(\%):80(\%) = 10$ (mL)$:x$ (mL) $x = 40$ mL of 20% finished solution

To make the solution place 10 mL of 80% solution into a container and add enough water to obtain a total of 40 mL of finished solution. To find the amount of diluent that would be used, subtract the lesser volume (the amount of the concentrated drug) from the greater volume of solution (the final amount of solution) (40 − 10 = 30 mL of diluent).

Another formula that can be used to solve this type of problem is:

$$\frac{\text{Desired strength}}{\text{Available strength}} \times \frac{\text{Total quantity}}{\text{of desired solution}} = \frac{\text{Amount of undiluted drug}}{\text{needed to make solution}}$$

This formula may be abbreviated as $\frac{D}{A} \times Q = q$

EXAMPLE: Make 1000 mL of 2% solution using a 60% solution. Substitute into the above formula.

$$\frac{2(\%)}{60(\%)} \times 1000 \text{ (mL)} = 33.3 \text{ mL of 60\% solution}$$

In each method, both the strength of the solution or solid drug used, and that being prepared, must be expressed as either a percent or a ratio. When necessary, convert percent to ratio or ratio to percent.

EXERCISE 4 *(answers on page 313)*

Solve the following problems:

1. Prepare 250 mL of a 2% sodium bicarbonate solution.

2. Prepare 0.5 L of a physiologic salt solution.

3. Prepare 1 L of a 1:250 potassium permanganate solution from a 1:10 solution.

4. Prepare 500 mL of a 5% sodium chloride solution.

5. Prepare 1 L of a 0.9% saline solution. Use NaCl or table salt.

6. Prepare 1 glassful (240 mL of water) of physiologic salt solution.

7. Prepare 1000 mL of a 1:1000 potassium permanganate solution from 0.33 g tablets.

8. Prepare 500 mL of a 5% sodium bicarbonate solution from a 20% solution.

9. Prepare a 0.5% hydrogen peroxide solution using f℥ii of a 3% solution.

14

Insulin Dosage

HYPOGLYCEMIA AND HYPERGLYCEMIA

Health care providers who administer insulin to patients have a responsibility to teach them about living optimally with diabetes mellitus. This includes the accurate measurement and administration of the prescribed insulin. Unless insulin is measured accurately the patient may receive an insufficient amount, leading to hyperglycemia, or an excess amount, producing hypoglycemia. Hyperglycemia is evidenced by certain signs and symptoms and can lead to diabetic coma. Hypoglycemia also presents with many signs and symptoms and can lead to insulin shock. Unless treated, either reaction can result in death. The symptoms of each condition vary considerably from one individual to another. Table 14-1 gives common causes for the occurrence of these conditions.

Hypoglycemia is the most frequently experienced adverse effect of insulin dosage. Box 14-1 lists signs and symptoms that occur with hypoglycemia. Commonly, hypoglycemia results when an individual has received more insulin than needed. This may be related to a patient having missed or delayed meals, worked or exercised more than usual, or having experienced vomiting, diarrhea, or emotional stress. Interactions between some drugs may also cause hypoglycemia. Box 14-2 lists signs and symptoms that may be experienced with hyperglycemia. Hyperglycemia may result from omitting an insulin dose, receiving too little insulin, overeating, insufficient exercise, or drug interactions. The signs and symptoms of either condition vary widely among individuals. Most diabetics are able to recognize symptoms of the impending conditions and intervene quickly and appropriately.

Table 14-1. Causes of hypoglycemia and hyperglycemia.

Causes of hypoglycemia	Causes of hyperglycemia
Too much insulin	Omitting insulin
Too little food intake	Too little insulin
Too much exercise or work for food and insulin intake	Too much food intake
Vomiting, diarrhea	Too little exercise
Emotional stress	Infection or fever

> **Box 14-1. Symptoms of Mild to Moderate Hypoglycemia.**
> Note that the severity of the symptoms increase with the depth of hypoglycemia.
>
> | | |
> |---|---|
> | Hunger | Drowsiness or fatigue |
> | Tremor | Inability to concentrate |
> | Lightheadedness or dizziness | Palpitation or tachycardia |
> | Headache | Tingling or numbness in hands, feet, lips, tongue |
> | Sweating | Blurred vision |
> | Irritability | Slurred or incoherent speech |
> | Restlessness or nervousness | Abnormal behavior |

> **✚ THINK CRITICALLY**
>
> Does the patient know
> - The name of the prescribed insulin?
> - The biologic source of the prescribed insulin?
> - The dose to be taken?
> - Time the dose is to be taken?
> - How to recognize hypoglycemia and hyperglycemia?
> - How to treat hypoglycemia and hyperglycemia?
> - How to regulate insulin dosage?
> - Measurement and injection techniques?

> **Box 14-2. Signs and Symptoms of Hyperglycemia and Diabetic Acidosis.**
>
> | | |
> |---|---|
> | Thirst | Unsteady movement |
> | Frequent urination | Disorientation |
> | Drowsiness | Dehydration |
> | Flushed face | Hypotension |
> | Loss of appetite | Fruity odor on breath |
> | Nausea and vomiting | Hyperventilation or heavy breathing |
> | Abdominal pain | Unconsciousness |
> | Malaise | Death |
> | Visual disturbances | |

Insulin preparations and dosage are prescribed by the physician to treat insulin-dependent diabetes mellitus. Insulin-dependent diabetics are unable to control the disease with diet and oral hypoglycemic agents. Choice of preparation and dose depend upon the requirements of the patient. Using the same brand of insulin consistently is often recommended to patients. Increasingly, human insulin is being prescribed because of its low antigenicity. With only one exception all insulin products are now manufactured in a concentration of 100 U/mL. The exception is Regular Insulin, Iletin II, (Concentrated) Pork, manufactured by Lilly, which is used only when the patient requires very high doses of insulin. Another product, Humulin BR, available in 100 U/mL, is used in external insulin pumps only (Fig. 14-1).

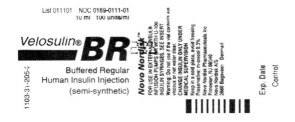

Fig. 14-1. Humulin BR is used in external insulin pumps only. It contains 100 units of insulin/mL.

SOURCES OF INSULIN

The source of insulin, called the species, is either human or animal. Human insulin is like the insulin produced by human beings. It is made in the laboratory by using recombinant DNA technology or chemically altering pork insulin. Human insulin is being prescribed with increasing frequency because of its low antigenicity. Insulin derived from animal sources continues to be used. If insulin is derived from cattle it is termed *beef insulin; porcine or pork insulin* is derived from pigs. Combinations of both beef and pork insulin are available.

STRENGTH OF INSULIN

Rather than using metric/SI measures, the unit is used to measure the strength of insulin. Insulin concentration is labeled and measured in units per milliliter. Insulin is always prescribed in units. Note that the potency of an insulin unit remains the same. However, one milliliter of 500 units/mL contains 5 times more units of insulin than one milliliter of 100 units/mL.

INSULIN SYRINGES

Special syringes are used for the measurement and administration of insulin. These syringes, called insulin syringes, approved by the American Diabetes Association, are calibrated for the measurement of U-100 insulin only. The design of the syringes makes it easier to measure small amounts of insulin accurately. Using insulin syringes calibrated for U-100 insulin to measure the prescribed dose of U-100 strength insulin eliminates calculation and helps avoid measurement errors. Fig. 14-2 illustrates three insulin syringes calibrated for measuring U-100

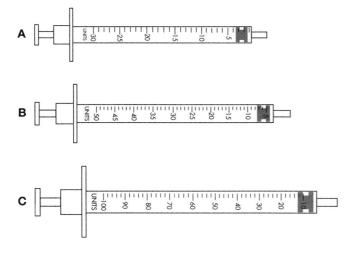

Fig. 14-2. 3 sizes of insulin syringes for measuring U-100/mL strength of insulin. A, The 0.3 mL syringe is recommended for measuring 30 units or less of insulin. B, The 0.5 mL syringe is recommended for measuring 31 to 50 units of insulin. C, The 1 mL syringe is recommended for measuring 51 to 100 units of insulin.

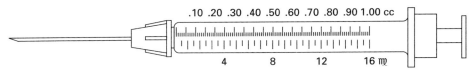

Fig. 14-3. Tuberculin syringe. The tuberculin syringe is graduated in 0.01 mL. It may be used to measure 1 mL or less of concentrated (500 U/mL) insulin.

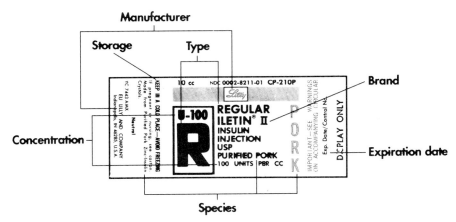

Fig. 14-4. The information provided on an insulin label.

insulin. Note that both the 0.3 mL and 0.5 mL syringes are calibrated in increments of single units, and the 1.0 mL syringe is calibrated in increments of 2 units. As a guide, the 0.3 mL syringe is used to measure doses of 30 units or less of U-100 insulin, the 0.5 mL syringes is used to measure amounts between 30 and 50 units of insulin, and the 1.0 mL syringe is used to measure amounts between 50 and 100 units of insulin.

Insulin syringes must not be used to measure other medications, including those prescribed in units, such as heparin and antibiotics. Other syringes should not be used to measure insulin, with the exception of U 500/mL. Because insulin syringes are calibrated to measure only insulin in a strength of U-100/mL, these syringes cannot be used to measure insulin in a concentration of U-500/mL. When the prescribed dose requires using insulin U-500/mL another type of syringe must be used. If 1 mL or less is required for the dose of U-500, a tuberculin syringe is used. Fig. 14-3 illustrates a tuberculin syringe. Remember to use the appropriate size of insulin syringe calibrated for U-100 to measure U-100/mL.

INSULIN LABELS

Each bottle of insulin is labeled with information about the insulin product. Fig. 14-4 indicates information found on the label. The large letter on the label is an abbreviation for the type of insulin. Table 14-2 gives abbreviations for the various types of insulin.

Table 14-2. Common abbreviations for types of insulin and activity of each.

ABBREVIATION	TYPE OF INSULIN	ACTIVITY
R	Regular	Rapid and short
N	NPH	Intermediate
L	Lente	Intermediate
U	Ultralente	Slow and long

ACTIVITY TIME SPANS

Each insulin product has its own activity time span. The time spans given in Table 14-3 are broad estimates only. For estimates specific to a particular brand and preparation of insulin, consult the package insert. Note that activity time spans vary by manufacturer.

Table 14-3. Estimated ranges of activity for insulin preparations. Considerable variation may occur with the product and patient.

	Onset of Action	Peak Action	Duration of Action

Short-Action
  Regular
  Velosulin
	15 to 30 minutes	2 to 5 hours	5 to 8 hours

Intermediate Action
  NPH
  Lente
	1 to 3 hours	6 to 12 hours	18 to 26 hours

Long-Action Ultralente	4 to 8 hours	14 to 24 hours	28 to 36 hours

Variations among individuals for the time of onset, peak action, and duration of effect are considerable. These variations result from many factors including the species of insulin used, site of injection, amount of exercise, body temperature, insulin antibodies, and brand of insulin. Generally, short-acting insulins act quickly, usually within 15 to 30 minutes, and last approximately 5 to 8 hours, with peak action occurring approximately 2 to 5 hours after injection. On the average, intermediate-acting insulins have an onset of action between 1 and 3 hours, peak action between 6 and 12 hours, and duration of effect lasting 18 to 26 hours. When mixtures are used to obtain both rapid and intermediate action, the onset is rapid, usually within 15 to 30 minutes. Long-acting insulins have an onset of approximately 4 to 8 hours, peak action between 14 and 24 hours and duration of action lasting 28 to 36 hours. Approximations for each specific product are given in package inserts.

> ### ✚ THINK CRITICALLY
> Is this the prescribed brand of insulin?
> Is this the prescribed formulation (R, N, L, U, or mixture)?
> Is this the correct strength?
> Is this the correct dose?
> Is this the customary type of syringe used for measuring the dose?
> Is this the appropriate size syringe to measure the dose?

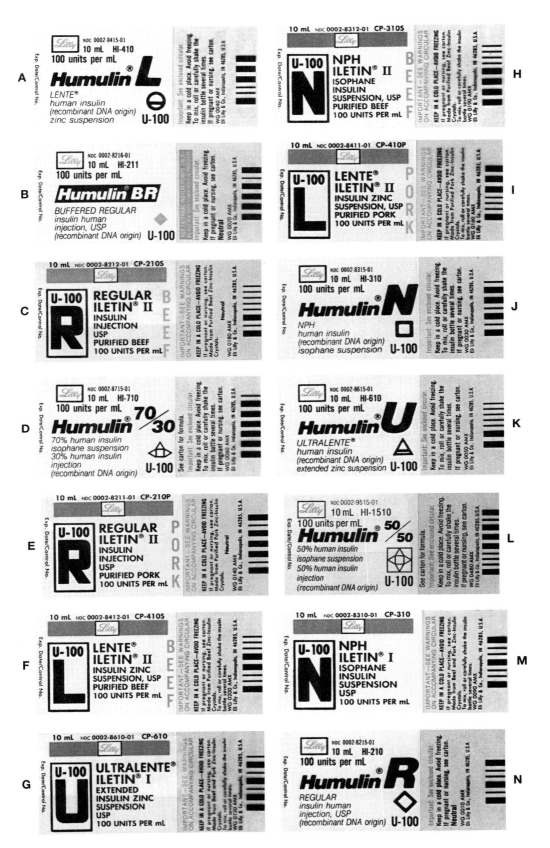

Fig. 14-5. Insulin labels.

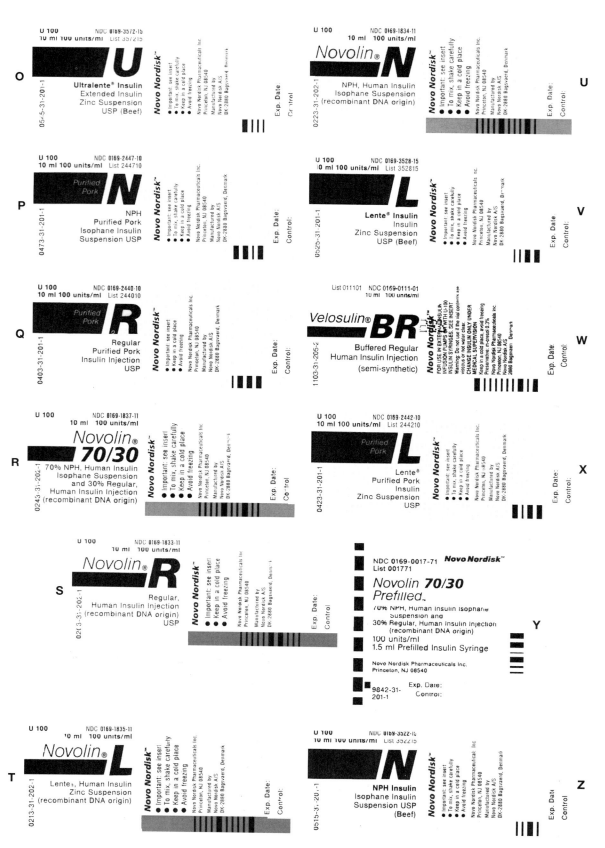

Fig. 14-5, cont'd. Insulin labels.

EXERCISE 1

(answers on page 314)

For each of the following problems **(a)** select the insulin solution that is to be used from the labels shown in Fig. 14-5 (p. 207-208) and indicate your choice by placing the letter for the insulin product in the space provided. **(b)** Read labels carefully and indicate the species of origin by circling the appropriate choice. **(c)** Indicate whether the preparation is short, intermediate or long-acting, (see Table 14-2) (p. 206) or 14-3 (p. 206) circling the correct choice. **(d)** Shade the area on the syringe to show the amount of insulin needed for the prescribed dose. For additional practice, identify the correct dose on the syringes shown in Fig. 14-2, p. 206.

For example, if the order is to give 25 U of Humulin N, **(a)** select the preparation lettered "F" and write "F" in the space provided. **(b)** Circle the correct choice to indicate the species of origin. **(c)** Indicate whether the preparation has a short, intermediate or long action by circling the correct choice. **(d)** Shade the area representing a dose of 25 units on the syringes.

1. Give 2 U Regular Iletin II Beef insulin.
   a. C
   b. human
      beef
      beef-pork
      pork
   c. *short action*
      intermediate action
      long action
   d. Shade syringe to show correct dose.

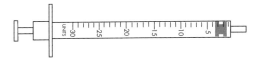

2. Give 84 U of Velosulin BR insulin.
   a. W
   b. *human*
      beef
      beef-pork
      pork
   c. *short action*
      intermediate action
      long action
   d. Shade syringe to show correct dose.
   e. How is this administered?
      In external insulin infusion pumps or U100 insulin syringes

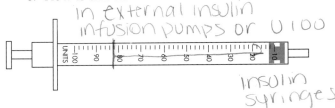

3. Give 24 U of Lente Purified Pork insulin (Novo Nordisk).
   a. X
   b. human
      beef
      beef-pork
      pork
   c. short action
      intermediate action
      long action
   d. Shade syringe to show correct dose.

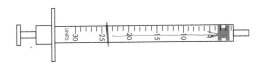

4. Give 66 U NPH Iletin I insulin.
   a. M
   b. human
      ~~beef~~
      beef-pork
      pork
   c. short action
      intermediate action
      long action
   d. Shade syringe to show correct dose.

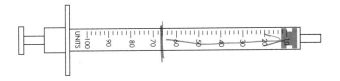

5. Give 18 U L human insulin (Novo Nordisk).
   a. T
   b. **human**
      beef
      beef-pork
      pork
   c. short action
      intermediate action
      long action

6. Give 7 U Regular Iletin II Pork insulin.
   a. E
   b. human
      beef
      beef-pork
      pork
   c. **short action**
      intermediate action
      long action

7. Give 32 U Ultralente Iletin I insulin.
   a. q
   b. human
      beef
      beef-pork
      pork
   c. short action
      intermediate action
      long action
   d. Shade syringe to show correct dose.

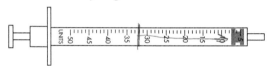

8. Give 88 U Novo Nordisk Ultralente insulin.
   a. O
   b. human
      beef
      beef-pork
      pork
   c. short action
      intermediate action
      long action
   d. Shade syringe to show correct dose.

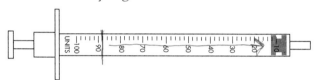

9. Draw up and give 42 U 70/30 Novolin insulin.
   a. P
   b. **human**
      beef
      beef-pork
      pork
   c. short action
      intermediate action
      long action
   d. Shade syringe to show correct dose.

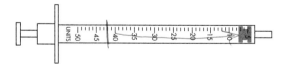

10. Give 14 U Humulin U insulin.
    a. K
    b. **human**
       beef
       beef-pork
       pork
    c. short action
       intermediate action
       long action
    d. Shade syringe to show correct dose.

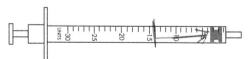

11. Give 34 U Humulin N insulin.
    a.
    b. human
       beef
       beef-pork
       pork
    c. short action
       intermediate action
       long action

12. Give 15 U Novolin N insulin.
    a.
    b. human
       beef
       beef-pork
       pork
    c. short action
       intermediate action
       long action

13. Give 56 U Humulin 50/50 insulin.
    a.
    b. human
       beef
       beef-pork
       pork
    c. short action
       intermediate action
       long action

14. Give 20 U Humulin 70/30 insulin.
    a.
    b. human
       beef
       beef-pork
       pork
    c. short action
       intermediate action
       long action

15. Give 8 U Regular Purified Pork Insulin (Novo Nordisk).
    a.
    b. human
       beef
       beef-pork
       pork
    c. short action
       intermediate action
       long action
    d. Shade syringe to show correct dose.

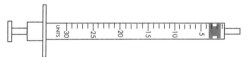

16. Give 60 U Lente Iletin II pork insulin.
    a.
    b. human
       beef
       beef-pork
       pork
    c. short action
       intermediate action
       long action
    d. Shade syringe to show correct dose.

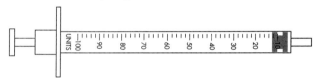

17. Give 46 U NPH Iletin II beef insulin.
    a.
    b. human
       beef
       beef-pork
       pork
    c. short action
       intermediate action
       long action
    d. Shade syringe to show correct dose.

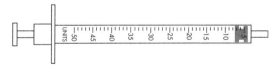

18. Give 25 U NPH beef insulin (Novo Nordisk).
    a.
    b. human
       beef
       beef-pork
       pork
    c. short action
       intermediate action
       long action
    d. Shade syringe to show correct dose.

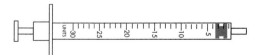

19. Give 12 U Humulin R insulin.
    a.
    b. human
       beef
       beef-pork
       pork
    c. short action
       intermediate action
       long action

20. Give 16 U Lente beef insulin (Novo Nordisk).
    a.
    b. human
       beef
       beef-pork
       pork
    c. short action
       intermediate action
       long action

21. Give 52 U Lente Iletin II beef insulin.
    a.
    b. human
       beef
       beef-pork
       pork
    c. short action
       intermediate action
       long action

22. Give 40 U Novolin R insulin.
    a.
    b. human
       beef
       beef-pork
       pork
    c. short action
       intermediate action
       long action

23. Give 18 U NPH purified pork insulin.
    a.
    b. human
       beef
       beef-pork
       pork
    c. short action
       intermediate action
       long action

24. Give 94 U Humulin L insulin.
    a.
    b. human
       beef
       beef-pork
       pork
    c. short action
       intermediate action
       long action
    d. Shade syringe to show correct dose.

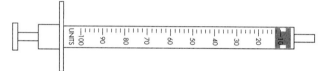

25. Give 72 U Novolin 70/30 insulin using prefilled syringe.
    a.
    b. human
       beef
       beef-pork
       pork
    c. short action
       intermediate action
       long action

26. The insulin preparations used in insulin pumps *only* are named (a) _____ and the labels are identified with the letters (b) _____ in Fig. 14–5.

27. Calculate the volume needed in hundreths of a milliliter; then shade the tuberculin syringes to show the measurement of Regular Insulin, Iletin II (Concentrated) Pork insulin, U-500/mL for orders of these amounts:
    a. 300 U

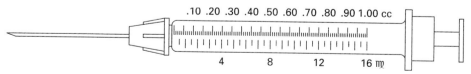

    b. 150 U

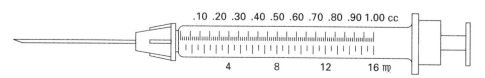

15

Intravenous Fluids and Medications

The health care professional has a major responsibility in the administration of IV fluids and medications. The physician orders the type, amount of solution, and medications to be given intravenously over a stated period of time. The order may indicate that a certain amount of solution is to be given over a specific time period such as 24 hours, 8 hours, 4 hours, or 1 hour. Similarly, an order that specifies the rate in mL/h and frequency provides essentially the same information. Often the order includes the addition of medications, including electrolytes, antibiotics, and other drugs.

Because IV solutions and their additives act immediately, it is imperative that all orders for IV therapy be carried out accurately. Careful reading of the orders and labels is essential. Giving the correct drug in the correct amount, type, and strength of solution is critical, because any product given intravenously acts immediately and the effects may be difficult or impossible to counteract. IV solutions that contain additives may be prepared in the pharmacy or added on the health care unit. In either case, labels must be read carefully to verify that the correct solution and additives are prepared and administered to the right patient, beginning at the right time, and over the right length of time. Additives with the same name are manufactured for different routes of administration. **Only those drugs that are labeled for intravenous use are to be administered intravenously.** Not all drugs are appropriate for intravenous infusion. Although the same drug may be available for intramuscular (IM) or subcutaneous (SC) administration, it may not be suitable for IV administration.

Labels must be read carefully to determine if the preparation is suitable for IV use. As a guide, preparations that are not true solutions or contain certain substances such as preservatives, oils, or particulate matter are not given intravenously. However, specially formulated lipid emulsions are given intravenously to help meet nutritional needs.

The compatibility of any mixtures of drugs and/or solutions must be known. Information about compatibilities is available in many reference books. Whenever such information is not available, it is wise to assume noncompatibility among the

> **Box 15-1. Strengths and tonicity of some commonly prescribed intravenous solutions.**
>
> Isotonic solutions are used to replace extracellular fluid. Hypotonic solutions, which are used to aid the kidney in the excretion of solutions, can cause serious problems; their use requires careful, frequent monitoring for early detection of complications. Hypertonic solutions are used to shift fluid from the extracellular space and can cause complications of either circulatory overload or dehydration if given too rapidly.
>
> ### Isotonic, Hypotonic, and Hypertonic Solutions
>
> **Isotonic solutions**
>
> Saline—0.9% NaCl
> 5% dextrose in water
> 5% dextrose in either 0.2% or 0.3% saline
> Ringer's solution
> Lactated Ringer's solution
>
> **Hypotonic solutions**
>
> Saline solutions containing less than 0.9% NaCl, usually 0.33% or 0.45%
>
> **Hypertonic solutions**
>
> Saline solutions that contain more than 0.9% NaCl, usually 3% or 5%
> 5% dextrose in either 0.45% or 0.9% saline
> 10% to 70% dextrose in water or saline
> 5% dextrose and lactated Ringer's solution

drugs and/or solutions. Awareness that solutions can be isotonic, hypotonic, or hypertonic is helpful for assessing whether the order is reasonable for a particular patient. Some common IV solutions, and their strengths and tonicity are given in Box 15-1. The label on the IV solution will tell you both the type and strength of the solutions.

> **✚ THINK CRITICALLY**
>
> Is this the correct type of solution?
> Is this the correct strength of solution?
> Is this the correct amount of solution?
> Does this solution contain the correct type and amount of electrolytes?
> Is the solution sterile?

READING ORDERS FOR INTRAVENOUS THERAPY

Abbreviations are used extensively in orders for IV therapy. For example, an order for a solution of 5% dextrose in water might be written as (a) D5W, (b) D-5-W, or (c) 5/0. In examples a, b, and c the letter "D" is used rather than writing out the word *dextrose*. Similarly W is used to symbolize water. In example c, O is used to symbolize water. In the other examples, 5 indicates that the strength of the solution is 5%. The rate at which the solution is to be administered is also indicated in the order. This might be stated in number of hours or milliliters per hour. The time that the infusion is to be started will also be indicated. There are too many different IV solutions and additives to include all of them in this book. However, an appreciation of the general approach to reading orders for IV therapy can be gained from working the problems in the following exercises.

EXERCISE 1
(answers on page 317)

Answer the questions following each order.

1. Infuse 1000 mL 5/0 over 8 hours beginning at 8 AM.
   a. What kind of IV fluid was ordered?
   b. Is the solution isotonic, hypotonic, or hypertonic?
   c. How much IV fluid was ordered?
   d. Are additives included in the order? If so, what is the name and dose of each?
   e. When is this IV solution to be started?
   f. Does the order state how long this solution is to run? If yes, how long?
   g. Does the order state the rate of flow to be used? If yes, what is it?

2. Give 2000 mL D5W over first 24 hours postop.
   a. What kind of IV fluid was ordered?
   b. Is the solution isotonic, hypotonic, or hypertonic?
   c. How much IV fluid was ordered?
   d. Are additives included in the order? If so, what is the name and dose of each?
   e. When is this IV solution to be started?
   f. Does the order state how long this solution is to run? If yes, how long?
   g. Does the order state the rate of flow to be used? If yes, what is it?

3. Give 5% dextrose in 100 mL water with 900 mg clindamycin over 30 minutes q12h. Start postsurgery.
   a. What kind of IV fluid was ordered?
   b. Is the solution isotonic, hypotonic, or hypertonic?
   c. How much IV fluid was ordered?
   d. Are additives included in the order? If so, what is the name and dose of each?
   e. When is this IV solution to be started?
   f. Does the order state how long this solution is to run? If yes, how long?
   g. How frequently is this order to be administered?
   h. Does the order state the rate of flow to be used? If yes, what is it?

4. Give Ringer's Lactate 1000 mL over 8 h Start at 9 AM
   a. What kind of IV fluid was ordered?
   b. Is the solution isotonic, hypotonic, or hypertonic?
   c. How much IV fluid was ordered?
   d. Are additives included in the order? If so, what is the name and dose of each?
   e. When is this IV solution to be started?
   f. Does the order state how long this solution is to run? If yes, how long?
   g. Does the order state the rate of flow to be used? If yes, what is it?

5. Give 5% dextrose in 0.45% NaCl 1000 mL with 20 mEq KCl q12h.
   a. What kind of IV fluid was ordered?
   b. Is the solution isotonic, hypotonic, or hypertonic?
   c. How much IV fluid was ordered?
   d. Are additives included in the order? If so, what is the name and dose of each?
   e. When is this IV solution to be started?
   f. Does the order state how long this solution is to run? If yes, how long?
   g. Does the order state the rate of flow to be used? If yes, what is it?

6. Continuously infuse Lactated Ringer's solution in 5% dextrose, 1000 mL over 8 hours. Start at 1700.
   a. What kind of IV fluid was ordered?
   b. Is the solution isotonic, hypotonic, or hypertonic?
   c. How much IV fluid was ordered?
   d. Are additives included in the order? If so, what is the name and dose of each?
   e. When is this IV solution to be started?
   f. Does the order state how long this solution is to run? If yes, how long?
   g. Does the order state the rate of flow to be used? If yes, what is it?

7. Give Lactated Ringer's solution in 5/O IV NGR (nasogastric replacement) mL/mL.
   a. What kind of IV fluid was ordered?
   b. Is the solution isotonic, hypotonic, or hypertonic?
   c. How much IV fluid was ordered?
   d. Are additives included in the order? If so, what is the name and dose of each?
   e. When is this IV solution to be started?
   f. Does the order state how long this solution is to run? If yes, how long?
   g. Does the order state the rate of flow to be used? If yes, what is it?

8. Infuse 3000 mL 5D/W for 24 hours with 40 mEq potassium chloride in each 1000 mL.
   a. What kind of IV fluid was ordered?
   b. Is the solution isotonic, hypotonic, or hypertonic?
   c. How much IV fluid was ordered?
   d. Are additives included in the order? If so, what is the name and dose of each?
   e. When is this IV solution to be started?
   f. Does the order state how long this solution is to run? If yes, how long?
   g. Does the order state the rate of flow to be used? If yes, what is it?

9. Give 2500 U heparin in 0.45% NaCl 250 mL at 10 mL/h.
   a. What kind of IV fluid was ordered?
   b. Is the solution isotonic, hypotonic, or hypertonic?
   c. How much IV fluid was ordered?

d. Are additives included in the order? If so, what is the name and dose of each?
e. When is this IV solution to be started?
f. Does the order state how long this solution is to run? If yes, how long?
g. Does the order state the rate of flow to be used? If yes, what is it?

Computerized orders

Orders for IV therapy may be computerized by the pharmacist. The computerized orders are derived from the physician's orders, and contain the same information as the written order. The form may vary, and additional information may be included. For example, the physician's order may state that the IV solution is to be administered over an 8-hour period. In addition to this information, the computer order may state the rate of flow in milliliters per hour and milliliters per minute. This is a time-saving measure for the person administering the IV solution. Because the calculations have been done, setting for the flow rate is easily determined. This information can be used to make a time-strip for the IV container (Fig. 15-1). An alternate method for estimating the rate of flow is presented in Fig. 15-2.

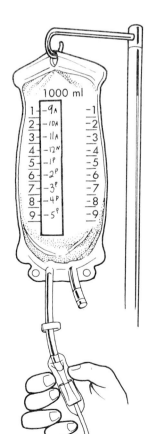

Fig. 15-1. The time at which the solution should reach a specific level is marked on tape. If 1000 mL is to be given at a rate of 100 mL, tape would be marked at 100 mL intervals as shown, beginning 1 hour after infusion is started. Note that the number 1 followed by a short line on IV bag represents 100 mL of fluid, number 2 represents 200 mL, etc. Preprinted adhesive tapes marked for a specific number of milliliters per hour are available commercially. The number of drops per minute can be written on the label by the health care provider.

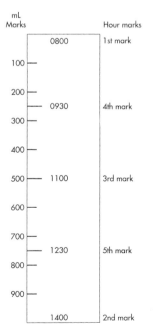

Fig. 15-2. An alternative method of estimating the rate of flow to be used if the number of mL/h are uneven and do not align easily with numbers on the container of IV solution. The marked tape shows that 1000 mL are to be delivered in 6 hours and the infusion is to start at 8 AM (0800) hours. Initially, the tape was marked to show that the infusion started at 0800 and is to end at 1400. Calculations done to place the next mark: ½ the total time of 6 hours = 3 hours and ½ the total solution of 1000 mL = 500 mL. A line is drawn on the tape at the 500 mL mark and 1100 written beside it. The 3-hour period is divided in half equaling 1½ hours and occurs at 0930. The 500 mL of solution (amount to be delivered in 3 hours) was divided in half to obtain 250. A line is placed at 250 mL and the time (0930) written beside it. Both the time between 11 AM (1100) and 2 PM (1400) and amount of solution to be delivered between 1100 and 1400 are divided and marked. Further subdivisions can be made, if desired.

The reading and interpretation of computerized orders is usually included in the orientation of new employees. The original orders are sent from the care unit to the pharmacy, processed promptly, and returned to the care unit within a short period of time. The format, abbreviations, and punctuation used for computerized orders varies. Even though derived from the physician's order, the computerized order is verified by a health professional on the patient unit. After checking the computerized order against the physician's order, the health professional initials the order, certifying that it was verified as correct. Any order about which there is a question should also be rechecked. In some institutions all capital letters are used on computerized orders because they are thought to be easier to read. Clock time or 24-hour time may be used, commas are sometimes used in orders of 1000 mL or more, and a variety of abbreviations may be used. For example, FD may be used to abbreviate first dose and LD for last dose. In most systems, a series of continuous IV solutions is separated from infusions that are intermittent. Each of the solutions in a series may be lettered or numbered to indicate the order of administration. A notation of whether the infusions are to be given continuously or intermittently may also be included. Identifying information and notations about allergies precede the orders.

EXERCISE 2

(answers on page 317)

Answer the questions following each of the computerized orders.

1. Lactated Ringer's in 1000 mL 5/O   Start: 1800   01/21
   Run 8 h Flow rate: 125 mL/h   Stop: 0200   01/22
   a. What kind of IV fluid was ordered?
   b. Is the solution isotonic, hypotonic, or hypertonic?
   c. How much IV fluid was ordered?
   d. Are additives included in the order? If so, what is the name and dose of each?
   e. When is this IV solution to be started?
   f. Does the order state how long this solution is to run? If yes, how long?
   g. Does the order state the rate of flow to be used? If yes, what is it?

2. 5% dextrose in 1000 mL 0.45% NaCl & 20 mEq KCl   Start: 1830   04/27
                                                      Stop: 0230   04/28
   a. What kind of IV fluid was ordered?
   b. Is the solution isotonic, hypotonic, or hypertonic?
   c. How much IV fluid was ordered?
   d. Are additives included in the order? If so, what is the name and dose of each?
   e. When is this IV solution to be started?
   f. Does the order state how long this solution is to run? If yes, how long?
   g. Does the order state the rate of flow to be used? If yes, what is it?

3. 5% normal serum albumin 500 mL   Start: 1300   06/23
   Run: 1 h   Flow-rate 500 mL/h   8.3 mL/min   Stop: 1400   06/23
   a. What kind of IV fluid was ordered?
   b. How much solution was ordered?

c. Are additives included in the order? If so, what are the name and dose of each?
d. When is this IV solution to be started?
e. Does the order state how long this solution is to run? If yes, how long?
f. Does the order state the rate of flow to be used? If yes, what is it?

4. 20 mg famotodine in 50 mL 0.9% NaCl   Start: 1900   05/04
Run: 15 min   Flow rate: 200 mL/h   3.3 mL/min
Give: q8h   2 doses only
   a. What kind of IV fluid was ordered?
   b. Is the solution isotonic, hypotonic, or hypertonic?
   c. How much IV fluid was ordered?
   d. Are additives included in the order? If so, what are the name and dose of each?
   e. When is this IV solution to be started?
   f. Does the order state how long this solution is to run? If yes, how long?
   g. Does the order state the rate of flow to be used? If yes, what is it?
   h. Is this order to be repeated? If yes, (a) when and (b) how many times is this order to be implemented?

5. 1 g cefazolin sodium (Ancef) in 50 mL 5% dextrose
Run: 15 min   Flow rate: 200 mL/h   3.3 mL/min
Give: q12h   First dose: 2100   01/12   Last dose: open
   a. What kind of IV fluid was ordered?
   b. Is the solution isotonic, hypotonic, or hypertonic?
   c. How much IV fluid was ordered?
   d. Are additives included in the order? If so, what are the name and dose of each?
   e. When is this IV solution to be started?
   f. Does the order state how long this solution is to run? If yes, how long?
   g. Does the order state the rate of flow to be used? If yes, what is it?

6. 25,000 U heparin in 0.45% in 250 mL NaCl (100 U/mL) Start: 0900   09/18
Run: 24 h   Flow rate: 10 mL/h   0.17 mL/min   Stop: 0900   09/19
   a. What kind of IV fluid was ordered?
   b. Is the solution isotonic, hypotonic, or hypertonic?
   c. How much IV fluid was ordered?
   d. Are additives included in the order? If so, what are the name and dose of each?
   e. When is this IV solution to be started?
   f. When is this order to be stopped?
   g. Does the order state how long this solution is to run? If yes, how long?
   h. Does the order state the rate of flow to be used? If yes, what is it?

7. 5% Dextrose in water 500 mL with 10,000 U heparin   Start: 1000   12/23
                                                                   Expires: 1000   12/24

Run: 10 h   Flow rate: 50 mL/HR   0.8 mL/min   1000 U/50 mL/h
   a. What kind of IV fluid was ordered?
   b. Is the solution isotonic, hypotonic, or hypertonic?
   c. How much IV fluid was ordered?

d. Are additives included in the order? If so, what are the name and dose of each?
e. When is this IV solution to be started?
f. When does this order expire?
g. Does the order state how long this solution is to run? If yes, how long?
h. Does the order state the rate of flow to be used? If yes, what is it?

8. 1 g aztreonam In 50 mL D5W   Start: 1100   10/14
Give: q12h   Stop: open
Run: 1 h   Flow rate: 100 mL/h   1.7 mL/min
   a. What kind of IV fluid was ordered?
   b. Is the solution isotonic, hypotonic, or hypertonic?
   c. How much IV fluid was ordered?
   d. Are additives included in the order? If so, what are the name and dose of each?
   e. When is this IV solution to be started?
   f. Does the order state how long this solution is to run? If yes, how long?
   g. Does the order state the rate of flow to be used? If yes, what is it?
   h. Is the order to be repeated? If yes, how often?

9. 10 mg prochlorperazine in 50 mL D5W   Time: q4h prn
                                                     First dose: 11 AM   11/02
Run: 15 min   Flow rate: 200 mL/h   3.3 mL/min Last dose: open
   a. What kind of IV fluid was ordered?
   b. Is the solution isotonic, hypotonic, or hypertonic?
   c. How much IV fluid was ordered?
   d. Are additives included in the order? If so, what are the name and dose of each?
   e. When is this IV solution to be started?
   f. Does the order state how long this solution is to run? If yes, how long?
   g. Does the order state the rate of flow to be used? If yes, what is it?
   h. When is the last dose to be given?

10. 500 mg vancomycin in 100 mL D5W   Time: q12h
    Run: 1 h   Flow rate: 100 mL/h   1.7 mL/min   First dose: 11 AM   11/02
                                                         Last dose: open
   a. What kind of IV fluid was ordered?
   b. Is the solution isotonic, hypotonic, or hypertonic?
   c. How much IV fluid was ordered?
   d. Are additives included in the order? If so, what is the name and dose of each?
   e. When is this IV solution to be started?
   f. Does the order state how long this solution is to run? If yes, how long?
   g. Does the order state the rate of flow to be used? If yes, what is it?
   h. When is the last dose to be given?

CALCULATING THE RATE OF FLOW

The health care provider is responsible for setting the rate at which IV solution is administered. The flow rate must be reasonably uniform if the patient is to receive the right amount of fluid over the right amount of time. Very rapid infusion may lead to serious complications such as circulatory overload, which leads to congestive heart failure. If the infusions are administered too slowly, dehydration and other serious problems may occur. Often this requires the health professional to calculate the rate of flow so that the solution is given over the amount of time specified by the physician. Whether it is necessary to set the flow rate in drops per minute or milliliters per hour depends upon the equipment used. The flow rate is controlled by gravity or a pump. Although computerized pumps and electronic regulators contain alarms to alert the health provider when problems occur in the system, periodic monitoring may detect problems before the alarm sounds. Such monitoring is usually scheduled q1h.

When IV solutions are delivered by gravity, the healthcare provider must calculate the number of drops per minute. The number of drops per milliliter of solution depends upon the drip chamber. This is referred to as the *drip factor* or the *drop factor*. The choice of a particular brand of tubing will determine whether the number of drops per milliliter of solution delivered will be 10, 12, 15, or 20. A minidrip (microdrip) chamber that delivers 60 drops/milliliter is available and is used when the rate is very slow, often 50 to 80 mL/h or less. Labeling on the package of the tubing will state the number of drops per milliliter that will be delivered (Fig. 15-3). When removing tubing from its box, it is important to read the labeling information to learn the approximate number of drops per 1 mL as well as other information and directions for using the tubing.

> ### ✚ THINK CRITICALLY
> Is this the right rate and is it reasonable?
> Is the IV solution being delivered on time?
> Are there signs or symptoms that indicate changes in IV therapy?

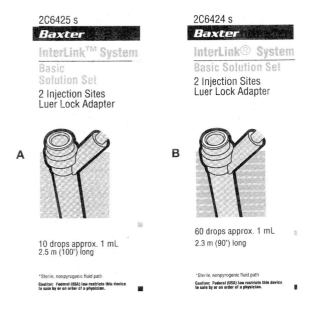

Fig. 15-3. IV tubing. A, 10 drops per mL (macrodrip), B, 60 drops per mL (microdrip).

(Courtesy Baxter Healthcare Corporation, Round Lake, Ill.)

The flow rate is controlled with clamps or an electronic flow-regulation device that counts the drops per minute. If clamps are used, the health professional counts the drops per minute. The electronic flow-regulator counts the drops per minute after it is set at the desired rate. Like all electronic devices, it must be installed correctly and monitored to be sure that it is working properly.

Computerized infusion pumps may be used to regulate the flow of solutions (Fig. 15-4). These pumps maintain the flow rate at a preset amount by controlling the pressure in the line needed to deliver the solution at the desired rate. Although the features of computerized pumps vary with the manufacturer, the pumps are set to deliver the solution in milliliters per hour. These can be set for whole milli-

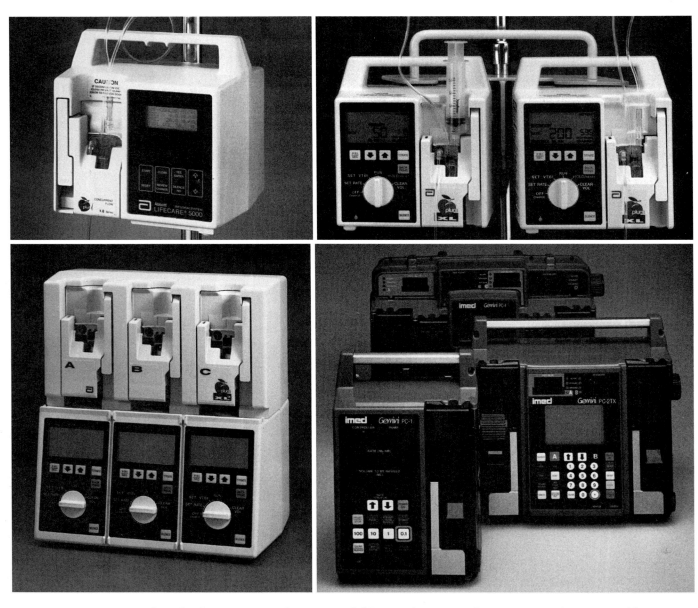

Fig. 15-4. Examples of infusion pumps that are available. **A,** Plum 1.6 Infusion System (Courtesy Abbott Laboratories, Abbott Park, Ill.) **B,** Plum XL. Note delivery of medication by syringe in addition to delivery of fluids on the left (Courtesy Abbott Laboratories, Abbott Park, Ill.) **C,** Plum XL3 (Courtesy Abbott Laboratories, Abbott Park, Ill.) **D,** Gemini PC-1, Gemini PC-2TX, Gemini PC-4 (Courtesy IMED Corporation, San Diego, Calif.)

liters; some accept decimal numbers. The correct tubing must be used for proper functioning of the pump.

Calculating the rate of flow in milliliters/hour

To calculate the rate of flow in milliliters per hour, it is necessary to know the total number of milliliters of solution that are to be given and the time in hours over which this amount of solution is to be given. Divide the total number of milliliters of solution by the total time in hours to find the number of milliliters per hour. This can be stated as the following formula:

$$\frac{\text{Total number of milliliters ordered}}{\text{Total hours for administration}} = \text{milliliters/hour}$$

This formula can be abbreviated even further to

$$\frac{\text{Total milliliters}}{\text{Total hours}} = \text{milliliters/hour} \quad \text{or} \quad \frac{\text{mL}}{\text{h}} = \text{mL/h}$$

EXAMPLE: Give 3000 mL in 24 hours.

Substitute into the formula $\frac{\text{mL}}{\text{h}} = \text{mL/h}$

$$\frac{3000}{24} = 24\overline{)3000}^{\,125 \text{ mL/h}}$$
$$\underline{24}$$
$$60$$
$$\underline{48}$$

EXERCISE 3 *(answers on page 318)*

Find the rate of flow in number of milliliters/hour for each of the following problems.

1. Give 1 L of 0.9% saline over 8 hours.

2. Give 100 mL of 5/O containing 500 mg vancomycin in 1 hour.

3. Give 500 mL of 5% serum albumin in 1 hour.

4. Give 1000 mL 0.9% saline in 12 hours.

5. Give 3000 mL D5W in 24 hours.

6. Give 500 mL D5W in 4 hours.

7. Give 1000 mL D5 0.45 NS with 40 mEq KCl at rate in 8 hours.

8. Give 50 mL D5W with 10 mg prochlorperazine in 15 minutes.

9. Give 50 mL of 5% dextrose in water with 12.5 mg promethazine in 10 minutes.

10. Give 100 mL D5W with 900 mg clindamycin in 30 minutes.

Calculating the rate of flow in drops

The rate of flow in drops per minute is often referred to as the drip rate. There are two major approaches to calculating the rate of flow in drops per minute. One method starts by using milliliters/hour and the other uses the volume in milliliters and time span. Both methods require knowledge of the drip factor for the tubing that will be used to deliver the solution.

Using the rate of flow when milliliters/hour is known

If the rate of flow in milliliters/hour is known, the number of milliliters/minute can be found by dividing the number of milliliters/hour by 60, the number of minutes in 1 hour. Then milliliters/hour is multiplied by the drop factor to find the number of drops per minute. Finding the number of milliliters per minute if the number of milliliters per hour is known can be stated as a formula.

$$\frac{mL/h}{60} = mL/min$$

EXAMPLE: Calculate the flow rate in milliliters/minute. The flow rate is 125 mL/h.

$$\frac{125 \ (mL/h)}{60 \ (min/h)} = 60 \overline{)125.00} \quad 2.08 \text{ or } 2.1 \ mL/min$$

Next, the number of milliliters/minute is multiplied by the drop factor, which depends upon the type of tubing used. The formula for this is:

$$mL/min \times drop \ factor = drops \ per \ minute$$

EXAMPLE: Find the flow rate in drops per minute if the flow rate is 2.1 mL/h and the drop factor is approximately 10 drops/mL.

Substitute into the formula:

$$mL/min \times drop \ factor = drops/min$$
$$2.1 \times 10 = 21 \ drops/min$$

EXERCISE 4
(answers on page 318)

Calculate the flow rate in milliliters/minute and drops/minute for each of the following flow rates, which are given in milliliters/hour.

1. If the flow rate is 125 mL/h and the drop factor is 10 drops/mL, what is the flow rate in (a) milliliters/minute? (b) drops minute?

2. If the flow rate is 200 mL/h and the drop factor is 10 drops/min, what is the flow rate in (a) milliliters/minute? (b) drops minute?

3. If the flow rate is 100 mL/h and the drop factor is 60 drops/mL, what is the flow rate in (a) milliliters/minute? (b) drops minute?

4. If the flow rate is 100 mL/h and the drop factor is 15 drops/mL, what is the flow rate in (a) milliliters/minute? (b) drops minute?

5. If the flow rate is 250 mL/h and the drop factor is 12 drops/mL, what is the flow rate in (a) milliliters/minute? (b) drops minute?

6. If the flow rate is 333 mL/h and the drop factor is 20 drops /mL, what is the flow rate in (a) milliliters/minute? (b) drops minute?

7. If the flow rate is 80 mL/h and the drop factor is 60 drops/mL, what is the flow rate in (a) milliliters/minute? (b) drops minute?

8. If the flow rate is 60 mL/h and the drop factor is 60 drops/mL, what is the flow rate in (a) milliliters/minute? (b) drops minute?

Using volume in milliliters, drop factor, and time span. This method may be used for calculating the flow rate when the flow is controlled by a manually regulated clamp. Knowledge of the total volume of fluid in milliliters, the total time for the infusion in minutes, and the drip factor is needed. If the total volume is ordered in liters, this number is multiplied by 1000 (the number of milliliters/liter) to convert it to milliliters. If the time is stated in hours, it is changed to minutes by multiplying the number of hours by 60 (the number of minutes in 1 hour). This may be stated as a formula:

$$\frac{\text{total mL} \times \text{gtts/mL}}{\text{total h} \times 60(\text{min})} = \text{gtts/min}$$

To solve problems that require calculation of the rate of flow, the known facts are substituted into the formula, and the problem is solved using arithmetic.

EXAMPLE: Give 3 L of IV solution during the first 24 hours postoperatively. Information on the container states that there are 10 gtts × per milliliter of solution.

METHOD 1. Substitute directly into the formula:

$$\frac{3000(\text{mL of solution}) \times 10(\text{gtt per milliliter})}{24(\text{hr}) \times 60(\text{min})} = x(\text{gtt per minute})$$

$$\frac{3000 \times 10}{24 \times 60} = \frac{30000}{1440} = 1440\overline{)30000.0} \quad 20.8 \text{ or } 21 \text{ gtts/min}$$

2880
1200 0
1152 0
48 0

✔ *The decimal is usually rounded off to the whole number.* In the above problem rounding off 20.8 tells the health care provider that the rate of flow should be approximately 21 drops per minute.

Either short or long division or cancellation may be used to find x:

$$x = 480\overline{)10000.0} \quad \text{20.8 or 21 gtts/min}$$
960
400 0
384 0
16 0

or

$$\frac{10000}{480} = \frac{125}{6}$$
$$= 20.8 \text{ or } 21 \text{ gtts/min}$$

x = 20.8 or 21 drops per minute rate of flow in order to administer 1 L, or 1000 mL, solution within 8 hours

METHOD 2. A similar approach to the problem may be used to determine the amount of solution to be given in a particular amount of time if it is less than the total time during which the total amount of solution is to be administered. This method is convenient when several units of solution are ordered or when it is necessary to recalculate the rate of flow. This is an alternate method of working the problem. In the previous example, the total time over which the solution was to be administered was 24 hours, which is divided by 3, the number of liters to be administered. This determines the amount of solution that would be administered in three equal time periods, every 8 hours. *A proportion may be used to determine the amount of solution that is to be given and would be established as follows:*

Amount of solution:time in hours = amount of solution:time in hours

EXAMPLE: If 3 L of solution are to be given in 24 hours, how much would be given in 8 hours?

$$3(L):24(hr) = x(L):8(h)$$
$$24x = 24$$
$$x = 1 \text{ L per 8-hour period}$$

Following this, the rate of flow can be determined by substituting into the formula previously given or by establishing a second proportion as follows:

total amount of solution in drops : total time of administration in minutes = amount of solution : 1 minute in drops

✔ *The total amount of solution in drops is found by multiplying the total number of milliliters of solution by the number of drops delivered with the equipment in use. The total time of administration in minutes is determined by multiplying the number of hours by 60, the number of minutes in an hour.*

If 1 L of solution is to run 8 hours and there are 10 drops in each milliliter, the proportion would be as follows:

total solution in drops : total minutes for administration = amount of solution in drops : 1 minute

$$1000(mL) \times 10(gtts/mL) : 8(h) \times 60(min/h) = x(gtts/mL) : 1 (min)$$

equals 10,000 mL of solution   equals total of 480 minutes

$$10,000 \text{ (mL)}:480 \text{ (min)} = x(gtt):1(min)$$
$$480x = 10,000$$
$$x = 10,000 \div 480 \text{ or } \frac{10,000}{480} = 20.8 \text{ gtt/min}$$

EXERCISE 5   (answers on page 318)

For each of the following problems, determine the rate of flow per minute unless the problem specifically asks for another unit of measure:

1. Give 1000 mL in 8 hours. There are 10 drops in each milliliter.

2. Give 1 L in 8 hours. There are 15 drops in each milliliter.

3. Give 1000 mL in 8 hours. There are 20 drops in each milliliter.

4. Give 1500 mL in 8 hours. There are 20 drops in each milliliter.

5. Give 1500 mL in 8 hours. There are 15 drops in each milliliter.

6. Give 1 L in 6 hours. There are 15 drops in each milliliter.

7. If 1 L is to be given in 8 hours, how many milliliters are to be administered per hour?

8. Give 3500 cc in 24 hours. There are 10 drops in each milliliter.

9. Give 1 L in 7 hours. There are 10 drops in each milliliter.

10. Give 500 mL in 3 hours. There are 60 minidrops in each milliliter.

11. Give 1000 mL of IV solution in an hour to test kidney function. There are 10 drops in each milliliter.

12. If 1000 mL are to be given in an hour, how many milliliters are to be given in a minute?

13. Give 3000 cc in 24 hours. There are 10 drops in each milliliter.

14. Give 1000 mL in 12 hours. There are 60 drops in each milliliter.

15. Give 3000 mL in 24 hours. There are 20 drops in each milliliter.

16. Give 2 L in 24 hours. There are 20 drops in each milliliter.

ESTIMATING THE RATE OF FLOW

In addition to calculating the rate of flow, it is helpful to mark the container of solution to determine quickly if the solution is infusing at the correct rate. This is done by placing a strip of tape lengthwise on the container of solution and marking the tape in hourly intervals. The tape should not cover the milliliter markings that are printed on the container. Times are written on the tape to indicate the level at which the solution should be at a stated time (see Fig. 15-1 on p. 217). This does not negate the importance of calculating and regulating the rate of flow. It provides only a rough estimate and may alert the health care provider that recalculation and further regulation of the rate of flow are indicated. (See Fig. 15-2 on p. 217.

When the IV preparation is labeled by the pharmacist to indicate the number of drops per minute that must be infused to administer the solution over a given period of time, this is regarded as a guide only. Many factors may influence the rate of flow and necessitate the recalculation and adjustment of the flow rate. This is a professional responsibility. Factors that alter the rate of flow include position of the needle in the vein, position of the extremity into which the IV needle is inserted, the condition of the vein, administration of medications, and other interruptions in the rate of flow. The latter may occur because of infiltration or obstruction in the tubing or needle.

INCREASING THE RATE OF FLOW BY A SPECIFIED PERCENT

Theoretically, careful calculation and regulation of the rate of flow ensure that the IV solution will be administered over the period that is specified. Realistically, there are many reasons why the rate of flow may be slower than was intended. A major reason for this occurrence is that the IV infusion infiltrates the tissue because the needle is displaced. When this happens, it becomes necessary to recalculate the rate of flow in order to deliver the amount of fluids necessary within a given time. **Caution:** The rate of flow for total parenteral nutrition (TPN) solutions is *always* tapered when increasing or decreasing the rate of flow. It is *never* increased to "catch up" because it must be well-diluted and time must be allowed for the endogenous insulin to control the additional load of glucose supplied by the parenteral nutrition solution.

Increasing the rate of flow is accompanied by hazards. For this reason, some agencies have established policies and guidelines that control the relative rate of increase of flow whenever careful monitoring does not prevent the slowing of the rate of flow. The following guidelines are permitted in some agencies as a method of catching up when the IV solution is flowing at a rate that causes the administration of the prescribed volume to be behind schedule.

First assess the patient carefully for signs of circulatory overload and other contraindications for increasing the rate of flow, such as the addition of selected medications to the IV solution, and the osmolarity of the solution.

✔ *If there are no contraindications and the patient is receiving continuous IV therapy, the infusion rate may be increased as much as 25% of the base rate of flow. The patient is reassessed to determine tolerance to this increased rate of flow. The patient's age and condition and other factors that may affect tolerance to increased fluids must be assessed carefully. On rare occasions, the rate of flow can be increased by another 25% of the base rate. This may require a physician's order.* This rate of flow is continued until the IV solution is on schedule. If these two percentage increases are insufficient to achieve the original schedule, it may be necessary to alter the original schedule for infusion. To do this, collaboration with the physician is required. A medical order prescribing further increases may be written following the physician's assessment of the patient.

EXAMPLE: An IV solution scheduled to flow at a rate of 125 mL/h is behind schedule. Agency policy states that you can, after assessing the patient for any contraindications, increase the flow rate by 25%. If the patient tolerates the new flow rate, another increase of 25% of the base rate may be allowed. The patient must be assessed carefully in making the determination to allow the second increase. At this time, it will probably be necessary to recalculate the rate of flow in order to maintain the desired schedule.

a. By what amount in milliliters can the flow rate be increased initially when a 25% increase is allowed?
   To find **the amount of the first increase, multiply the infusion rate by 25% or ¼.**

   $$\text{Infusion rate} \times 25\% = \text{amount of increase}$$
   $$125 \text{ (mL/h)} \times 25\% = 125 \times 0.25 = 31.25 \text{ or } 31 \text{ (mL/h)}$$
   or
   $$\text{Infusion rate} \times \tfrac{1}{4} = \text{amount of increase}$$
   $$125 \text{ (mL/h)} \times \tfrac{1}{4} \text{ or } 125 \div 4 = 31.25 \text{ or } 31 \text{ (mL/h)}$$

b. What is the total number of milliliters/hour that will be delivered when this increase is put into effect?
   Add the amount of the increase to the original rate of flow to find the new rate of flow.

   Base rate of flow + 25% increase = New rate of flow
   $$125 \text{ (mL/h)} + 31 \text{ (mL/h)} = 156 \text{ mL/h}$$

c. If the drop factor for the tubing used is 10 gtts/mL, how many drops per minute are needed to deliver this amount (156 mL/h) of solution?
   Use the formula:

   $$\frac{\text{mL/h} \times \text{drop factor}}{60 \text{ (min/h)}} = \text{gtts/min}$$
   $$\frac{156 \times 10}{60} = \frac{1560}{60} = 26 \text{ gtts/min}$$

d. Calculate the total number of milliliters/hour if a second increase of 25% is allowed.
   To find this, add the amount of the first increase of 25% (found in a) to the total current rate of flow (found in b).

   Rate of flow with 25% increase + 25%
   = Rate of flow after second increase.
   $$156 \text{ (mL/h)} + 31 \text{ (mL/h)} = 187 \text{ mL/h}$$

   Alternatively, the formula for this step can be stated as:

   Base rate in milliliters/hour + 50% of base rate
   = rate of flow after second increase of 25%.
   $$125 \text{ (mL/h or base rate)} + 62.5 \text{ (50\% of base rate)}$$
   $$= 187.5 \text{ or } 188 \text{ mL/h}$$

e. Calculate the number of drops per minute needed to deliver this rate of flow if the approximate drop factor is 10 drops/minute.
   Use the same formula that was applied in part c of this example.

   $$\frac{\text{milliliters/hour} \times \text{drop factor}}{(60 \text{ min/h})} = \text{gtts/min}$$
   $$\frac{188 \times 10}{60} = \frac{1880}{60} = 31.3 \text{ or } 31 \text{ drops per minute}$$

EXERCISE 6 *(answers on page 319)*

Work each of the following problems in which the rate of flow of IV solution is less than desired, and agency policy allows a 25% increase of the base rate to occur twice if there are no contraindications. For each problem, state the following answers:

    a. Amount in milliliters per hour by which flow rate can be increased each hour initially if a 25% increase is allowed.
    b. Total number of milliliters that will be delivered each hour when the initial increase of 25% is put into effect.
    c. Number of drops per minute of IV solution that delivers the amount of solution after the initial increase is in effect.
    d. Total number of milliliters that may be given hourly if a second increase of 25% is to be put into effect.
    e. Number of drops per minute needed to deliver solution after second increase of 25% is to be put into effect.

1. The IV solution was originally scheduled to flow at a rate of 60 mL/h. There are 60 drops in each milliliter.
   a.
   b.
   c.
   d.
   e.

2. The IV solution was originally scheduled to flow at a rate of 50 mL/h. There are 60 drops in each milliliter.
   a.
   b.
   c.
   d.
   e.

3. The IV solution was originally scheduled to flow at a rate of 100 mL/h. There are 15 drops in each milliliter.
   a.
   b.
   c.
   d.
   e.

4. The IV solution was originally scheduled to flow at a rate of 200 mL/h. There are 10 drops in each cubic centimeter.
   a.
   b.
   c.
   d.
   e.

5. The IV solution was originally scheduled to flow at a rate of 3 L in 24 hours. There are 10 drops in each milliliter.
   a.
   b.
   c.
   d.
   e.

6. The IV solution was originally scheduled to flow at a rate of 1 L in 8 hours. There are 60 drops in each milliliter.
   a.
   b.
   c.
   d.
   e.

7. The IV solution was originally scheduled to flow at a rate of 2 L in 24 hours. There are 15 drops in each milliliter.
   a.   d.
   b.   e.
   c.

8. The IV solution was originally scheduled to flow at a rate of 150 mL/h. There are 10 drops in each milliliter.
   a.   d.
   b.   e.
   c.

9. The IV solution was originally scheduled to flow at a rate of 75 mL/h. There are 60 drops in each milliliter.
   a.   d.
   b.   e.
   c.

KEEP OPEN RATE OF FLOW

The physician may order a flow rate for IV solution that is called *keep open*. This may be written in the order as *KO* (keep open), *TKO* (to keep open), or *KVO* (keep vein open). For this, the solution is given very slowly. The principle is to run the solution fast enough to keep the vein open. Rate of flow is more easily controlled if a minidrip tubing that supplies 60 gtts/mL is used. Agency policies regarding the rate of flow and use of minidrippers for keep open rate vary. The following may be used as a general guide if not contraindicated by agency policy. If tubing with a drop rate factor of 10, 12, or 15 drops per minute is used, the keep open rate may be as much as 25 mL/h, or 4 drops a minute, or 1 drop every 15 seconds for tubing with a drop rate factor of 10. Thus to give 25 mL/h using tubing with a macrodropper that has a drop factor of 10, the equation would be:

$$\frac{mL/h \times gtt\ factor}{60\ (min/h)} = gtts/minute$$

$$\frac{25 \times 10}{60} = \frac{250}{60} = 4\ drops/minute$$

60 seconds/minute ÷ 4 (drops per minute) = 1 drop every 15 seconds

If the order reads to administer 8 mL/h to keep the vein open, substitution into the above formula would be:

$$\frac{mL/h \times minidrops/minute}{60\ min/h} = minidrops/minute$$

$$\frac{8\ mL \times 60\ minidrops/minute}{60\ min/h} = \frac{480}{60} = 8\ drops/minute$$

using a *minidropper* with a factor of 60

Thus for a keep open rate of 8 mL/h, the minidrop factor would be 8 minidrops per minute.

INTRAVENOUS MEDICATIONS

Medications may be added directly to the primary container of solution by the manufacturer, the pharmacist, or the health care provider. Fig. 15-5 illustrates the addition of medications to the primary solution. When added by the manufacturer, the name and amount of medication will be indicated on the label. If added by the pharmacist or health care provider, a label indicating this informa-

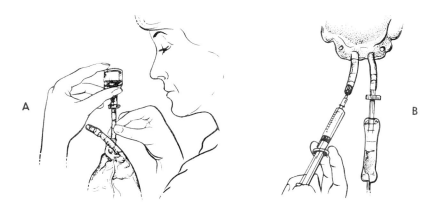

Fig. 15-5. Adding medication to IV solution. **A,** The spike of a vial is inserted into the port of an IV bag. **B,** Injection of medication into the IV solution using a syringe.

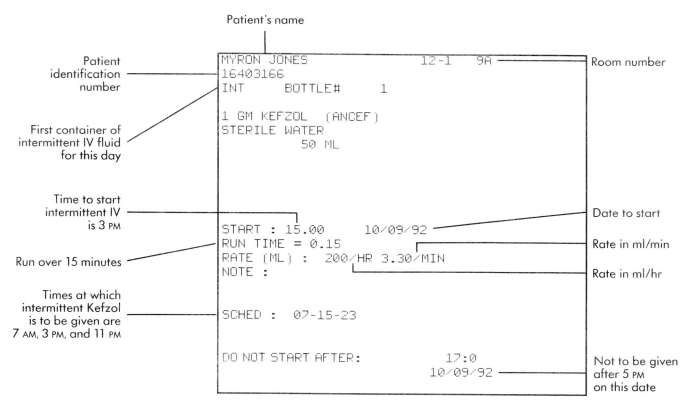

Fig. 15-6. Example of a computerized label. The amount and kind of information will vary by institution.
(Copyright Mayo Foundation for Medical Education and Research. Used with permission.)

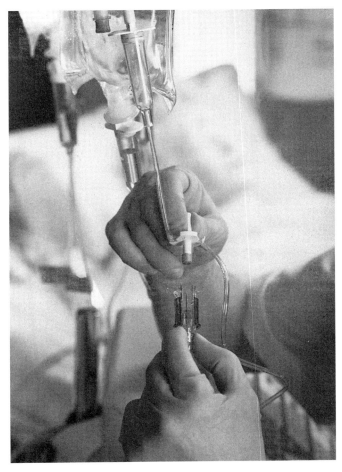

Fig. 15-7. Lifeshield Connector and Docking Station. This is an example of a connector developed to prevent needle sticks.
(Courtesy Abbott Laboratories, Abbott Park, Ill.)

tion must be applied to the container of solution. Fig. 15-6 on p. 232 illustrates an example of a computerized label that is applied to an intermittent solution of IV medication.

Medications can also be given by adding a secondary container of solution containing the medication. This is attached to the primary solution by connecting it to a special port on the tubing that is attached to the primary container of solution (Fig. 15-7). This is described as a piggyback, or intermittent method of administering the solution (Fig. 15-8). Sometimes the secondary container is referred to as a *rider* or *IVPB* (intravenous piggyback).

Compatibility of medications with each other and intravenous solutions

It is essential to know whether medications that are to be added to an IV solution are compatible with each other and with the solution. Some drugs are compatible with many solutions while others may be compatible with only a few solutions. As

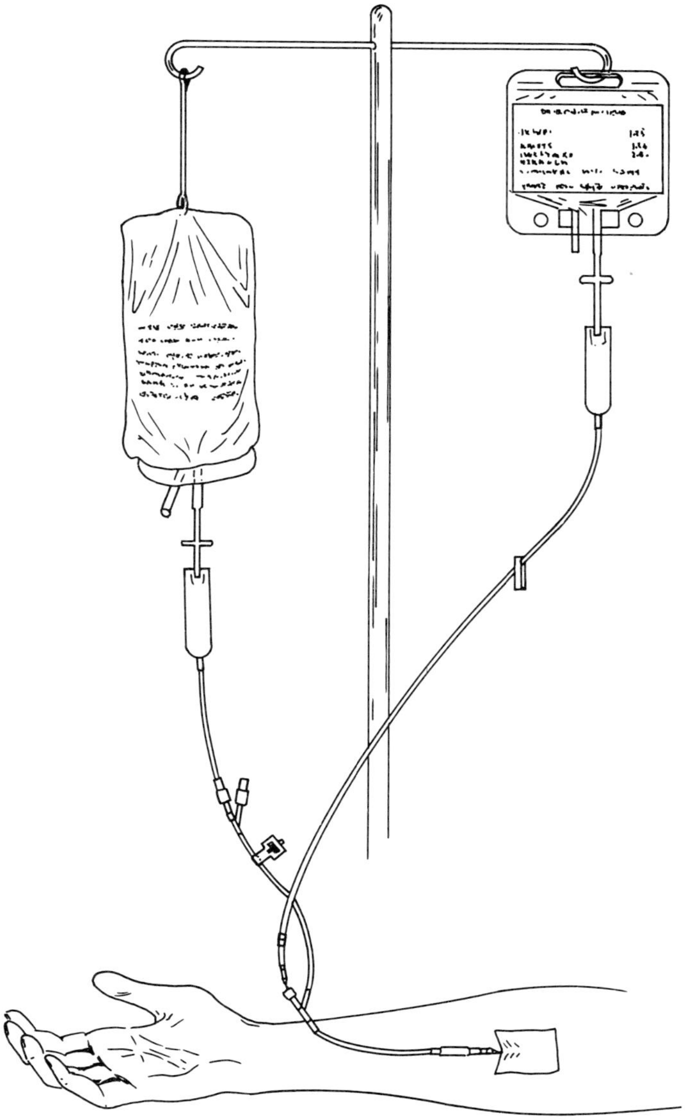

Fig. 15-8. IV piggyback (IVPB) administration setup. Note that the smaller bottle is hung higher than the primary bottle.

a guide, drugs that differ greatly in pH will be incompatible. If mixed, drugs that are incompatible with each other, or with an IV solution, will react, producing a solution that is unsafe for administration. The changes that occur when incompatibles are mixed may be visible in the form of color change or precipitation. *However, incompatibility can occur without any visible changes in the mixture. Whenever information on compatibility is unavailable, the health professional should assume that the medications and solutions are incompatible.*

It is necessary to know whether drugs are compatible with each other and with the IV solution being administered. Incompatible drugs must not be given simultaneously because this may inactivate one or both of the drugs so that the patient receives no benefit from either drug. Adverse reactions, including life-threatening ones such as anaphylaxis and infarctions, can occur following the administration of incompatible drugs or solutions. Drugs that are incompatible with each other or with an IV solution can be given if the heparin lock or IV tubing is flushed with normal saline between doses. A new or separate piece of tubing is used for each medication given intermittently. Note that when more than one medication is given in a volume control device, the medications must be compatible with each other.

> ### ✚ THINK CRITICALLY
> Is this medication suitable for IV administration?
> Is it compatible with the IV solution?
> Is it compatible with other drugs administered at the same time?
> Is it the correct dose?
> Is it compatible with other solutions that are in the IV line?
> Is its tonicity appropriate for the patient's condition?
> Is the rate reasonable for the dose?

Intermittent administration of medications

Containers of solution for intermittent administration of IV drugs contain relatively small amounts of solution. Common amounts are 50, 100, and 250 mL of solution. The intermittent solution may be given very rapidly. Often 50 to 100 mL of solution is given over a period of 15 minutes to an hour. The rate is influenced by the nature of the drug and the volume of solution. *When fluid balance is critical or large volumes of intermittent doses of drugs are given intravenously, the total amount of solution that is to be given is considered when calculating the rate of flow.* Thus, if the physician specifies that the patient is to receive 1000 mL of fluid intravenously over an 8-hour period of time, the amount of the secondary fluid containing the medications is subtracted from the total of 1000 mL of solution before calculating the rate of flow for the primary solution.

EXAMPLE: The physician orders 50 mL of cefazolin (Ancef) to be given at 8 AM, 100 mL of ranitidine (Zantac) to be given at 12 noon, and another 50 mL of cefazolin to be given at 4 PM. The order also specifies that the patient is to be given a total of 1000 mL of 5% dextrose in water solution over 8 hours. The volume of solution containing the drugs is 200 mL (50 mL of cefazolin + 100 mL of ranitidine + 50 mL cefazolin = 200 mL of solution). This amount would be subtracted from 1000 mL, the total amount of solution to be given over 8 hours. 1000 mL − 200 mL = 800 mL or the amount of 5% dextrose in water that is to be administered over the 8 hours in addition to cefazolin and ranitidine. The flow rate would then be calculated for 800 mL that is to be given over an 8-hour period of time. Thus the patient would receive 100 mL/h in addition to the medications.

When the physician specifies a total amount of solution to be given within a certain period, such as 24 hours, and writes orders for additional amounts of solution containing medications, the health professional should calculate the total for the amount of solution ordered for a stated period of time before calculating the rate of flow. If the total amount obtained exceeds the total amount of solution ordered for that period of time, calculations are necessary to ensure that the patient receives only the prescribed amount of IV fluid, including piggybacked medications. For example, if 3 L of IV solutions were ordered for 24 hours and 4 piggyback containers of 100 mL each were added, the total amount would be 3400 mL, not 3000 mL. The health professional would subtract the 4 piggyback solutions, or 400 mL, from the 3000, obtaining a total of 2600 mL. The total, 2600 mL, is the amount of the IV solution that is to be administered in addition to the piggyback medications.

Volume control chambers

Another method of controlling the amount of solution administered is to attach a special volume control chamber in the tubing (Fig. 15-9). When used, the rate of flow is calculated for the amount of solution in the volume control chamber. If medication is being given using a volume control chamber, a label stating the type and amount of drug should be attached to the chamber.

All medications given using volume control chambers **must** be compatible with each other. It is nearly impossible to flush all medications from an in-line device.

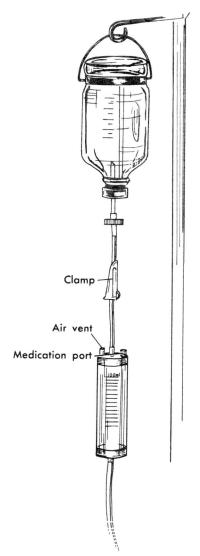

Fig. 15-9. Volume control chamber. The volume control chamber is located between the container of IV fluid and the IV line for the administration of small amounts of solution or medication. Clamp above the chamber controls the flow of IV solution into the chamber. Medication may be injected through the medication port after it is cleansed with a suitable antiseptic.

(Courtesy Travenol Laboratories, Inc., Deerfield, Ill.)

Heparin lock

A heparin lock may be used when access to a vein is needed for intermittent administration of medications or fluids (Fig. 15-10). IV medications may be given using the heparin lock by the IV push method or by the drip method. Before giving a medication, the health care provider must know of any special precautions that must be followed. For example, some medications must be given at a specified rate. Observation for symptoms of adverse reactions is imperative when IV drugs are being administered.

The heparin lock is attached to the indwelling IV needle and flushed periodically to prevent clotting. Because the frequency for flushing heparin locks and the solution used may vary, it is important to know the agency's policies.

Saline flush. Flushing with saline has largely replaced the so-called *heparin flush.* For this, 2.5 mL to 5 mL of sterile normal saline is injected into the heparin lock.

Heparin flush. Although it has largely been replaced by the saline flush, heparin continues to be used in some agencies. Instilling 1 mL of solution containing 10 U of heparin into a peripheral site is called *heparinization.* More solution is required for central lines.

Heparin is incompatible with many medications and must not be allowed to come into contact with incompatible medications. The lock must be flushed with a heparin-compatible solution, usually sterile normal saline, before and after an incompatible drug is administered. The amount of saline used to flush a heparin lock is usually 2½ mL. The letters "**SISH**," which represent Saline, Intravenous medication, Saline, Heparin may be helpful for remembering this. To reduce the amount of heparin needed, it is recommended that the auxiliary port that is nearest to the needle site on the main tubing be used for infusing medication.

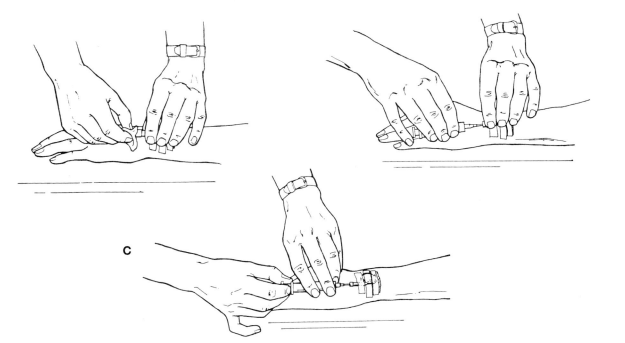

Fig. 15-10. Heparin lock for injection of drug. **A,** Injection site is cleansed. **B,** A syringe containing prescribed drug is inserted into the heparin lock. **C,** Following gentle aspiration, the drug is injected slowly. Heparin is usually injected at a rate of no more than 1 mL per minute.

Flushing intravenous lines

Usually, separate or new tubing is used for incompatible solutions or medications. However, if an IV line requires flushing, approximately 3 times the amount of fluid that the tubing will hold is necessary to clear the line of incompatible solution. Because the volume held varies with the brand of tubing, this must be determined by measuring the amount of liquid needed to fill 1 foot of tubing. The length of the tubing is multiplied by this amount and by a factor of 3 (times the amount of fluid held by the tubing).

DETERMINING FLOW RATE FOR ADMINISTERING SPECIFIC AMOUNT OF DRUG IN A SPECIFIED AMOUNT OF TIME

Prescribed medications are added to many IV solutions. The physician's order may specify that a specific amount of a drug be added to a certain amount of solution that is to be administered over a given period. This controls the amount of drug that is administered so that it is infused at a regular rate. Another method of prescribing IV drug therapy is to state that a particular dose of medication is to be placed in a specific amount of solution, and that the solution is to be administered at a rate that delivers a fractional amount of the total drug dosage to the patient within a particular time. For example, the order may state that 40 milliequivalents (mEq) of potassium chloride is to be added to 1000 mL of IV solution and that it is to be administered at a rate that will deliver 4 mEq of potassium chloride to the patient during each 1-hour period. It is necessary to calculate the rate of flow of the solution needed to deliver the prescribed amount of drug over the time span ordered.

EXAMPLE A: Give 4 mEq of potassium chloride each hour using 1000 mL of solution that contains 40 mEq of potassium chloride. *A proportion may be established as follows:*

$$\frac{\text{total amount}}{\text{of drug}} : \frac{\text{total volume}}{\text{of solution}} = \frac{\text{prescribed}}{\text{dose of drug}} : \frac{\text{needed volume}}{\text{of solution}}$$

Substituting into the proportion would be as follows:

40 (mEq):1000 (mL) = 4 (mEq):x (mL)

$40x = 1000 \times 4$
$40x = 4000$

$x = 100$ mL of solution needed to give 4 mEq of potassium chloride

Determination of the rate of flow can be done by substituting into the formula given earlier in this chapter. Thus, if 100 mL of solution containing 10 drops per milliliter is to be delivered over a 1-hour (or 60-minute) period, the problem would be worked as follows:

$$\frac{100 \text{ (mL)} \times 10 \text{ (gtt)}}{1 \text{ (h)} \times 60 \text{ (min)}} = \frac{1000}{60} = \begin{array}{l} 16.6 \text{ or } 17 \text{ gtt/min} \\ \text{would deliver 4 mEq of} \\ \text{potassium chloride each} \\ \text{hour from this solution} \end{array}$$

If the solution is to be administered over a period less than 1 hour, the problem may be solved by substituting into the following formula:

$$\frac{\text{total number of drops (mL} \times \text{gtt)}}{\text{total number of minutes}} = \text{drops/minute}$$

EXAMPLE B: Give 40 mL of solution over 10 minutes. Each milliliter of solution contains 15 drops.

$$\frac{40 \text{ (mL)} \times 15 \text{ (gtt)}}{10 \text{ (min)}} = \frac{600 \text{ (gtt)}}{10 \text{ (min)}} = 60 \text{ gtt/min}$$

DETERMINING THE AMOUNT OF DRUG THAT HAS BEEN ADMINISTERED IN A PARTICULAR AMOUNT OF SOLUTION

A similar calculation is necessary whenever the amount of drug that has been delivered intravenously in a particular amount of solution requires documentation. This commonly occurs at the end of a 24-hour shift and when infusions are interrupted or discontinued. Such problems can be solved using the proportion method.

The proportion method can be used to determine the amount of drug that has been administered in a specified amount of solution.

EXAMPLE: An IV solution is discontinued after the patient receives approximately 500 mL of the original volume of 1000 mL of solution that contained 80 mEq of potassium chloride. How much potassium chloride did the patient actually receive?

$$80 \text{ (mEq)}:1000 \text{ (mL)} = x \text{ (mEq)}:500 \text{ (mL)}$$
$$1000x = 80 \times 500$$
$$1000x = 40{,}000$$
$$x = \frac{40{,}000}{1000} = 40 \text{ mEq of potassium chloride was received by the patient}$$

EXERCISE 7 (answers on page 319)

1. The IV solution contains 40 mEq of potassium chloride in 1000 mL of solution. How much potassium chloride will have been given when 600 mL of solution has been infused?

2. A 50 mL bag of IV solution contains 1.5 million U of ampicillin. How many million units of the drug will have been given when 25 mL of solution has been infused?

3. A 50 mL bag of solution contains 1.5 million U of ampicillin and is to be infused over 20 minutes. (a) What should the rate of flow per minute be if each milliliter contains 15 gtt of solution? (b) When the IV solution has infused at the correct rate for 12 minutes, how much ampicillin will the patient have received?

4. An IV solution contains 80 mEq of potassium chloride in 1 L of solution. (a) How much potassium chloride will the patient have received when 800 mL of solution remains to be given. (b) How much potassium chloride remains to be given?

16

Heparin Dosage and Administration

HEPARIN ADMINISTRATION

Administration of heparin may be ordered either intravenously or subcutaneously. Heparin is prescribed for the prevention of clot formation. It does not dissolve clots. Low doses may be given subcutaneously to prevent the formation of thrombi in those at risk, such as patients undergoing thoracic or abdominal surgery. A common dose for this purpose is 5000 U every 8 to 12 hours until the patient is ambulatory. However, the dose may range between 8000 and 10,000 U every 8 hours or 15,000 to 20,000 U every 12 hours. When ordered subcutaneously, the dose is injected into the deep subcutaneous (intrafat) tissues of the abdomen or above the iliac crest. Injection into muscle should be avoided because it is likely to cause a hematoma. The amount of heparin solution injected subcutaneously should not exceed 1 mL. Extremely low doses (10 U/mL) are also prescribed to maintain the patency of an indwelling needle when a heparin lock is in place. Instillation of heparin into the heparin lock is sometimes referred to as a *heparin flush*. Because it is used to administer medications other than heparin and IV fluids, information on the heparin lock is found in Chapter 15, Intravenous Fluids and Medications. When large doses of heparin are prescribed, either continuous or intermittent IV infusion is used. Because intermittent infusion provides large doses of heparin over a relatively short period of time, the risk of bleeding is greater than when heparin is given more slowly. Therefore many physicians prefer to prescribe a continuous infusion of heparin. IV infusion also eliminates the need for frequent injections. Intermittent infusion usually begins with an initial IV dose of 10,000 U in 50 to 100 mL of isotonic solution followed by an infusion of 5000 to 10,000 U in 100 mL of isotonic solution every 4 to 6 hours. Continuous infusion is often begun with 5000 U in 50 to 100 mL of isotonic solution followed by 20,000 to 40,000 U of heparin in 1000 mL of isotonic sodium chloride each day. Sometimes units per hour are prescribed. The previously given dosage ranges are intended as guides only and are based on recommended doses for most people who weigh approximately 68 kg.

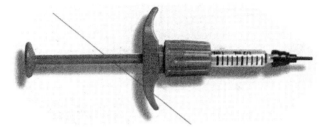

Fig. 16-1. A 1 mL prefilled needleless Tubex cartridge. Each calibration represents a tenth of a millimeter. The cartridge has been placed in a special holder provided by the manufacturer. The unit is designed as a closed system and prevents needlesticks.

(Courtesy of Wyeth-Ayerst Laboratories, Philadelphia).

Agency policies may state which health professionals may add heparin to IV solutions. Often heparin is added to the IV solution in the pharmacy. The person adding or administering heparin must read the labels very carefully. Different sizes and strengths of heparin are available and are often stored in the same location. Different strengths of heparin include:

10 units/mL	5000 units/mL
100 units/mL	10,000 units/mL
1000 units/mL	

The amount of heparin solution in a syringe or vial also varies. Vials may contain 1, 4, 10, or 30 mL. Heparin is also available in a variety of strengths in prefilled syringes and cartridges. Because heparin prevents coagulation of the blood, the importance of providing the correct amount of drug to the patient must be emphasized.

In an effort to standardize the strength of heparin solution used and lessen chances for error in the dosage of heparin, some institutions have policies requiring that the same strength of heparin solutions be used for all doses other than heparin flushes. Even if such a policy is in effect, careful reading of the label remains important.

Measurement of heparin

Prefilled syringes of heparin solutions are often used. These may be calibrated in tenths of a milliliter (Fig. 16-1). When using vials, small amounts of heparin solution, (1 mL or less of solution) may be measured using a tuberculin syringe. A regular syringe may be used to measure larger doses. Although calibrated in units, insulin syringes must *never* be used to measure heparin doses.

CALCULATIONS FOR INTRAVENOUS ADMINISTRATION OF HEPARIN

When adding a large number of units of heparin to an IV solution, it is useful to know how many units are contained in a particular vial of heparin.

To find the number of units of heparin in a vial, multiply the number of milliliters in the vial by the number of units in each milliliter:

mL/vial × U/mL = total units/vial

EXAMPLE: How many units of heparin are in a 4 mL vial of heparin that contains 10,000 U/mL?

mL/vial × U/mL = total units/vial
4 × 10,000 = 40,000 units in the vial

If the number of units in a vial of solution and the number of milliliters of solution in the vial are known, the number of units in a milliliter of solution can be calculated.

To find the number of units in 1 mL of solution, divided the total number of units in the vial by the number of milliliters of solution.

Sometimes the physician's order will specify administration of a certain number of units of heparin each hour. If the number of units of heparin in each milliliter of solution is known, the number of milliliters of solution needed to give the prescribed dose can be determined.

To calculate the number of milliliters to be administered in 1 hour in order to give a specific number of units, establish a proportion with the known facts (also referred to as labeling information or strength of the solution) as one ratio and the orders (prescribed or desired dose) as the other ratio. In abbreviated form, the formula is:

$$\text{Labeling information} = \text{Prescribed dose}$$
$$(\text{Known}) \quad\quad\quad (\text{Desired})$$

EXAMPLE: Give 1200 U each hour. How many milliliters are needed to give this number of units each hour if there are 40 U of heparin in each milliliter of solution?

$$\text{Labeling information} = \text{Prescribed dose}$$
$$(\text{Known}) \quad\quad\quad (\text{Desired})$$

Units:milliliters = units:milliliters
40:1 = 1200:x

$$40x = 1200$$
$$x = 1200 \div 40$$
$$x = 30 \text{ mL of solution is needed to give}$$
1200 units of heparin each hour

It is helpful to know whether the dose is within the usual dosage range. If the dose falls outside the usual dosage range, an instructor, supervisor, or the physician should be consulted. Remember the usual range of dosage for heparin is 20,000 to 40,000 U per day.

To find whether the dose is within the normal range, multiply the number of milliliters of solution that is given each hour by the number of units of drug in each milliliter of solution times 24 hours. This equation may be stated as:

$$\text{mL/h} \times \text{U/mL} \times 24\text{h} = \text{24-hour dose}$$

EXAMPLE: The patient is receiving 30 mL of heparin each hour. There are 40 U of heparin in each milliliter of solution. How many units will the patient receive in 24 hours? Is this within the usual range of dosage?

$$\text{mL/h} \times \text{U/mL} \times 24\text{h} = \text{24-hour dose}$$
$$30 \times 40 \times 24 = 28{,}800 \text{ units (dosage being given in 24 hours)}$$

This is within the normal range of 20,000 to 40,000 units/day.

When institutional policy requires use of the same strength of heparin solutions, a solution of 40 U per milliliter is commonly used. Thus 1000 mL of solution would contain 40,000 U of heparin, the upper limit of the normal daily dosage range.

> ### ✚ THINK CRITICALLY
> Is the dose within the normal range for heparin dosage?
> Is the dose appropriate to the purpose for giving the heparin and appropriate for the patient's condition?
> Is the strength of the heparin solution appropriate to the physician's order?
> Is the dose to be given as a flush, deep subcutaneous (intrafat) injection, or an intermittent or continuous IV infusion?
>   If flush, what precautions must be followed?
>   If deep subcutaneous (intrafat), what site is to be used?
>   If IV, is it to be given intermittently, continuously, or IV flush?
>   If IV, is the amount and kind of diluent specified?
>   If IV, over what period of time is the dose to be given?
>   If IV, is a separate site needed because of incompatibility with other drugs and solutions?

EXERCISE 1
(answers on page 320)

1. How many units of heparin are contained in a 10 mL vial if the solution contains 1000 U/mL?

2. If there are 10,000 U/mL of solution, how many units of heparin are there in a 4 mL vial?

3. How many units of heparin are contained in a 30 mL vial if there are 1000 U/mL?

4. If there are 100 U/mL **(a)** how many units are there in a 10 mL vial? **(b)** in a 30 mL vial?

5. Mrs. Kallatty, age 65, is scheduled for abdominal surgery. The physician orders 5000 U heparin SC to be given q12h to prevent thrombi from forming.
   (a) If the following amounts are available in multiple dose vials, which is appropriate?
   10 U/mL (10 mL and 50 vials)   5000 U/mL (1 and 10 mL vials)
   100 U/mL (2, 10, 30 mL vials)   10,000 U/mL (1, 4, and 10 mL vials)
   1000 U/mL (10 and 30 mL vials)

   (b) Which of the following prefilled cartridges would provide this exact dose?
   10 U/mL   1000 U/mL   7500 U/mL
   25 U/2.5 mL   2500 U/0.5 mL   10,000 U/mL
   100 U/mL   5000 U/0.5 mL   20,000 U/mL
   250 U/2.5 mL   5000 U/mL

6. 5000 U of heparin are to be given using a tuberculin syringe. Mark the syringes to show how much solution is needed if the multiple dose vial contains:
   (a) 5000 U/0.5 mL

   (b) 5000 U/mL

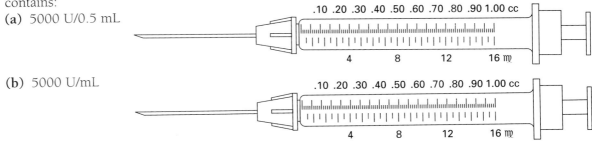

7. If the only solution available contained 10,000 U of heparin/mL, how much would be needed for a dose of 5000 U?

8. An order given for SC heparin is for 2500 U. Which strength of solution available in prefilled cartridges would be appropriate and why?

10 U/mL	1000 U/mL	5000 U/0.5 mL	7500 U/mL
25 U/mL	2500 U/mL	5000 U/mL	10,000 U/mL

9. If there are 40,000 U of heparin in 1 L of solution, how many units of heparin are there in each milliliter of the IV solution?

10. If the order is to run a solution at the rate of 1000 U/h, how many milliliters of solution containing 40,000 U/L will deliver this dose?

11. If there are 40,000 U/L, how many milliliters of solution are needed to deliver 1200 U/h?

12. 500 mL solution is being administered intravenously. The medication label on the container indicates that 40,000 U of heparin have been added to the solution. The physician's order is to administer 1100 U of heparin per hour.
    (a) How many units of heparin are contained in each milliliter of solution?
    (b) At what rate in milliliters per hour should the solution be delivered?
    (c) If the current flow rate is 14 mL/h, is the above dosage within the normal range?

13. If the physician orders 900 U of heparin to be given each hour, and 500 mL of solution contains 10,000 U, (a) what should the hourly flow rate be? (b) Is it within the normal range?

14. A solution for IV administration that contains 10 U/mL is required. If the heparin preparation available contains 5000 U/mL, how much heparin will be added to 1000 mL of solution?

15. If 100 U/mL of heparin is needed, how much heparin preparation containing 5000 U/mL would be added to 1000 mL of IV solution?

17

Critical Care Dosages

Drugs that are used in critical care may be ordered in micrograms/kilogram/hour or micrograms/kilogram/minute. Micrograms may be abbreviated as mcg or µg. In some institutions the drug will be prepared by the pharmacist. At times, qualified health care professionals are responsible for preparing solutions of the drugs just before administration. The health care professional is expected to prepare such solutions of drugs in emergency situations.

Drugs that are ordered by micrograms/kilograms/minute may need frequent titration because of the patient's rapid physiologic responses. Titration refers to the adjustment of the dose of a drug based on the physiologic responses of the patient to that drug. Accurate calculations are critical. Computer programs are available for calculating doses for individual patients requiring critical care. The accuracy of a computer-calculated dose depends upon the accuracy of the information that is put into the computer. If a computer is not available or is disabled, the health care provider, physician, or another qualified person calculates the dose. The person doing the calculations and/or administering the drug should always recheck the calculations. Always think through the entire process and decide whether the amount represents a reasonable dose. This helps to prevent errors. It is important to have another qualified person recheck the calculations. Knowing the usual range for doses of the prescribed medication is very helpful. This information can be found in a variety of drug references including drug formularies, the *Physician's Desk Reference,* and package inserts. The pharmacist may be consulted for this information also.

Before doing any calculations, read the order carefully. Determine whether the order is for micrograms or milligrams of drug. Milligram is abbreviated *mg.* Microgram is abbreviated as either *mcg* or *µg.* Careful reading will prevent misinterpretation of the abbreviations *mg* and *mcg.* Some prefer to use the abbreviation *µg,* which is less easily confused with the abbreviation for milligram. It is also necessary to know whether the rate of flow of the IV solution will be regulated manually or if an IV pump is to be used in order to infuse the correct amount of the drug. The agency policy may name specific drugs for which use of an IV pump is mandatory.

Mastery of the following calculations is necessary to compute micrograms/kilogram/hour and micrograms/kilogram/minute:

1. How to find the number of milligrams per milliliter
2. How to change milligrams/milliliter to micrograms/milliliter
3. How to convert weight in pounds to kilograms
4. How to convert micrograms/kilograms/minute to micrograms/kilograms/hour
5. How to find the number of milliliters of solution per hour needed for the prescribed dose
6. How to change milliliters/minute to milliliters/hour

EXAMPLE: The physician prescribes 2 mcg/kg/min of sodium nitroprusside intravenously to maintain the blood pressure between 100/60 and 130/85. The patient weighs 189.2 lb.

Step 1. Before beginning any calculations, determine if the prescribed dose is within the usual dosage range for this medication. Check the hospital formulary, *Physician's Desk Reference,* or the package insert to find that the usual dosage range for sodium nitroprusside is 0.5 to 10 mcg/kg/min.

Is the prescribed dose of 2 mcg/kg/min within the recommended dosage range?

Yes, 2 falls between 0.5 and 10.

Step 2. How many milligrams are there in each milliliter of this IV solution? The label states that there are 50 mg of sodium nitroprusside in 250 mL of IV solution. To find the milligrams in 1 mL of solution establish a proportion using the labeling information as one of the ratios and unknown (x) mg/1 mL as the other ratio.

Rule: mg:mL = x mg:1 mL

Labeling information   Unknown number of mg/mL
Milligrams:milliliters = x milligrams:1 milliliter

$50:250 = x:1$ $x = 50 \div 250$
$250x = 50$ $x = 0.2$ mg sodium nitroprusside in 1 milliliter of IV solution

Step 3. Find the number of micrograms in each milliliter of sodium nitroprusside. To do this multiply the number of milligrams/milliliter by 1000. This gives the number of micrograms/milliliter.

Rule: mg/mL × 1000 = mcg/mL

The previous calculation shows that there are 0.2 mg of sodium nitroprusside in each milliliter of solution.

mg/mL × 1000 = mcg/mL
0.2 × 1000 = 200.0 or 200 mcg/mL

Step 4. Find the patient's weight in kilograms. The patient weighs 189.2 lb. To find this patient's weight in kilograms divide the number of pounds by 2.2.

Rule: Pounds ÷ 2.2 = kg

$189.2 \div 2.2$ or $2.2\overline{)189.0}^{\,86} = 86$ kg

Step 5. Find how many micrograms/kilogram/minute of sodium nitroprusside are to be given. The physician prescribed 2 mcg/kg/min. Multiply the weight of the patient in kilograms by the prescribed number of micrograms/kilograms/minute to find the number of micrograms/minute of drug.

Rule: kilograms × mcg/kg/min = mcg/min

86 (kilograms) × 2 (mcg/kg/min prescribed) = 172 mcg/min

Step 6. Find the number of milliliters of solution per minute needed to deliver 172 mcg of drug each minute. Set up a proportion using the number of micrograms of drug in 1 mL of solution as one ratio and the prescribed dose in micrograms/kilograms/minute in x mL as the other ratio. You know from *Step 3* that there are 200 mcg of drug in each milliliter of solution. You also know that the amount ordered (see *Step 5*) is 172 mcg/min.

Available solution   Prescribed dose
$$\text{mcg:1 (mL)} = \text{mcg/kg/min}: x \text{ (mL)}$$
$$200:1 = 172:x$$
$$200x = 172$$
$$x = 172 \div 200$$
$$x = 0.86 \text{ mL/min (needed to deliver the prescribed dose).}$$

```
      0.86
200)172.00
    160 0
     12 00
     12 00
```

Step 7. Determine the number of mL/h that will deliver the desired dose. This is necessary if an IV pump calibrated for milliliters/hour is being used to infuse the solution. To change the milliliters/minute to milliliters/hour, multiply by 60 minutes in 1 hour.

Rule: mL/h = mL/min × 60

In *Step 6*, we found that 0.86 mL/min was needed to provide the prescribed dose. Substitute into the formula:

$$\text{mL/h} = 0.86 \times 60 = 51.6 \text{ or } 52 \text{ mL/h}$$

✚ THINK CRITICALLY
Is the order for micrograms or milligrams?
Is the calculation to be in milliliters/minute or milliliters/hour?

✚ THINK CRITICALLY
Is the prescribed amount within the usual dosage range for this drug?
How many milligrams of drug are in each milliliter of solution?
How many micrograms of drug are in each milliliter of solution?
What is the patient's weight in kilograms?
How many micrograms/kilograms/minute were prescribed?
How many milliliters/minute will deliver the prescribed dose?
How many milliliters/hour will deliver the prescribed dose when an IV pump is used?

EXERCISE 1   *(answers on page 320)*

The usual dosage range for sodium nitroprusside is 0.5 to 0.1 mg/kg/min. The order reads to give 3 mcg/kg/min of sodium nitroprusside intravenously to maintain the blood pressure between 100/60 and 120/80 mm Hg. The available solution contains 50 mg of drug in 250 mL of D$_5$W.

(a) How many milligrams of sodium nitroprusside are contained in each milliliter of solution?
(b) How many micrograms of drug are contained in each milliliter of solution?
(c) How many milliliters per hour will deliver 3 mcg/kg/min if the patient weighs 149.6 lb?

```
| mcg × kg = mcg/min       |  mcg/h
|--------------------------|  ------ = mL/h
| mcg/min × 60 min = mcg/h | mcg/mL
```

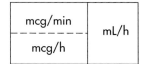

Fig. 17-1. Derivation of the cell contents. To find mcg/min, multiply mcg × kg. To find mcg/h, multiply mcg/min × 60 minutes. To find mL/h, divide mcg/h by mcg/mL.

Fig. 17-2. Contents of individual cells.

	Weight in Kilograms				
mcg/min	54	56	58	60	
0.5	27 / 1620	8.1			
1		56 / 3360	16.8		
2			116 / 6960	34.8	
3				180 / 10,800	54

Fig. 17-3. Sodium nitroprusside (Nipride) 100 mg in 500 mL D$_5$W (Concentration: 1 mL = 200 mcg).

A table such as the one that is shown in Fig. 17-3 may be constructed by personnel working in critical care units. The table is useful because rapid changes in the patient's condition require repeated calculations. Once a table is completed, it allows the health care provider to respond quickly to changes in the patient's condition. The table given as an example is for sodium nitroprusside (Nipride). Variations of this table can be constructed for drugs that are ordered by microgram/kilogram/minute. Construction of the cells is illustrated in Fig. 17-1 and 17-2. Fig. 17-1 shows the calculations done to complete the first cell of Fig. 17-3 (Exercise 2, problem 1).

EXAMPLE: Construct the cell found in the upper left hand corner of Fig. 17-3 using the information provided.

Step 1. mcg × kg = mcg/min
0.5 × 54 = 27

Step 2. mcg/min × 60 = mcg/h
27 × 60 = 1620

Step 3. mcg/h ÷ mcg/mL = mL/h
1620 ÷ 200 = 8.1 mL/h

EXERCISE 2 *(answers on page 320)*

1. Complete the cells in Fig. 17-3.

2. Use the completed table as a reference to find the dose for a patient who weighs 127.6 lb. The physician's order is for sodium nitroprusside (Nipride), intravenously, 2 mcg/kg/min. What rate in milliliters/hour would deliver this dose if an IV pump is being used?

3. The physician orders the rate to be set at 3 mcg/kg/min if the blood pressure decreases by 10 mm Hg. What flow rate in milliliters/hour would be needed for a person weighing 58 kg, to deliver this amount of drug? Refer to the completed table.

4. The physician has ordered sodium nitroprusside (Nipride) 4 mcg/kg/min for a patient who weighs 123.2 lb. 250 mL of D_5W containing 100 mg of sodium nitroprusside is flowing at a rate of 34 mL/h. Is the flow rate set correctly?

5. The doctor requests that a solution of 100 mcg/mL of sodium nitroprusside be used instead of 200 mcg/mL. If the sodium nitroprusside is to be instilled in 500 mL of D_5W, how many milligrams of drug is needed?

EXERCISE 3 *(answers on page 321)*

Dopamine hydrochloride (Intropin) is ordered to stimulate cardiac outflow and renal flow. There are 400 mg of dopamine in 500 mL of IV solution. The patient weighs 132 lb. The physician's order reads "Give dopamine 4 mcg/kg/min IV."

1. Calculate the number of milligrams of dopamine in 1 mL (mg/mL) of IV solution.

2. Calculate the number of micrograms of dopamine in each milliliter (mcg/mL) of IV solution.

3. Convert the patient's weight to kilograms.

4. How many micrograms per minute (mcg/min) were prescribed for this patient?

5. How many milliliters per minute (mL/min) will deliver the prescribed number of micrograms?

6. How many milliliters will deliver the prescribed amount of drug in an hour (mL/h)?

EXERCISE 4 (answers on page 321)

1. Mr. Leonard has been diagnosed with congestive heart failure. The drug that will be used to relieve this condition is called amrinone lactate (Inocor). The patient weighs 198 lb. The physician's order reads "Inocor 7 mcg/kg/min." Careful reading of the IV solution label shows that there are 400 mg amrinone lactate in 250 mL of solution. An IV pump is in use. At what rate will the IV pump be set in milliliters/hour in order to administer the correct dose?

2. Following a mild heart attack, Mr. Anderson develops dysrhythmia due to cardiac irritability. To control this condition, the physician orders a maintenance infusion of lidocaine hydrochloride to be given at a rate of 2 mg/min. The IV solution available contains 2 g of lidocaine in 500 mL of solution. At what rate in milliliters per hour should the IV pump be set?

3. Although used less than inhalants because of its toxicity, aminophylline may be needed for some who experience a severe attack of asthma. When the prescribed inhalants do not help Mrs. Bobery, the physician orders aminophylline 15 mg/h IV. The available solution contains 1 g of aminophylline in 1000 mL of solution. Calculate the hourly rate at which the IV pump should be set in milliliters/hour.

4. Procainamide hydrochloride (Pronestyl) 5 mg/min IV has been ordered to treat a cardiac arrhythmia that developed subsequent to Mrs. Kalang's heart attack. The IV solution contains 3 g of procainamide hydrochloride in 500 mL of IV solution and is set at a rate of 40 mL/h. (a) Is this setting correct? (b) If not, what is the correct setting?

18

Pediatric Dosages

When prescribed for children, the dosage of many drugs is less than the dosage of the same drug for an adult. As a general guide, pediatric dosages are given to children who weigh 40 kg (88 lb) or less. The most accurate methods of calculating children's dosage are based on the amount of drug per kilogram of body weight or on body surface area. The range of dosage suitable for children is published for some drugs as milligrams/kilograms/day. This information is used to determine whether the prescribed dose is within the safe range for a specific medicine. Whenever the prescribed dose exceeds the recommended safe range of doses, the physician should be consulted. Situations arise when it may be necessary to exceed the safety range. Other tables for children's dosage have been developed by some manufacturers. The older methods of basing the calculation of the child's dose on the average adult dose are unsatisfactory because of wide variations in the size of children, the development of the organs that metabolize the drug, and the maturity of the enzyme systems. *Although the formulas for these methods are included, it is emphasized that these methods of calculating children's dosage provide very rough estimates only. Other more accurate methods should be used whenever possible.*

Regardless of the method used to determine the prescribed dose, observation of the child's response to the dose is critical in assessing whether the dosage needs to be adjusted for the benefit of the individual child. The degree of illness may indicate a dosage of certain drugs, such as antibiotics and anticonvulsants, that approximates the dose given to an adult. Computing a child's dose from a total daily dose will require dividing the total daily dose into individual doses. This can be done before or after computing the child's dose by dividing the total daily dose by the number of doses to be given daily.

CALCULATION OF DOSAGE BASED ON WEIGHT IN KILOGRAMS

Calculating dosage based on the child's weight in kilograms is a very accurate method. Calculations are based on the recommended dose of the drug per kilogram of body weight. Often the dose is computed for a 24-hour period of time and then divided into an equal number of doses. The number of doses in a 24-hour period is determined by the desired frequency of administration. If the recommended dose is 30 mg/kg/day in four divided doses, this means that the amount of drug needed for the 24-hour period would be 30 multiplied by the weight of the child in kilograms. To learn the amount of drug needed for each individual dose, the total daily dosage would be divided by 4.

EXAMPLE: Give 30 mg/kg/day in four divided doses to a child who weighs 44 lb.

Step 1. Determine the child's weight in kilograms.
$$44 \div 2.2 = 20 \text{ kg}$$

Step 2. Multiply the child's weight in kilograms by the dose/kilogram/day.
$$20 \text{ (kg)} \times 30 \text{ (mg)} = 600 \text{ mg/day}$$

Step 3. Divide the total daily dose by the number of doses needed (four doses).
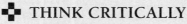
$$600 \div 4 = 150 \text{ mg q6h}$$

✚ THINK CRITICALLY

Is this a single or a total daily dose?
Is the dose based on body surface area or on weight?
Is the dose based on kilograms or pounds?
Is the calculated dose reasonable for this child?

EXERCISE 1 *(answers on page 321)*

Solve the following problems by calculating the dosage based on the amount of drug per kilogram of body weight:

1. If the recommended dose of phenytoin (Dilantin) is 5 mg to 7 mg/kg/day, **(a)** What would be the range in milligrams for a total daily dose if baby Kari weighs 8⅘ lb? **(b)** If the medicine is to be given in two divided doses, how much phenytoin is needed for each dose? **(c)** If each 5 mL contains 125 mg phenytoin, how much will be needed for one dose of 30 mg? **(d)** Is the dose 30 mg within the normal range for this child?

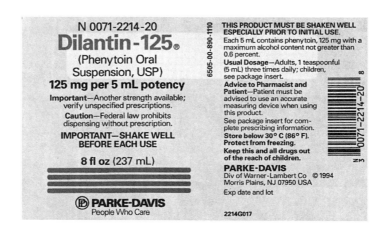

2. Amoxicillin is to be given to Terry who has an infection and weighs 11 lb. The recommended dose is 20 mg/kg/day in divided doses q8h. (a) How much is the total daily dose? (b) How many milligrams would be given every 8 hours? (c) If the amoxicillin suspension contains 50 mg of drug in each milliliter of solution, what would the total daily dose be in milliliters? (d) What would be the total volume of suspension for each dose? (e) If the available suspensions contain either 125 mg/5 mL or 250 mg/5 mL, how much of each is needed for a dose of 50 mg?

3. Harriet, a 44-lb child, is to be given 20 mg/kg/day of erythromycin suspension (EryPed) in four equally divided doses to treat streptococcal pharyngitis. (a) How many milligrams are needed for the total daily dose? (b) How many milligrams are needed for each individual dose? (c) If the solution contains 200 mg/5 mL, what volume would supply one individual dose? (d) Select the correct label.

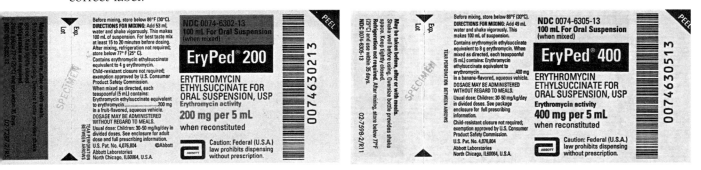

4. If the recommended dose of sulfisoxazole (Gantrisin) is 150 to 200 mg/kg/day, (a) What would be the range of dosage if a child weighs 66 lb? (b) If the maximum dose is to be given in four divided doses, how much drug is necessary for each dose?

5. Oxacillin is to be given to a 5.5-lb child. (a) Based on the recommended dose of 25 mg/kg/day, what would the total daily dose be? (b) This dosage is to be equally divided and administered q6h. How much drug would be used for each individual dose? (c) Each dose would be approximately how many milliliters if there are 250 mg/5 mL?

6. Ted weighs 42.5 lb. He is diagnosed with herpes simplex encephalitis. Acyclovir (Zovirax) is prescribed. The recommended total daily dose is 30 mg/kg/day. It is to be given q8h.

(a) How many kg does 42.5 pounds equal?

(b) What will the total daily dose of acyclovir for Ted equal?

(c) How much acyclovir is required for one dose?

(d) If the first dose is given at 7 AM, schedule the times for the other doses.

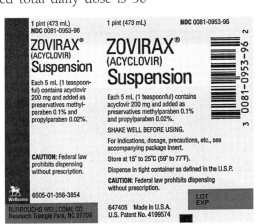

7. Digoxin elixir is ordered to improve cardiac output for Alyson, age 3. The recommended digitalizing dose for children ages 2 to 5 years is 30 to 40 mcg/kg. Half of the digitalizing dose is to be given immediately and the remainder is to be divided into two doses which are to be given at 8-hour intervals. Alyson weighs 48 lb.

   (a) Her weight in pounds is equal to how many kilograms?
   (b) The recommended dosage range for Alyson is between _____ and _____ .
   (c) The first dose will fall in the range of _____ to _____ .
   (d) The second and third doses will range between _____ and _____ micrograms.
   (e) The physician orders 350 mcg digoxin for the first dose. How many milliliters of elixir provide this dose?
   (f) If the first dose is given at 0600 hours, when should the next two doses be scheduled?
   (g) What would this schedule be in clock hours?

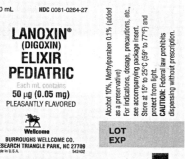

8. Bradley, age 5, is to receive acetaminophen as three tablets of Chewable Children's Tylenol to reduce his fever and discomfort. The usual dose for a child, age 5, is three tablets. If each Chewable Children's Tablet contains 80 mg of acetaminophen, what dose will Bradley receive by chewing and swallowing all three tablets?

9. Ashley weighs 66 lb and has congestive heart failure. She is to have furosemide (Lasix) for treatment of edema. The usual initial dose is calculated as 2 mg/kg.
   (a) What is Ashley's weight in kilograms?
   (b) What dose would you expect to be prescribed for Ashley?

10. Scott, who weighs 35 kg, has 50 mg meperidine (Demerol) ordered for pain that he is experiencing following trauma from an accident. The recommended dose of meperidine is 0.5 mg to 0.8 mg per pound, up to the adult dose of 50 to 100 mg.
    (a) How many pounds does Scott weigh?
    (b) What is the recommended dosage range for someone of Scott's weight?
    (c) Is the ordered dose within the recommended range?
    (d) If the prescribed dose were to exceed the dosage range for adults what action should be taken?

11. The following information is provided with cephalexin (Keflex suspension).

Child's weight	125 mg/5 mL	250 mg/5 mL
10 kg (22 lb)	½ to 1 tsp qid	¼ to ½ tsp qid
20 kg (44 lb)	1 to 2 tsp qid	½ to 1 tsp qid
40 kg (88 lb)	2 to 4 tsp qid	1 to 2 tsp qid
	or	
10 kg (22 lb)	1 to 2 tsp bid	½ to 1 tsp bid
20 kg (44 lb)	2 to 4 tsp bid	1 to 2 tsp bid
40 kg (88 lb)	4 to 8 tsp bid	2 to 4 tsp bid

A child weighing 10 kg is given ½ tsp qid of cephalexin (Keflex suspension) 250 mg/5 mL.
(a) How many milligrams of cephalexin is the child receiving in each dose?
(b) How many milligrams of cephalexin is the child receiving for the total daily dose?
(c) How far apart, in hours, should the doses be scheduled?

12. If the usual recommended dose of cephalexin is 25 to 50 mg/kg/day, what is the dosage range for a child weighing 44 lbs?

13. Robert, who weighs 66 lb, has otitis media. The recommended dosage range of cephalexin for this condition is 75 to 100 mg/kg/day, divided into four doses.
(a) What does Robert weigh in kilograms?
(b) What is the recommended total daily dosage range for a child of this weight?
(c) What is the recommended dosage range for each dose if given qid?
(d) If the first dose was given at 1800 hours, when should the other doses be given?

14. Maria weighs 46 lb. Cephalexin (Keflex suspension) is being considered as a treatment for an infection that she is experiencing.
(a) What does Maria weigh in kilograms?
(b) Using the chart provided in problem 11, what is the recommended dosage range for the total daily dose for a child of this weight?
(c) What is the recommended individual dose if the total daily dose is divided into four doses?
(d) What is the dosage range for one of the four doses when measured in milliliters?

15. The usual recommended dose of cephalexin (Keflex) is 25 to 50 mg/kg in divided doses. Emma, who weighs 38 lb, has streptococcal pharyngitis. Keflex 250 mg bid is prescribed.
(a) What is Emma's weight in kilograms?
(b) What is the total daily dosage range for Emma?
(c) If the drug is administered bid, what will the dosage range for each dose be?
(d) Is the prescribed dose within the recommended dosage range?
(e) If the suspension contains 125 mg/5 mL, how many mL are needed for one dose?

16. Clindamycin (Cleocin Pediatric) is available in water soluble granules and must be reconstituted. After reconstitution, each 5 mL of solution contains 75 mg clindamycin.
(a) How many milliliters are needed to give a dose of 90 mg?
(b) How many milliliters of Cleocin Pediatric, reconstituted to 75 mg/5 mL would be needed for a dose of 150 mg?

17. Mark weighs 76 lb. He has a serious staphylococcal infection for which the pediatrician prescribed Clindamycin (Cleocin Pediatric) 90 mg qid. If the recommended dose is 8 to 12 mg/kg/day, determine whether the prescribed dose is within the normal range.

   (a) How many kilograms does Mark weigh?

   (b) What is the recommended dosage range per day?

   (c) What is the recommended dosage range per dose?

   (d) Is 90 mg qid within this range?

   (e) If there are 75 mg/5 mL, how many milliliters of oral solution of clindamycin is needed for a 90 mg dose?

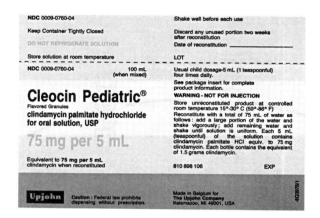

18. During an outbreak of meningitis, several people in one community are hospitalized in serious or critical condition and two deaths have occurred. The decision is made to give all people who may be carriers of the causative organism an antibiotic, rifampin (Rifadin). Adults will receive 600 mg twice daily for 2 days. The pharmacist prepares a syrup of rifampin (Rifadin) which contains 10 mg/mL for administration to young children. The dose for children under 1 month of age is 5 mg/kg q12 hours for 2 days.
   (a) How many capsules of the following preparation are required for one adult dose?
   (b) How many capsules are needed for 2 day's dosage for adults?
   (c) Compute one dose in milligrams for an infant weighing 9.9 lb.
   (d) What is the total daily dose in milligrams for a 9.9-lb infant?
   (e) How many milliliters of the prepared syrup will provide one dose for this child?
   (f) How many milliliters of the prepared syrup are needed for 2 days' dosage?

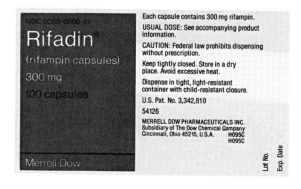

19. A child who weighs 66 lb is also being treated with rifampin (Rifadin). However, the dose for children over 1 month of age is 10 mg/kg q12 hours for 2 days.

   (a) What amount of rifampin will this child receive at each dose?

   (b) This child is able to swallow capsules. For the child to take as few capsules as necessary, what size capsule would be appropriate?

   (c) How many capsules should the child take for each dose?

CALCULATION OF DOSAGE BASED ON BODY SURFACE AREA

Methods of determining the child's dose based on body surface area (BSA) are also used. Three steps are used to determine the child's dose based on calculation of body surface area. These are:

Step 1. Obtain the child's weight in kilograms.
Step 2. Determine the body surface area in square meters.
Step 3. Calculate the dosage using the formula that is based on the assumption that an adult weighing 140 lb has a body surface area of 1.7 m².

✔ *A simple formula may be used to provide a reasonably accurate estimate of body surface area in square meters (m²) when the child's weight (W) in kilograms is known. It is considered accurate for patients weighing between 1.5 and 100 kg.*

Formula for Estimating BSA in m²

$$\frac{\text{four times child's weight in kilograms} + 7}{\text{child's weight in kilograms} + 90} = \text{body surface area (BSA) in square meters (m}^2\text{)}$$

In its abbreviated form, the formula for BSA is stated as follows:

$$\frac{4W + 7}{W + 90} = \text{BSA in m}^2$$

✔ *To compute dosage (based on the assumption that an adult weighing 140 lb has a body surface area of 1.7 m²) use this formula:*

$$\frac{\text{Body surface area in m}^2}{1.7} \times \text{adult dose} = \text{child's dose}$$

EXAMPLE: Using body surface area, calculate how much drug would be given to a child weighing 30 lb if the adult dose is 2 g.

Step 1. Convert 30 lb to kilograms (there are 2.2 lb in 1 kg):

```
         1 3.6  kg in 30 lb
   2.2.)30.0.0
         22
         ‾‾
          8 0
          6 6
          ‾‾
          1 4 0
          1 3 2
```

Step 2. Substitute into formula for BSA in m²:

$$\frac{(4 \times 13.6) + 7}{13.6 + 90} = \frac{54.4 + 7}{13.6 + 90} = \frac{61.4}{103.6}$$

or

```
            0.59  BSA in m²
     103.6.)61.4.00
            51 8 0
             9 6 00
             9 3 24
               2 76
```

Step 3. Calculate the dose:

$$\frac{\text{BSA in square meters}}{1.7} \times \text{adult dose} = \text{child's dose}$$

$$\frac{0.59}{1.7} \times 2 \text{ (g, the adult dose)} = \text{child's dose}$$

```
         0.34+ × 2 (g) = 0.68 g or 680 mg (child's dose)
    1.7.)0.5.90
          5 1
            80
            68
            12
```

EXERCISE 2 *(answers on page 321)*

Calculate the following dosages for children based on BSA:

1. Child weighs 50 lb; adult dose is 30 mL.

2. Child weighs 30 lb; adult dose is 1 mL.

3. Child weighs 75 lb; adult dose is gr x.

4. Child weighs 44 lb; adult dose is 2 mg.

5. Child weighs 96 lb; adult dose is 20 mcg.

6. Child weighs 102 lb; adult dose is 15 mL.

7. Child weighs 12 lb; adult dose is 40 mcg.

8. Child weighs 17 ⅗ lb; adult dose is ℨiv.

9. Child weighs 20 lb; adult dose is 2 g.

10. Child weighs 80 lb; adult dose is 1000 mg.

ESTIMATING BODY SURFACE AREA USING THE WEST NOMOGRAM

The body surface area can be estimated using standard charts or a nomogram. Fig. 18-1 illustrates the West nomogram, which may be used to estimate the body surface area of children. The nomogram is more accurate when used with children of normal proportion (see column called "For children of normal height and weight"). To use the nomogram, first determine the height and weight of the child, then draw a line between the height and weight. The point at which the line crosses the surface area column, labeled SA, is read and recorded as the estimated body surface area.

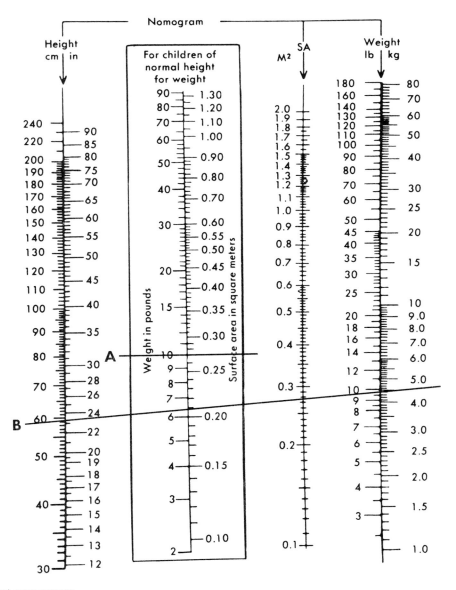

Fig. 18-1. West nomogram.
(Modified from data of Boyd E by West CD. In Behrman RE, Vaughn VC, editors: *Nelson's textbook of pediatrics*, ed 14, Philadelphia, 1992, WB Saunders.)

CLARK'S FORMULA

Clark's formula may be used to determine whether the prescribed dose seems reasonable. It is based on the weight of the child and is stated as follows:

$$\frac{\text{weight of the child in pounds}}{150} \times \text{adult dose} = \text{child's dose}$$

As stated previously, Clark's rule is less accurate than calculations based on the body surface area or recommended dose per kilogram of body weight.

EXAMPLE: Using Clark's rule, estimate the dose for a child weighing 30 lb if the adult dose is 2 g.

$$\frac{30}{150} = \frac{30}{150} = \frac{1}{5} \times 2 = \frac{2}{5} \text{ or } 0.4 \text{ g or } 400 \text{ mg}$$

EXERCISE 3
(answers on page 322)

Using Clark's formula calculate the following dosages for children:

1. Child weighs 50 lb; adult dose is 30 mL.

2. Child weighs 8 kg; adult dose is 10 mL.

3. Child weighs 22 lb; adult dose is 40 mcg.

YOUNG'S FORMULA

The formula for Young's rule, which is based on the age of the child in years, follows:

$$\frac{\text{age of the child in years}}{\text{age of the child} + 12} \times \text{adult dose} = \text{child's dose}$$

EXAMPLE: Using Young's rule, estimate the drug dosage for an 8-year-old child if the adult dose is 40 mg.

$$\frac{8}{8+12} \times 40 = \frac{8}{20} \times \frac{40}{1} = 16 \text{ mg}$$

This rule is seldom used because children of the same age vary greatly in size.

EXERCISE 4
(answers on page 322)

Using Young's formula calculate the following dosages for children:

1. Child is 6 years old; adult dose is 10 mg.

2. Child is 8 years old; adult dose is gr xx.

3. Child is 4 years old; adult dose is gr xx.

19

Geriatric Dosages

Most people who are 65 years of age or older have one or more chronic health problems. Many of these conditions are treated with prescription drugs. In addition, individuals may use over-the-counter (OTC) medicines. Frequently-used OTC medications include laxatives, aspirin and other pain relievers, cough medicines, and antacids. For maximum benefits from drugs, it is important to consider physiologic factors, drug interactions, compliance, and opportunities to teach persons about their drug therapy. In addition, measures that lessen or eliminate the need for some drugs are useful.

PHYSIOLOGIC FACTORS

Different responses to drug therapy may occur because of genetic and physiologic factors. Genetic factors are present from birth and remain throughout the lifespan. People age at different rates, and the rate at which an individual will age is not predictable. Physiologic change that occurs with aging affects the way drugs are used by the body. For example, a drug may have toxic effects in an elderly person that would not have occurred in the same individual at a younger age. Therefore adjustment of drug dosage is required if therapeutic effects are to be obtained safely. Changes in diet or health may warrant changes in medications or dosages. Allergic responses to drugs, ranging from mild reactions to those that are life-threatening, may occur at any age. Always withhold the drug and consult the physician when an allergic reaction is suspected.

Physiologic variations among the aging helps explain why drug references rarely recommend specific doses for the geriatric patient and why there are no formulas for calculating geriatric doses of drugs. Adjustment of drug dosage to the individual's requirements is often necessary for safe and therapeutic effects.

DRUG INTERACTIONS

Drug interactions should always be a consideration. Interactions may increase or decrease the effects of the drugs or cause dangerous reactions. Interactions can result from taking incompatible drugs at the same time, or by mixing them before ingestion. Interactions include contradictory effects so that neither drug works as intended, gastrointestinal effects such as nausea and vomiting, increased reaction to the drug, motor incoordination, or depression of the central nervous system. Interactions can occur between other prescription drugs and some antibiotics, oral antidiabetic agents, cardiac drugs, antihypertensive agents, cholesterol-lowering agents, corticosteroids, bronchodilators, thyroid preparations, tranquilizers, and others. Interactions sometimes occur because people share their prescription drugs. This is a dangerous practice and should be prevented through education.

The number of drug interactions tends to increase as drug intake increases. Misuse of drugs also increases the number of drug interactions and other unwanted effects. For this reason, it is recommended that the minimum number and dose of drugs be used to obtain the desired effects. Use of nonprescription drugs that can interact with each other is to be discouraged. This can happen with such drugs as antacids, vitamin preparations, and potassium supplements.

Older adults commonly use the following groups of drugs: laxatives, pain medications, cardiac and diuretic drugs, sedative-hypnotic drugs, and tranquilizers. Other frequently-used over-the-counter medications include cough medicines and antacids. Aspirin and other pain-relievers, sedative-hypnotic drugs, and tranquilizers are most likely to be misused. Because these three groups of drugs depress the central nervous system, overdoses occur when drugs from these groups are taken together. Alcohol also increases depression of the central nervous system.

DRUG COMPATIBILITY

Whenever a person takes more than one medication, compatibility between and among medications should be considered. Medications are compatible if they do not interact with each other. Compatibility of medications is determined by reading current drug information or by consulting a pharmacist. Drug references are available in many public libraries and book stores.

All prescriptions should be filled at the same pharmacy to allow the pharmacist to check for drug compatibilities whenever a new medication is prescribed. If asked, the pharmacist will share information about the safety of taking over-the-counter drugs with the prescribed ones.

Another safeguard in preventing problems with medications involves seeing the same doctor, who knows which medications the patient is taking. It is wise for patients to take their medications with them when consulting their physician. Some patients carry a complete list of the medicines that they take, including the doses and times. This information is helpful to health care providers.

OLDER ADULTS' COMPLIANCE WITH DRUG THERAPY

The compliance of older adults with a drug therapy program is influenced by their knowledge, understanding, and acceptance of how the treatment is to be implemented. Noncompliance is said to occur if a patient takes too much or too little drug, uses it inconsistently, takes it for purposes other than those for which the drug was prescribed, or does not complete the course of drug therapy. Often noncompliance indicates that people do not understand the therapy or need a scheme for remembering to take their medicines. Most older adults can learn effectively if teaching is done well and is timely and appropriate for their needs.

Sometimes noncompliance occurs because the drug therapy is complex. Drug schedules that are planned in accordance with people's life styles are more likely to be followed. It is desirable to simplify drug therapy as much as possible. It is not uncommon for people to stop taking medications that cause unpleasant effects. This is less likely to occur if they know which side effects to expect, what measures they can use to relieve them, and when it is appropriate to contact their physician.

> **THINK CRITICALLY**
> Can the patient read the label?
>   Is the print large enough?
>   Is patient's language used, or is an interpreter available?
> Can patient open the container and remove the drugs?
>   Are childproof caps necessary?
>   Do seals need to be removed?
>   Does cotton filler need to be removed from bottle?

It is important to assess the patient's learning needs, styles, abilities, and resources in designing medication therapy. The following should be considered: (1) Can the person for whom the medication is being prescribed financially afford to buy the medications? (2) Does the person have transportation to get the medications, or is a delivery service available? (3) Is the person able to read the label (is the print large enough and are the instructions in the person's native language?) and (4) Can the person open the container and remove the drug? Childproof containers can be difficult or impossible for older adults to open because of decreased muscle strength or arthritis. The size of the containers may also make it difficult to remove the medications. Protective seals and the packing on top of tablets or capsules can be very difficult to remove. Tweezers, forceps, small pliers, or a pickle fork facilitate the removal of the packing.

> **THINK CRITICALLY**
> Will insurance pay for the patient's drugs?
> Can the patient afford the drugs if insurance does not pay?
> Does the patient have transportation, or can the drugs be delivered?

Remembering to take the appropriate drugs at the correct times can also be a problem. This may happen because the older person may have a less structured lifestyle, does not know which drugs to take or when to take them, or simply forgets to take them. Various methods may be used to help the person take the drugs correctly. It is important to work with the individual in designing a system for taking drugs. The best system is the one that works well and is used consistently by the individual. One system uses containers with multiple compartments for dispensing either a daily or weekly supply of drugs. Another system writes the names of the drugs, the times they are to be taken, and special directions on a daily calendar. The information is crossed off when the person takes the medicine. Some people will prefer to prepare the next dose immediately after taking a dose of medicine. Setting an alarm clock for the time that a medication is to be taken may be helpful. Others develop a system of recording which medications were taken and

✔ when they were taken. Some people maintain a daily drug diary. *Remember, the best results are achieved when written instructions are provided, the simplest possible routine is used, and the fewest drugs necessary to adequately treat the person's condition are prescribed.* Knowing the meaning of side effects and how to deal with them is important for every patient, but especially for older adults. For instance, if a drug is known to cause low blood pressure, the person is instructed to change positions slowly. Nausea and vomiting that occur may be relieved or prevented by taking some drugs with food. However, because food interferes with the effects of some drugs, it is important to know if the drug can be taken with food without changing its effects.

The following list of questions will assist patients who wish to test their knowledge of their drug therapy:

1. What is the name of each of my medicines?
2. When (specific time and frequency) am I to take each medicine?
3. How much of each medicine should I take?
4. May I take the medicine with food or drink?
5. Can this medicine be taken at the same time as my other medicines?
6. If I am to take the medicine on an empty stomach, how long must I wait before or after eating to take the medicine?
7. For how long should I take this medicine?
8. Are there circumstances when I should not take my medicine?
9. For what kinds of problems with my medicine should I contact my doctor?
10. How can I remember (or remind myself) to take my medicine at the right times?
11. Where and how should I store my medicine?
12. Can I have my prescription refilled?
13. What should I do if I forget to take my medicine?

✚ THINK CRITICALLY

Does the patient know the name of each of his or her medicines?
Does the patient know when to take each medicine?
Does the patient know how much of each medicine to take?
Does the patient know if the medicine can be taken with food or drink?
Does the patient know if the medicine is to be taken without food, and the amount of time that must elapse before or after eating?
Does the patient know how long to take this medicine?
Does the patient know what to do if a dose of medicine is forgotten?
Does the patient know when not take this medicine?
Does the patient know when and how to contact the doctor about problems with the medications?
Does the patient know how to remember to take the medicine at the correct times?
Does the patient know where and how to store the medicine?
Does the patient know whether the prescription can be refilled?

NURSING INTERVENTIONS THAT REDUCE DRUG THERAPY

Multiple factors must be considered when drug therapy is ordered. If the drug is ordered to be given as necessary, the health care provider must always consider care measures that may substitute for the drug or provide conditions under which the drug will act more effectively. For example, the use of laxatives can be reduced by increasing the intake of fiber and fluid, and by increasing physical activity. The need for analgesics and tranquilizers may be lessened by increasing patient comfort. Tightening bed linen, repositioning pillows, giving back-rubs, adjusting room temperature, changing soiled linen, and helping the person to a comfortable position may decrease or eliminate the need for drugs. Talking quietly with the person, reading aloud, holding the person's hand, or helping the person relax can have a calming effect. Some will respond favorably to a snack or a warm drink. Honoring usual bedtime routines also has a calming effect. It is very helpful to allow patients to follow their established bedtime routines.

STORAGE OF MEDICINES

Correct storage of medicines preserves them. Most medicines should be stored in a cool, dark, moisture-free place. Special storage instructions may be placed on the label of some medicines. A few, such as reserve supplies of insulin, are stored under refrigeration. As a general rule, medicines should be stored in their original containers. Medicines must be stored out of the reach of children. Ideally, medicines are kept in locked cabinets if children are in the home because childproof containers have been opened by children.

Always ask patients where and how they store their medicines. Places where medicines should not be stored, but frequently are, include window sills; medicine cabinets in bathrooms; the tops of stoves, microwaves, or heaters; or in refrigerators or freezers. These places may allow light, moisture, heat, cold, or condensation to alter the drug or make it ineffective.

DISPOSAL OF DRUGS THAT ARE NO LONGER NEEDED

When discontinued or outdated, unused medicines should be disposed of appropriately. The pharmacist can provide information on the proper method of disposal for specific drugs. Medicines and syringes should never be disposed of in waste baskets, garbage containers, or other places from which they might be retrieved.

COMPUTATION OF GERIATRIC DOSAGES

A brief review of three methods used to calculate dosage follows. The same dosage problem is used to illustrate each method. See Chapter 12, Computation of Oral Dosages, if more review of these methods is needed.

Before using any method, be sure the drug preparation and the prescribed dose are in the same units of measure. Convert within or between systems as necessary. It is customary to convert to the measure used on the drug preparation. When the dose is ordered in grams and the drug preparation is labeled in milligrams, convert the prescribed dose to milligrams. If the drug is ordered in the apothecaries' system and the drug preparation is labeled in metric/SI units, convert the apothecaries' unit to its metric/SI equivalent. For further review see Systems of Weights and

Measures, Unit II, which presents the various systems of measurement and conversions within or between systems.

EXAMPLE: The physician orders 650 mg of acetaminophen (Tylenol). The label on the bottle of acetaminophen indicates that there are 325 mg in each tablet.

METHOD 1. *Using 2 ratios established by drug label and prescribed dose.* Establish a proportion using the labeling information as one ratio and the prescribed dose as the other.

Label side of proportion   Prescribed dose
milligrams:tablet = milligrams:tablet
325 (mg):1 (tab) = 650 (mg):x (tab)

$325x = 650$
$x = 650 \div 325$

$x = 2$ tablets of acetaminophen, 325 mg/tablet

METHOD 2. *Using dosage formula.* Substitute into the following formula:

$\dfrac{\text{dose desired}}{\text{dose available}} \times 1$ (tab or unit of measure) = number of tablets or units needed to administer the prescribed dose

$\dfrac{650 \text{ (mg)}}{325 \text{ (mg)}} \times 1 \text{ (tab)} = \dfrac{650}{325} \times 1 = 2$ tablets, each containing 325 mg of acetaminophen

The formula may be abbreviated as:

$$\dfrac{D}{H} \times U = A$$

METHOD 3. *Using 2 ratios established by size.* Establish a proportion stating that lesser:greater = lesser:greater.

lesser:greater   =   lesser:greater
milligrams:milligrams = tablets:tablets
325 (mg):650 (mg) = 1 (tab):x (tab)

$325x = 650$
$x = 650 \div 325$

$x = 2$ tab, each containing 325 mg of acetaminophen

EXERCISE 1   *(answers on page 322)*

1. Mrs. Joan H., age 68, complained of swelling and extreme tenderness in her left great toe. Her physician diagnosed this condition as gouty arthritis and prescribed indomethacin (Indocin) 50 mg tid pc. 25, 50, and 75 mg tablets are available. **(a)** Which size tablet provides this dose? **(b)** How many tablets are required for one dose? **(c)** When is the medication to be taken?

2. Because Mrs. H. has difficulty swallowing tablets, the physician changes the order to an oral suspension that contains 25 mg/5 mL of indomethacin. How much of the suspension provides a 50 mg dose?

3. Her roommate also has gout, but takes 100 mg of allopurinol (Zyloprim) tid for a total daily dose of 300 mg. (a) Which size tablet provides one dose? (b) How many tablets does she need for a 30-day supply?

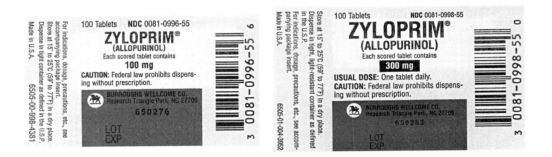

4. Martin M. has hypercholesterolemia. Despite following a strict dietary regimen, his blood cholesterol levels remain elevated. Pravastatin (Pravachol) 20 mg qd with the evening meal is ordered. 10, 20, and 40 mg tablets are available. Which one will provide the exact dose in one tablet?

5. Methyldopa (Aldomet) is prescribed to treat Muriel B.'s hypertension. The prescribed total daily dose is 500 mg. bid. 125, 250, and 500 mg tablets and an oral suspension containing 250 mg/5 mL are available. (a) How often is she to take this medicine? (b) Which size tablet provides one dose? (c) If the oral suspension were used, how much liquid would provide one dose?

6. Mrs. Suban, 80 years old, has had difficulty falling asleep and awakens frequently since the death of her husband 2 months ago. A 3-week trial of flurazepam hydrochloride (Dalmane) 15 mg hs is prescribed. Available capsules contain 15 mg or 30 mg of flurazepam. (a) Which capsule will provide one dose? (b) How many capsules will she receive when the prescription is filled?

7. Naomi C. had a large part of her pancreas removed in order to remove a benign tumor. She is to take one capsule pancrease MT 10 with each meal and with snacks. Four different preparations are available, containing different amounts of pancreatic enzymes. The following table shows the amounts of lipase, amylase, and protease in each preparation.

USP Units in Pancrease MT Capsules

	MT 4	MT 10	MT 16	MT 20
Lipase	4000	10,000	16,000	20,000
Amylase	12,000	30,000	48,000	56,000
Protease	12,000	30,000	48,000	44,000

If, on a normal day, she eats three meals and has two snacks, **(a)** how many capsules should Naomi take daily? **(b)** What is the total amount of lipase in her normal daily dose? **(c)** What is the total amount of amylase that she will normally receive daily? **(d)** What is the total amount of protease that she will normally take daily?

8. Emil G. has a history of congestive heart failure and has been taking a mild diuretic. When edema in his extremities worsens and he complains of shortness of breath, oral furosemide (Lasix), a diuretic available as 20, 40, and 80 mg tablets is prescribed. The initial prescription is for a daily dose of 20 mg. He receives 100 tablets. In a short time, the dose is increased to 40 mg/day. **(a)** How many tablets of the original prescription are needed for this new dose of 40 mg? **(b)** If the dose is increased to 60 mg, how would one dose be prepared?

9. When Laurena A. develops herpes zoster (shingles), acyclovir (Zovirax) is ordered to shorten the course of the infection and to relieve pain. The dose ordered is 800 mg five times a day for 10 days. **(a)** Ideally the size that would be used to provide the fewest possible number of tablets or capsules each day is the one that contains how many milligrams? **(b)** If she takes one tablet or capsule for each dose, how many should she receive in the prescription? **(c)** If the order is changed because she has difficulty swallowing, how much suspension is needed for one dose of 800 mg? **(d)** How much suspension is required for a 10-day supply of medication?

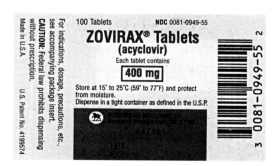

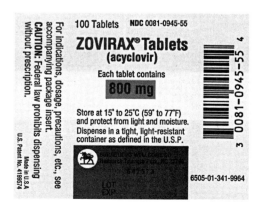

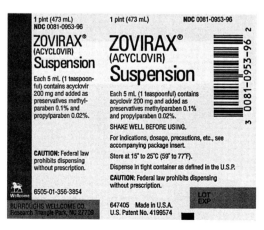

20

Home Care Considerations

Home care considerations are very important for the achieving of optimal health care and in providing for the comfort and well-being of the patient. Many people medicate at home. Some use only medicines prescribed by a physician, others use over-the-counter (OTC) drugs, and many use a combination of both. Although people have the right to self-medicate and to refuse medication, it is important that they understand the consequences of their actions. People are reluctant for a variety of reasons to take drugs. Fear of becoming dependent on or addicted to a drug or group of drugs is seen when people refuse to take medication for severe pain. Concern that taking the drug as often as prescribed may cause tolerance is sometimes expressed as "If I take a drug this often, soon it won't do me any good." Others may tend to overuse or abuse drugs. Cultural practices and ethnic values also influence drug therapy. Recent immigrants tend to continue customary practices although they may accept some medical therapy. Many people have traditional practices that they continue along with medical therapy. The amount and kind of knowledge needed by each person varies. Teaching specific to individual needs promotes following prescribed drug therapies. Everyone who needs to take a medication needs to know what the medicine is, why it is needed, when it is to be taken, the correct dose, and any precautions that are necessary.

TEACHING THE PATIENT AND FAMILY MEMBERS ABOUT DRUG THERAPY AT HOME

Both the patient and family members should be taught about the prescribed drug therapy and helped to develop the skills needed to carry it out. Effective teaching involving the patient and family members is a complex task. It involves much more than telling facts to patients or handing them a sheet of information. It is imperative that the health care professional have the necessary knowledge and skills related to the drug therapy and have a positive attitude. Many sources of information about drugs are available. Basic skills are presented in a variety of textbooks.

The health care professional who displays enthusiasm toward the subject being taught and believes that the patient or family member can learn the necessary knowledge and skills usually has a positive influence on learning. Several criteria should be considered in each teaching session. It is important to relate information to the person's current level of knowledge and ability, and particular needs. Even though highly educated, some patients may not have the knowledge or skills needed for personal drug therapy. Conversely, patients with limited formal education may be very knowledgeable. Young children and people with limitations respond well when the teaching is modified appropriately. Patients and family members are the best resources for telling the teacher what they need to know. Being able to respond to patients' needs as they arise helps promote learning. Stimulating curiosity often provides necessary motivation for learning. Active involvement in the learning process along with periodic reinforcement of both knowledge and skills is very important.

Practice is important because people learn what they do. Learning new motor skills such as those involved in preparation and administration of an injection is likely to cause stress, uncertainty and hesitancy, and awkwardness as evidenced by jerky, cautious movements. With encouragement and repetition, most people become proficient in the necessary skills. As teaching progresses, it is important to observe the patient or family member performing new skills. This allows the health professional to analyze difficulties and plan corrections in problem areas.

Discussing procedures and rationale may help the patient to learn more quickly. Explaining the information using different words and sequence of content is often helpful. Although teaching may begin during hospitalization or at a health clinic, plans for follow-up teaching in the home are often warranted. Few patients remain in the hospital or clinic long enough to allow for comprehensive teaching and learning. Usually, questions about implementing instructions occur only when the treatment is done at home. Written instructions that can be used as references are helpful. It is reassuring for patients to possess the names and phone numbers of resource people whom they may contact when questions arise. Follow-up telephone calls and referrals to home health agencies may be appropriate.

Evaluation of learning must be done very carefully. When told to take a written or oral examination on their knowledge of the drugs they are taking, many patients become apprehensive. Anyone who has constructed a written test knows that writing the test questions so that none are misinterpreted requires considerable knowledge and skill. The health care provider may elicit more information by telling the patient, "In order to be sure you understand your drug therapy, I would like you to tell me what you know about your drugs, when and how often to take them, and what you can expect them to do for you." The well-prepared health care provider will listen carefully, ask questions that cover important omissions, add necessary information, and praise the patient when appropriate.

PSYCHOLOGY OF MEDICATING

It is always important to conduct and document a complete drug history. This tells what the patient has taken and is currently taking, or if problems with medications are known. It also alerts the health care provider to the possibility of drug interactions. Some common over-the-counter drugs such as antacids and laxatives interfere with the actions of certain drugs. Other over-the-counter medications may increase the dose or action of prescribed drugs. Less well-known are the adverse effects of some drugs on physiology. For example, some of the common dietary aids and pain relievers are known to increase blood pressure. This effect, while serious in a healthy person, can be disastrous for someone with hypertension. Along with the patients' drug history, information should be obtained about the person's diet. A high-protein diet or a vegetarian diet will change the absorption rate for some drugs. This occurs because a high-protein diet makes the urine more acid, and a vegetarian diet makes it more alkaline. Smoking or drinking alcoholic beverages may change the rate at which some drugs are metabolized.

The belief that the prescribed drug therapy will produce the desired effects is essential. Expectation of obtaining certain results from medications is likely to influence the person's willingness to follow the prescribed regimen. The attitude and manner of approach exhibited by health professionals will have an impact on the effects of drug therapy. An attitude of "I think this will help" is more effective than "This probably won't work." Compliance with drug therapy is facilitated by knowledge and hope.

BASIC MEDICATION INFORMATION THAT THE PATIENT SHOULD KNOW

Basic information about prescribed medication therapy is required by most people. Everyone who takes a medication should know its name and be given this information in writing. Other commonly used names for the same drug should also be provided. For example, the person who is taking aspirin or is allergic to it needs to know that it has another name and is contained in many over-the-counter preparations. Knowing that aspirin is also known as acetylsalicylic acid, and reading labels of over-the-counter drugs could prevent overdosage and reactions.

A person's own understanding of the meaning of drug therapy requires consideration. For example, Richard, who has been on a medication to lower blood pressure for several years following a heart attack, was told that he no longer needs the medication. He believed this medicine was needed to prevent another heart attack and worried about discontinuing it. He found it helpful to learn that a planned slow reduction in dosage and close monitoring of his condition will allow early detection and correction of problems, should any occur.

Knowing the purpose of the drug is important. Why is the drug necessary? What can it realistically be expected to do? What are the undesirable and unintended effects of the drug? Some drugs may have undesirable effects that may be troublesome but not harmful. For example, some drugs may discolor the skin, some discolor body excreta, and some produce an unpleasant body odor. Suggestions by health professionals may help patients cope with undesirable effects. For example, although it may not be possible to completely cover discoloration of the skin, some brands of makeup are more effective than others for this purpose. Warning that discoloration of urine or feces will occur prevents unnecessary concern. Coping with unpleasant body odor presents a challenge to both patients and family members. Unless another drug that will produce the same therapeutic effects is available, counseling may be required for patients to accept and continue the drug therapy.

> ✚ **THINK CRITICALLY**
>
> Do the patient and family members know
>   the name of the drug?
>   the dose of the drug?
>   how to prepare the drug?
>   when to take it?
>   how much water to drink with an oral dose?
>   how to administer the drug?
>   the precautions when applicable?

Patients must also know if a medicine is known to have unintended effects. Rather than try to list all the unintended effects, it is often wiser to instruct patients and family members to contact the physician if new signs or symptoms develop, such as rashes and other unintended effects common to a particular drug. Although reportable signs and symptoms can be discussed, any disturbing or unusual symptom should be reported. If patients feel excessively tired or unable to perform usual daily activities, this could be a reaction to a drug and requires medical evaluation.

> ✚ **THINK CRITICALLY**
>
> Can the patient verbalize understanding of
>   the purpose of the drug?
>   the drug's expected effects?
>   the drug's nuisance effects?
>   unexpected effects of the drug that should be reported?
>   when and how to contact a health care provider if an adverse reaction occurs?

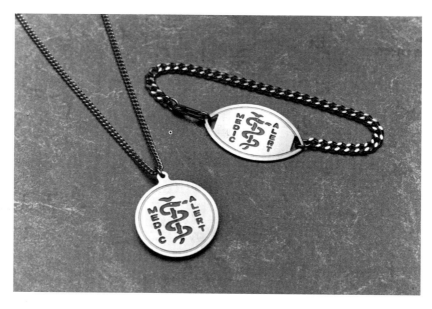

Fig. 20-1. A bracelet or necklace engraved with medical caduceus and personal medical facts such as allergies, medicines and medical conditions is worn to alert caregivers in an emergency. The jewelry shown is sold by Medic Alert, an organization with a 24-hour hot line that supplies the caller with additional information such as the name and phone number of patient's physician.
(Courtesy Medic Alert Foundation United States, Turlock, Calif.).

A printout of information about drugs may be made available to patients. Many hospitals distribute information that has been prepared in-house on drugs that are prescribed. In the community, the pharmacist may provide printed material and answer questions about drugs. Always encourage patients to consult a health care provider about drug therapy concerns.

As a guide, it is prudent to ask about adverse drug reactions and allergies. It is beneficial to learn what a patient experienced with an adverse reaction. Being non-judgemental is imperative when discussing drug reactions. It is never helpful to indicate disbelief. Not only may the health care provider be wrong in assuming that a particular reaction is impossible, but the patient is likely to become apprehensive and distrustful. When asked about drug allergies five years after he had experienced nearly fatal agranulocytosis, Mr. Jarold was incredulous and became distrustful and angry when the health care provider laughed and commented, "I've never heard of such a thing and I doubt that anyone else has."

People who have known allergies are wise to carry identification that states the allergies. A card can be carried in a billfold. Engraved necklace or bracelet medallions may be worn. These are available from a variety of sources. These contain a medical caduceus that alerts health care providers that the person has a particular medical problem or allergies. Medic-Alert (Fig. 20-1) also keeps records noting how to contact the person's physician. Caution must be used if information is written on paper because moisture may damage it.

Whenever a drug has caused an allergic reaction, the drug should be avoided in the future. If no other drug is available to treat a condition, patients are sometimes given a "challenge" dose of the drug. This is a small dose and is given to determine how the person will react to the drug. As a rule, a drug challenge is not done if a drug is known to have caused a life-threatening reaction. Related drugs may cause cross-sensitivity. For example, people who are allergic to penicillin may also be allergic to clindamycin. Caution is important whenever a new drug is added to a regimen, and is especially important when patients have a history of drug allergies. People with known allergies are more likely to exhibit additional allergies. It is also wise to remember that no drug can be guaranteed to be safe. Even the most commonly used drugs have caused serious and fatal allergic reactions.

Knowing the correct dose, and knowing how often and when to take the medication is essential. As a general rule, people are told how much drug to take for each dose. They must be told the time to take the drug, and told whether it is to be taken with food or taken a period of time after ingesting food. Ideally the schedule for taking medications is established with the patient. The schedule must consider the patient's underlying health problems and usual daily activities. Along with the schedule, the patient should know that variation in the time for taking the medicine (½ hour before or after the designated time) may be allowed. A greater time span may not alter the effects of some preparations, such as multivitamins. However, following a schedule consistently helps patients to remember to take medications. It is easier to remember a simple schedule than a complex one.

✚ THINK CRITICALLY

If the patient has known allergies, does he or she wear jewelry engraved with this information?

Is the drug prescribed related to any drugs to which patient is allergic?

A schedule that requires taking medicine only once a day is more likely to be followed, although some medicines must be taken more frequently. When medicine must be taken with meals away from home, this can be done discretely in restaurants and other public places. If patients travel long distances, it is appropriate to discuss how to adjust the dose when traveling across time zones. When traveling east, the time available is shortened and when traveling west, it is lengthened.

REMEMBERING AND COMPLYING WITH MEDICATION SCHEDULE

Remembering to take medicine is sometimes difficult. Many elderly people are treated each year either because they failed to take their medicine or overdosed. Many types of devices are used to help people remember to take their medicines promptly. Most drug stores display a variety of items for the administration of medications in the home. Compartmentalized boxes are available with a compartment marked for each day of the week or marked for several times each day (Fig. 20-2). Medicines for the entire week can be placed in the appropriate compartments. Boxes containing a series of compartments are available for multiple doses for a single day. Each series is labeled for 1 day of the week and the compartments within the series are labeled for AM, noon, PM, and bedtime. If more than one daily dose of a medicine is prescribed, a different colored box can be used for each time of day. For example, Mr. Hazlorny takes a dose of an oral antidiabetic drug each morning and evening. He uses a yellow medicine box for his morning doses and a blue box for his evening doses. Some people prefer to take the medicine directly from the container when required for a dose. Some like to place all the medicines needed for the next dose in a small container. Others use an alarm clock or a wristwatch alarm to remind them when the next dose of medicine is due. Leaving the lid of the compartment of a pill box open after taking the dose of the medicine helps some people to remember whether or not they took the previous dose. Others may find it helpful to write a notation on a calendar.

Mechanical devices are available that can be used to set up a weekly supply of medications (Fig. 20-3). Some devices have a buzzer that sounds to remind a person when to take a medicine. The medicine for a particular time can be removed and taken but the dose cannot be repeated. Mrs. Bilapen began using this device when she first experienced symptoms of Alzheimer's disease. Although the disease has progressed, she remembers to take her medicine when the buzzer sounds.

Learning to prepare a dose can be relatively simple if it only involves removing the medicine from a container. Adults often need help with or explanation about opening childproof containers. Adults should be informed that they can

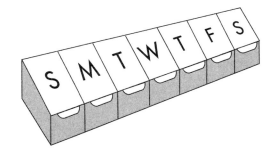

Fig. 20-2. Medicine box, with individual compartments for each day of the week. Other sizes and shapes are available.

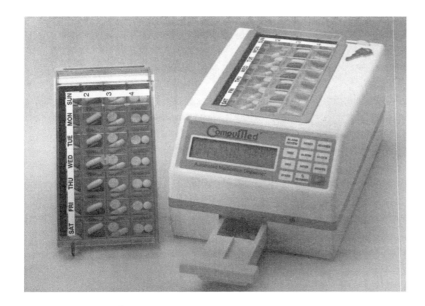

Fig. 20-3. The CompuMed automated medication dispenser with a tamper-proof lock. This machine can be programmed to automatically dispense doses of pill-form medications at preselected times. An alarm sounds when one or more medications are to be taken. The screen displays messages about how to take the medicine. Error messages are also displayed on the screen.
(Copyright CompuMed, Inc. Meeteetse, Wyo).

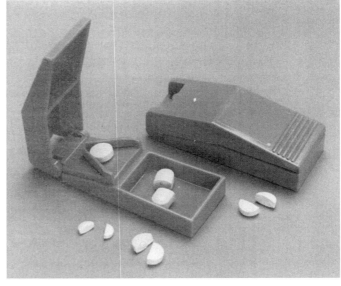

Fig. 20-4. Pill splitter. To divide a tablet, place pill splitter on a firm surface, place the tablet in the point of the pill splitter, aligning scored depression with blade, lower the lid, and press gently on it. A sharp blade in the lid will cut the tablet into two parts and the parts will be contained by the pill splitter.
(Courtesy Apex Medical Corporation, Sioux Falls, SD).

request caps that are not childproof be put on their bottles of medicine. When difficulty opening the bottle of medicine was experienced by Mrs. Zemieski, she had a friend open the bottle and then left the cap off so she could use the medicine as prescribed. If a medicine bottle is left open air and moisture may cause the medicine to deteriorate. If a tablet must be divided, a device called a pill-splitter, available at drug stores, may be used (Fig. 20-4). Other methods of dividing tablets are often frustrating, and some methods have caused injury.

Measuring solutions accurately may require instruction and supervision. Preparation and administration of injections requires knowledge and skill. In addition to learning to use aseptic technique, patients must also learn to measure the sterile solution and inject it into an appropriate area. This requires practice and follow-up. Whenever injectable medicines, such as insulin, must be mixed, patients must be taught to do this correctly. If patients cannot measure drugs such as insulin, a week's supply of syringes, each containing the required amount and type of insulin, can be prepared. These must be stored correctly.

Learning to administer IV solutions or medications can be frightening for patients and family members. They must be taught the procedures for aseptic technique, and for diluting, mixing, and injecting medications into the line or into the container of solution. Consideration must also be given to the obtaining of and proper storage of solutions such as those used in nutritional therapy.

The unpleasant taste of a drug may need to be disguised. Pharmacists may flavor medicines or they can be flavored at home. Because some flavors enhance rather than disguise unpleasant tasting medicines, a "taste-test" approach to flavoring may be necessary. As a rule, the taste of medicine should *never* be disguised with any food, juice, or milk that patients need for nutritional purposes. Alice D. was told that the liquid medicine she needed daily could be disguised with milk. She tried placing it in milk and found that the milk did disguise the taste. However, a few weeks later, Alice found she no longer liked the taste of milk.

Patients and family members must understand the reason for limits on the amount of drug per dose and per day. The temptation to overdose on pain medications, for example, greatly increases when pain is not relieved immediately. Doses of many over-the-counter medications are restricted, even for common drugs such as acetaminophen, (Tylenol). When restricted, the recommendation states that the total daily dose not exceed a specific number of grams or other amounts (teaspoonfuls, for example) of the drug. When a drug is to be taken prn, patients must be told that the medicine can be taken when needed for a symptom such as pain, but must not be taken more often than the time interval specified.

SAFEGUARDING THE WELFARE OF PATIENTS

The welfare of patients who need drug therapy can be safeguarded in several ways. The greatest protection for patients is their own knowledge. Not only do they need the information already covered in this chapter, but they also need to know about potential drug interactions. Some drugs are potentiated by other drugs. Patients must be cautioned to avoid such combinations. Caution should be given about drugs that increase blood pressure or otherwise adversely affect body functions. It may be necessary to tell patients not to drink alcoholic beverages or operate motorized vehicles when taking certain drugs.

Blood tests are necessary for monitoring the blood levels of some drugs. Examples include blood thinners such as warfarin (Coumadin), and lithium, which is used to treat manic depression. Frequency of the blood tests vary. When the therapeutic dose is being determined, daily blood level tests may be necessary. Usually less frequent blood tests are necessary once the maintenance dose is established.

Planning for emergencies also protects the welfare of patients. Helping patients understand how to handle situations that may arise enables them to react appropriately. Do patients who may travel know what to do if a prescription medication has been inadvertently left at home? Do patients who may develop gastrointestinal symptoms such as diarrhea or vomiting know what to do about taking their medications? Particular attention should be paid to instructing those who take medications such as insulin. Do patients know how to regulate their insulin? Do they know how to store it when traveling? The importance of taking antibiotic drugs at equally spaced intervals in order to keep the steady level of drug in the blood necessary to fight the disease-causing organism may need to be emphasized. Patients need to understand that the organisms causing the illness may become resistant to antibiotics if all the antibiotics in the prescription are not taken. Emphasize that resistance to antibiotics means that the drug will no longer be able to fight the organisms causing this or any other health problem. The only time that a course of antibiotic therapy should be stopped is when the physician asks that the drug be discontinued or an adverse reaction occurs.

Instructions about taking an oral drug with adequate amounts of fluid are usually necessary. Patients must be told exactly how much water is to be drunk with a dose of a drug such as sulfonamide or psyllium (Metamucil). Patients must also know whether the drug being used is compatible with other drugs or food. Ingestion of some foods will enhance the effects of certain drugs, some foods may lessen or destroy the effects of other drugs, and some food and drug combinations may cause toxic effects. For example, a drug commonly prescribed to relieve symptoms of allergy inactivates a common antibiotic. Bulk-forming laxatives such as psyllium (Metamucil) interfere with absorption if taken at the same time as other drugs. The key is to schedule the dose of psyllium at a time when other drugs are not being taken. For example, if drugs are taken before breakfast, the psyllium might be taken before the evening meal.

Adequate information and the habit of patronizing one pharmacy will help protect patients against many undesirable effects, and will aid in coordinating drug therapy if more than one health care professional is involved in a patient's care. Most pharmacies use computers for record-keeping. This provides pharmacists with knowledge about all the prescriptions that have been filled by that pharmacy. Pharmacists can warn people about common side effects of drugs and if an incompatibility exists between a prescribed drug and other drugs. Pharmacists will contact the physician for further orders. Pharmacists will provide information on drugs and will answer questions about drug therapy. People who have known allergies can ask to have these listed on their pharmacy records. This provides another safeguard against taking drugs that could cause problems.

> ### ✚ THINK CRITICALLY
> Does the patient have written information about the drug?
> Does the patient have a written drug schedule?
> Does the patient have knowledge about OTC drug interactions?
> Does the patient know other names for the prescribed drugs?

OVER-THE-COUNTER DRUGS

Many people take over-the-counter (OTC) drugs. These can be dangerous when taken together or added to prescription drugs. Careful reading of labels may help prevent the taking of medicines that increase or decrease the effect of a drug taken regularly. For example, a daily dose of aspirin may be prescribed by the physician. Knowledge that aspirin is also known as acetylsalicylic acid or ASA alerts people who see this on the label of another common preparation that this will increase the dose. If people are taking blood thinners, aspirin may be contraindicated. When selecting over-the-counter drugs, patients should ask the pharmacist if the preparations are compatible with other drugs they are taking. Patients should always carry with them a list of the names and doses of medications they take.

OBTAINING MEDICATIONS

Obtaining prescribed medications may present problems. If patients cannot afford prescribed medications they may be referred to a social agency for assistance. Insurance may pay for all or part of the cost. Some insurance policies cover the cost for generic brands only. Some insurers require that prescriptions be sent to a central place for processing, a practice which requires considerable planning. If prescriptions are sent too soon, they are returned unfilled. If sent late or mail delivery is slow, the drugs may not arrive by the time they are needed. Patients also need to know if, when, and how to obtain refills of prescription drugs. If prescriptions are being filled locally, do patients have transportation to obtain the drugs? Some pharmacies deliver prescriptions, taxicabs can be hired to deliver prescriptions, or neighbors or friends may be willing to pick up prescriptions. Most physicians will telephone prescriptions to their patients' pharmacy.

HOME STORAGE OF MEDICATIONS

Health professionals should instruct patients on the proper home storage of drugs. This is an important aspect of safety and ensures that the drugs retain their strength. Medicines should be kept in a locked cupboard. All medicines should be stored where they cannot be reached by children. The ingenuity of children in finding and opening medicine containers must never be underestimated. *Everyone should post the telephone number of the nearest poison center on their telephone along with other emergency numbers.* A bottle of ipecac should be kept in the home for emergency treatment of accidental poisoning.

The conditions under which medicines are stored is important. A few drugs require refrigeration. Many are never to be stored in the refrigerator. Most drugs are best stored in a cool, dark cupboard. Because heat and moisture cause deterioration of many drugs, storage in bathroom medicine cabinets, on window sills, above kitchen stoves, on radiators or microwaves, or in other areas that expose the medicine to strong light or heat is undesirable. The high temperature of car interiors during hot weather may cause deterioration of drugs left in cars for a short time. Drugs should not be allowed to freeze in cars during cold weather. Storing medicine in freezers is not recommended as moisture from condensation may adversely affect tablets.

Drugs should be stored in the original containers except when set up as daily or weekly doses. The dark brown color of some containers protects medicines from light. All drugs should be kept in closed containers. They should also be kept in the original container with the pharmacy label intact. When a health care provider asked to see the medicines Mrs. Casteel was currently taking, she extracted an unlabeled bottle containing a variety of tablets from her purse. She said it was too much trouble to carry several bottles of medicines. Instruction was needed to help her understand the danger of putting several medicines together in an unlabeled or incompletely labeled container. With help, Mrs. Casteel was able to understand the reasons for keeping medicines in their original, labeled containers. She was able to determine that she only needed to have one medicine with her at all times. The others could be stored at home.

> ### ✚ THINK CRITICALLY
> Is the medicine stored away from extreme temperature levels, light, and moisture?
> Is the cap secure and the medicine stored out of the reach of children?

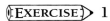 **1** (answers on page 322)

Some questions have more than one correct answer.

1. Mr. Binrad is being dismissed from the hospital. He will have several new medications to take at home. Which of the following are important considerations? Check all that apply.
   (a) Teaching him the purpose of his drugs
   (b) Providing him with a written schedule for taking the drugs
   (c) Telling him how to report adverse reactions
   (d) Advising him to skip his medications one day each week

2. Mrs. Walmith developed a near fatal agranulocytosis from the drug procainamide. What must she know if she is to avoid future reactions to this drug? Check all that apply.
   (a) To ask for a test or challenge dose of the medicine
   (b) To always wear a necklace or bracelet stating this and other allergies
   (c) The other names for the drug to which she is allergic
   (d) To avoid taking this drug

3. Mary P. developed acute respiratory distress after taking aspirin. What must she be taught?
   (a) To take aspirin with lots of water
   (b) Other names for aspirin such as acetylsalicylic acid, ASA, and Ecotrin
   (c) That many combination and OTC medicines contain aspirin
   (d) To read labels and inserts carefully to avoid aspirin.

4. Miss Benevtel keeps bottles of medications on the window sill above the kitchen sink. What three conditions for the correct storage of medications are being violated?

5. Nancy M. needs to take a life-saving medication that will cause her skin to have a bluish-grey cast. What does she need to know to cope with this?

6. Mr. Raspnuty had an allergic reaction to an injection of penicillin. He says he wants to try taking penicillin orally the next time he needs an antibiotic. What advice can you give him?

7. Name two methods that Mrs. Brenstan could use to remember to take her medications as ordered?

8. Mr. Gelbritsen complains that he has such bad arthritis that he cannot open bottles of medicine with childproof caps. What advice can you give?

9. The label on Mrs. Ferodel's medicine states "take 1 capsule q4-6h prn for severe headache." She asks you to explain the meaning of this statement. What will you tell her?

10. Mr. Dravert has a drug prescribed that decreases motor coordination. What precautions must he take while using this medicine?

Unit Three Posttest

EXPLANATION: The following posttest may be used to assess your understanding of dosages and solutions. If you experience difficulty solving any of the problems accurately, a review of the appropriate chapters may be helpful.

Directions: Work the following problems as indicated:

1. The physician orders 10 gr of enteric coated acetylsalicylic acid. The dose on hand is in 325 mg tablets. How many tablets would be given?

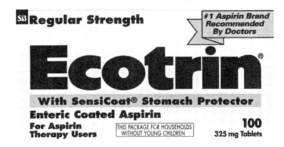

2. The physician orders 10 mg of morphine sulfate. The dose on hand is in 0.005 g tablets. How much would be given?

3. The physician orders 0.0005 g of digoxin (Lanoxin). The following preparations are available. (a) Which is appropriate? (b) How many tablets are needed for the dose?

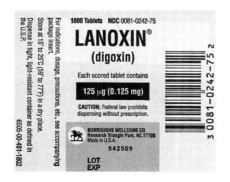 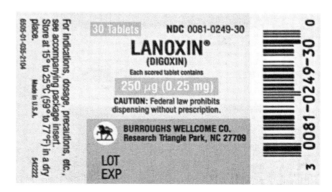

280

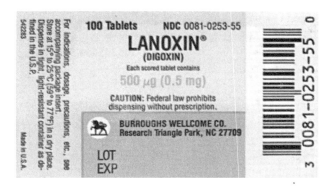

4. The physician orders 10 mg of morphine sulfate. The dose on hand is in 5 mg tablets. How many tablets are needed for the dose?

5. The physician orders 500 mg of amoxicillin q6h. The dose on hand is in 250 mg capsules. How many capsules are needed for the dose?

6. The physician orders ½ gr of phenobarbital. (a) Which size tablets are appropriate? (b) How many tablets are needed for the dose?

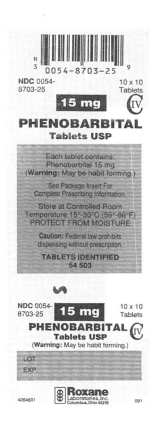
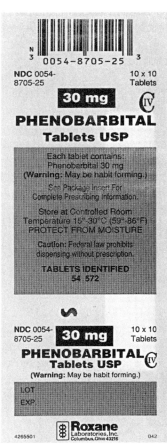

7. The physician orders 650 mg of acetominophen. It is available in regular strength (325 mg) and extra strength (500 mg) tablets. (a) Which size tablet is appropriate? (b) How many tablets are needed for one dose?

8. The physician orders 15 mg of morphine sulfate to be given by injection. The dose on hand contains 10 mg/mL. What amount of solution in milliliters is needed for this dose?

9. There are 5 mg of a drug in 4 mL of solution. How much solution is required to give 20 mg?

10. A 500 mg vial of antibiotic diluted with sterile bacteriostatic water yields 4 mL of solution. It is to be given in four divided doses. How much drug in milligrams would each dose contain?

11. If each vial contains 50 mg of drug and the dose ordered is 0.5 mg/kg, how many vials will be needed to give the correct dose to a person weighing 110 lb?

12. Find (a) The total daily dose if a child weighing 22 lb is to be given 60 mg/kg/day. (b) The amount for each individual dose if the total daily dose is to be given in six divided doses.

13. Using the BSA formula, compute the total daily dose for a child weighing 10 kg if the adult dose is 4 g/day.

14. If you wish to administer 1 L of IV solution in 8 hours and there are 60 gtt/mL, what would be the rate of flow per minute?

15. If you wish to administer 3 L of IV solution in 24 hours and there are 20 gtt/mL what would be the rate of flow per minute?

16. If you wish to administer 3000 mL of IV solution in 24 hours and each liter contains 40 mEq of potassium chloride, how much drug will the patient have received after 12 hours?

17. There are 5 g of vancomycin in 1000 mL of IV solution. (a) If the solution is to be given over an 8-hour period, how much solution should be delivered each hour? (b) How much drug would be delivered every hour?

18. How much 5% sodium bicarbonate solution can be made using 10 g of $NaHCO_3$?

19. Make 250 mL of 0.9% sodium chloride solution.

20. Make 500 mL of a 2% solution from a 1:4 solution.

Comprehensive Posttest

Express in Roman numerals:

1. 13 _____

2. 9 _____

Express in Arabic numbers:

3. XVI _____

4. IV _____

Change the following fractions to the higher terms indicated:

5. $\dfrac{7}{8} = \dfrac{}{56}$

6. $\dfrac{5}{9} = \dfrac{}{27}$

Reduce the following fractions to lowest terms:

7. $\dfrac{14}{20} =$

8. $\dfrac{9}{36} =$

Change the following improper fractions to whole or mixed numbers:

9. $\dfrac{14}{3} =$

10. $\dfrac{77}{8} =$

Change the following mixed numbers to improper fractions:

11. $2\dfrac{7}{8} =$

12. $5\dfrac{3}{7} =$

Circle the smallest fraction in each group:

13. $\dfrac{4}{5} \quad \dfrac{5}{8} \quad \dfrac{8}{40}$

14. $\dfrac{3}{10} \quad \dfrac{2}{3} \quad \dfrac{4}{5}$

Circle the largest fraction in each group:

15. $\dfrac{1}{4} \quad \dfrac{2}{3} \quad \dfrac{3}{5}$

16. $\dfrac{1}{2} \quad \dfrac{5}{8} \quad \dfrac{9}{16}$

Add the following fractions and mixed numbers (reduce answers to lowest terms):

17. $\dfrac{5}{6}$
    $\dfrac{2}{3}$
    $\dfrac{7}{8}$

18. $4\dfrac{3}{7}$
    $\dfrac{5}{6}$
    $5\dfrac{1}{2}$

Subtract the following mixed numbers (reduce answers to lowest terms):

19. $8\dfrac{7}{9}$
    $4\dfrac{2}{3}$

20. $2\dfrac{7}{64}$
    $1\dfrac{13}{64}$

Multiply the following fractions and mixed numbers (reduce answers to lowest terms):

21. $4\dfrac{1}{2} \times 7\dfrac{2}{3} =$

22. $\dfrac{5}{8} \times 2\dfrac{3}{4} =$

Write the words for the following:

23. 4.17 _____

24. 0.235 _____

Change the following fractions to decimals (round off at two places if necessary):

25. $\dfrac{8}{9} =$

26. $\dfrac{3}{5} =$

Change the following decimals to fractions (reduce to lowest terms):

27. 0.025 =

28. 0.0005 =

Add the following decimals:

29. 5.037
     0.4
    +1.25

30. 9.21
     0.0043
     8.72
    +4.5

Subtract the following decimals:

31. 14.001
    − 7.29

32. 9.435
    −0.689

Multiply the following:

33. 12.02
    × 3.04

34. 120
    × 70.2

Divide the following fractions and mixed numbers:

35. $7\frac{2}{3} \div 5\frac{1}{2} =$

36. $3\frac{3}{4} \div 5\frac{7}{8} =$

Divide the following numbers, rounding to hundredths when necessary:

37. $90 \div 0.078 =$

38. $732.6 \div 42.5 =$

Circle the larger of the two decimal numbers:

39. 0.2 or 0.04

40. 0.125 or 0.05

Change the following fractions and mixed numbers to decimal numbers, rounding to thousandths when necessary:

41. $7\frac{1}{8}$

42. $16\frac{3}{7}$

Rewrite the following fractions as ratios, percentages, and decimals:

	Fraction	Ratio	Decimal	Percentage
43.	$\frac{3}{4}$	= _____	= _____	= _____
44.	$\frac{7}{8}$	= _____	= _____	= _____

Solve the following percentage problems:

45. 6½% of 494 =

46. 12% of 88 =

Solve for x in the following problems:

47. $\frac{5}{8} = \frac{25}{x}$

48. $\frac{2}{3} = \frac{44}{x}$

Change the following units of measure to the indicated equivalents:

49. 5 mg = _____ g

50. 2000 g = _____ kg

51. 400 mL = _____ L

52. f℥ i = _____ mL

53. 4.9 lb = _____ g

54. 180 lb = _____ kg

55. 8 cm = _____ mm

56. 3 m = _____ yd

57. 100° F = _____ °C

58. 36.8° C = _____ °F

59. 4 in = _____ cm

60. 10 mL = _____ t

Change the following traditional clock times to 24-hour (military) times:

61. 3 PM _____

62. 2:30 AM _____

Change the following 24-hour (military) times to traditional clock times:

63. 1600 _____

64. 2200 _____

65. Answer the following questions based on information found on the label:

   a. What is the trade name of the drug?

   b. What is the generic name of the drug?

   c. What is the dosage unit?

   d. What is the dose per unit?

   e. What is the usual dose?

   f. What is the method of administration?

   g. Any special handling instructions?

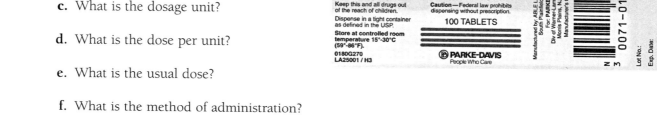

66. The physician orders warfarin sodium (Coumadin) 7 mg q AM for its anticoagulant effect. (a) Which strength preparation is appropriate? (b) How should the dose be prepared?

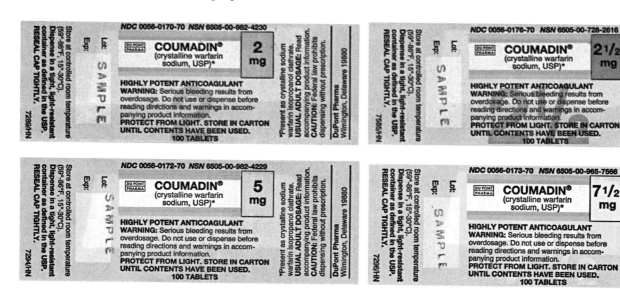

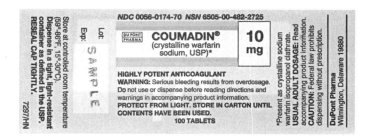

67. The physician orders diphenhydramine HCl (Benadryl) 50 mg bid to relieve itching. (a) Which size capsule will provide a dose? (b) How many capsules are needed each day? (c) How many capsules will be supplied if the prescription was written for 2 weeks?

68. If the physician orders aminophylline gr 3 and it is available in 200 mg tablets, how many tablets are needed for one dose?

69. The physician orders 0.5 mg digoxin (Lanoxin) (a) Which strength preparation is most appropriate to use? (b) How many tablets are needed for one dose?

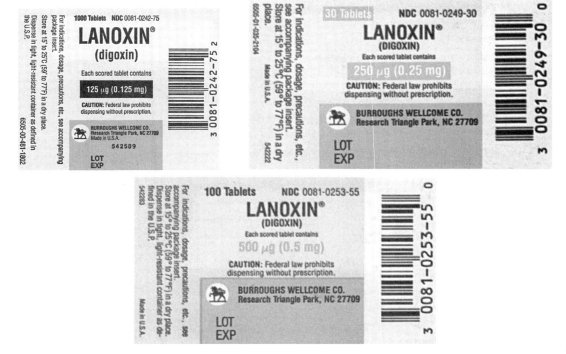

287

70. Captain Win has a tinea infection for which his physician has prescribed 500 mg of griseofulvin qd per os. (a) How often is Captain Win to take this medicine? (b) How many mL are needed for one dose? (c) how is the medicine to be taken? (d) How many doses are in one bottle of medicine? (e) Mark the appropriate medicine cup to show this amount.

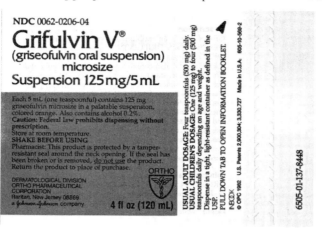
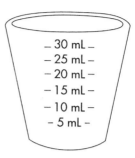

71. The physician's order is for penicillin V-potassium (V-cillin K) 200,000 units bid. Available solutions are labeled 125 mg (200,000 mcg)/5 mL and 250 mg (400,000 mcg)/5 mL. (a) Which solution is appropriate? (b) How many milliliters are needed for the dose? (c) Shade this dose on the appropriate medicine cup).

72. The physician orders a total dose of lithium carbonate 16 mEq. How many milliliters are needed for this dose if available preparations contain 8 mEq/5 mL or 16 mEq/5 mL?

73. The physician orders 75 mg of meperidine IM stat. How much solution is needed for this dose if there are 50 mg/mL? Mark the syringe to show this amount.

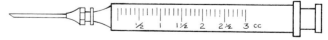

74. Atropine sulfate gr 1/120 is ordered. Strengths of available solutions contain 0.4 mg/mL, 0.5 mg/mL, and 1 mg/mL. (a) Which solution is most appropriate? (b) How much of this solution is needed for one dose? (c) Mark the syringe to show the correct dose.

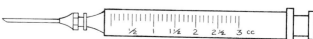

75. If morphine sulfate gr 1/6 IM is ordered and the strengths of the available injectable solutions are 10 mg/mL and 15 mg/mL, (a) which solution would you choose? (b) How much solution is needed for one dose? (c) Mark the syringe to show the correct amount.

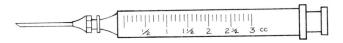

76. The physician orders cefoperazone (Cefobid) 4 g q 12 h in divided doses. (a) How much will be given in each dose? (b) If the following size vials are available, which is appropriate? (c) How much diluent is used to reconstitute the 1 g and 2 g vials?

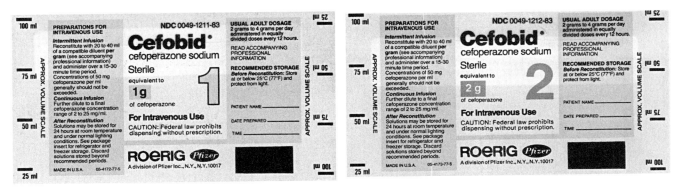

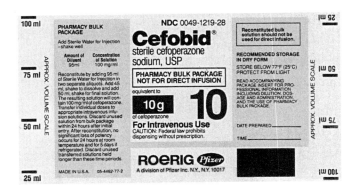

77. Mrs. Long has tuberculosis. Although it has known serious side effects, streptomycin sulfate IM has been prescribed because of suspected resistance of the causative organism to other drugs. The usual dose is 15 mg/kg/day for adults. However, the dose must not exceed 1 g/day. (a) If Mrs. Long weighs 121 lb, what will the daily dose be in milligrams? (b) in grams? (c) If there is 1 g/2.5 mL, how much solution will provide one daily dose?

78. Emil Moritell is to soak his feet for 20 minutes twice a day in a physiologic salt solution. If the foot basin holds 4 L of solution, how many grams of salt are needed to prepare one soak?

79. Myra N seeks to relieve a sore throat by gargling qid with physiologic saline solution. Each time, she prepares a glassful (240 mL) of the solution. (a) How many times a day is she gargling? (b) How much salt should she use each time? (c) To approximately how much is this equivalent, if she uses household measuring spoons? (d) What are the steps she should follow in preparing the solution?

80. Give 20 U of NPH Iletin I.
    a. Circle the label of the preparation to be used.

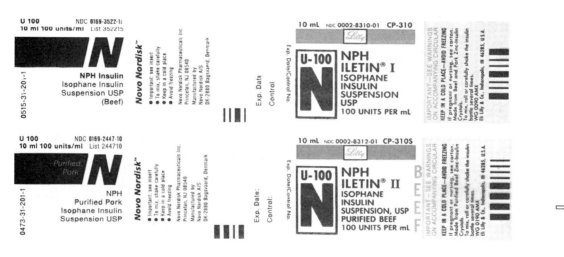

   b. Name the species of origin for this insulin.
   c. Is this preparation considered to be short-acting, intermediate-acting, or long-acting?
   d. Shade the area on the syringe to indicate the correct dosage.

81. Give 16 U of Humulin L insulin.
    a. Circle the preparation to be used.
    b. Name the species of origin.
    c. Is this preparation considered to be short-acting, intermediate-acting, or long-acting?
    d. Shade the area on the syringe to indicate the correct dose.

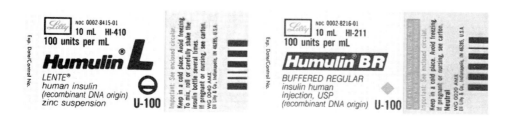
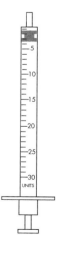

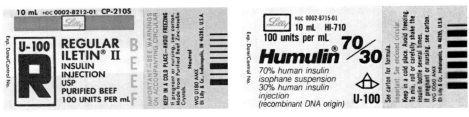
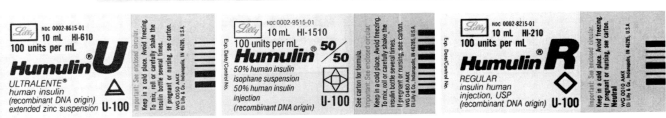

82. Read the following order for IV fluid therapy before answering the questions that follow.
    Give 5% dextrose in 0.45% NaCl 1000 mL with 20 meq KCl q 12 h. Start at 1800.
    a. What kind of solution was ordered?
    b. Is the solution isotonic, hypotonic, or hypertonic?
    c. How much IV solution was ordered?
    d. Are additives included in the order? If so, what is the name and dose of each?
    e. When is this IV solution to be started?
    f. Does the order state how long this solution is to run? If yes, what is the time span?
    g. Does the order state the rate of flow? If yes, what is it?

83. After reading the computerized order for IV therapy, answer the following questions.

    1 g cefazolin sodium (Ancef) in 50 mL 5% dextrose. Run 15 minutes. Flow rate 200 mL/h 3.3 mL/min
    Give q12h   First dose: 01/12   Last dose: open
    a. What kind of solution was ordered?
    b. Is the solution isotonic, hypotonic, or hypertonic?
    c. How much IV solution was ordered?
    d. Are additives included in the order? If so, what is the name and dose of each?
    e. How often is this to be administered?
    f. Does the order state how long this solution is to run? If yes, what is the time span?
    g. Does the order state the rate of flow? If yes, what is it?

84. Calculate the rate of flow in milliliters per hour if you are to administer 3 L of 5/0 that is to run for 24 hours.

85. If the flow rate for the IV solution is 60 mL/h and the drip factor is 60 gtts/mL, what is the flow rate in drops per minute?

86. If the flow rate is 125 mL/h and the drip factor is 10 gtts/minute, what is the flow rate in gtts/minute?

87. If the physician orders 1000 mL of IV solution to be given in one hour, how many mL are to be given each minute?

88. The IV solution that was originally scheduled to run at 125 mL/h is behind schedule because it infiltrated and had to be restarted. The drip factor for the tubing is 20 gtts/mL. Your agency policy allows a 25% increase in the base rate twice, if there are no contraindications.
    a. How much can the flow rate be increased initially?
    b. How many mL/h will be delivered when the initial increase is put into effect?
    c. How many gtts/min will deliver this amount?
    d. If a second increase in the flow rate is necessary, how many mL/h will be administered?
    e. How many gtts/min are needed to deliver this amount?

89. The IV solution contains 1.5 million U of ampicillin in 50 mL of solution. How many units of ampicillin will be delivered in the first 25 mL of solution?

90. An IV solution of 1 L of 5/0 contains 40 mEq of potassium chloride. How much potassium chloride will the patient have received when 700 mL of solution remains to be given?

91. How many units are in a 4 mL vial of heparin that contains 10,000 U/mL?

92. If there are 40 U of heparin in each milliliter of solution, how many milliliters/hour are needed to administer 1200 U/h?

93. What is the usual dosage range of heparin?

94. If there are 40,000 U of heparin in 1 L of solution, how many units of heparin are there in each milliliter of solution?

95. Mr. Jameran has congestive heart failure which is to be treated with amrinone lactate (Inocor). He weighs 198 pounds. The physician's order is: Inocor 7 mcg/kg/min. When the IV solution is delivered, the label states that there is 400 mg Inocor in 250 mL of solution. At what rate should the IV pump be set in milliliters/hour to administer the dose ordered?

96. The recommended daily dose of sulfisoxazole (Gantrisin) is 150 to 200 mg/kg/day. (a) What is the dosage range for a child who weighs 44 lb? (b) If the maximum total daily dose is to be given in four divided doses, how much drug is necessary for each dose? (c) If there are 0.5 g/5 mL of solution, how many milliliters are needed for a single maximum dose?

97. Kara who weighs 66 lb has a serious infection for which the drug clindamycin (Cleocin Pediatric) is prescribed qid. The recommended dosage range is 8 to 12 mg/kg/day.
    a. How many kilograms does Kara weigh?
    b. What is the daily dosage range that is appropriate for Kara?
    c. If the maximum dose is given qid, how many milligrams would she receive in each dose?
    d. If each 5 mL of reconstituted solution contains 75 mg of the drug, how much is needed for the maximum total daily dose?
    e. Each 5 mL of reconstituted solution contains 75 mg of drug, how much is needed for the minimum total daily dose?

98. Mrs. Greenbein asks you to help her plan a schedule for taking her medications. You know that calcium tends to bind with other drugs and should be taken an hour or two before or after other drugs. Her daily medications are:
    Pravastatin (Pravachol) 30 mg (1½ tablets)   Estrogen (Premarin) 0.625 mg (1 tablet)
    Benazepril (Lotensin) 10 mg (1 tablet)   Calcium 600 mg (1 tablet, 600 mg)
    Aspirin (Ecotrin) 325 mg (1 tablet)   Multivitamin
    Psyllium (Metamucil), 1 t with a full glass of water

99. Using body surface area, calculate the dose for Andy who weighs 11 lb. The adult dose is 600,000 U.
    a. What is Andy's weight in kilograms?
    b. What is his body surface area in square meters (rounded to hundredths)
    c. How many units are needed for Andy's dose?

100. Mrs. Beinameier is to take 0.15 g of chlorpromazine (Thoraxine) tid.
    a. Which strength preparation should she use?
    b. How many tablets are needed for one dose?
    c. How many tablets will be needed for a total daily dose?
    d. She comments that it is very difficult to break the tablets. Although she has been able to cut them, the pieces are not equal in size and sometimes "fly away." What might you suggest as a possible solution to this problem?

Answer Key

Unit I Pretest

1. V
2. XXXVIII
3. XVIII
4. LVI
5. XLIX
6. LXV
7. CXV
8. XXIX
9. XII
10. 33
11. 15
12. 24
13. 14
14. 94
15. 104
16. 1100
17. 113
18. 58
19. $\frac{1}{2}$
20. $\frac{2}{9}$
21. $\frac{5}{8}$
22. $\frac{1}{20}$
23. $\frac{1}{5}$
24. $\frac{2}{7}$
25. 75
26. 20
27. 35
28. 13
29. 6
30. 35
31. 4
32. $7\frac{3}{5}$
33. $14\frac{1}{4}$
34. $18\frac{2}{3}$
35. $5\frac{5}{6}$
36. $12\frac{1}{11}$
37. $3\frac{3}{5}$
38. $8\frac{5}{9}$
39. $4\frac{1}{7}$
40. $\frac{7}{2}$
41. $\frac{23}{5}$
42. $\frac{13}{3}$
43. $\frac{119}{9}$
44. $\frac{44}{7}$
45. $\frac{347}{8}$
46. $\frac{1}{3}$
47. $\frac{2}{9}$
48. $\frac{4}{9}$
49. $\frac{3}{5}$
50. $1\frac{41}{50}$
51. $1\frac{23}{40}$
52. $14\frac{41}{45}$
53. $18\frac{11}{28}$
54. $\frac{1}{24}$
55. $\frac{11}{36}$
56. $\frac{4}{7}$
57. $4\frac{5}{6}$
58. $\frac{7}{10}$
59. $5\frac{1}{3}$
60. $\frac{39}{56}$
61. $4\frac{1}{40}$
62. $1\frac{4}{21}$
63. $\frac{1}{34}$
64. 10
65. $1\frac{10}{31}$
66. Three and twenty-five hundredths
67. One and five tenths
68. Two hundred one and sixteen hundredths
69. Four hundred thirty-two and eight hundred sixty-eight thousandths
70. 0.833
71. 0.875
72. 0.857
73. 0.9
74. 0.3
75. 0.625
76. 5.25
77. 3.8
78. $\frac{2}{5}$
79. $\frac{3}{50}$
80. $\frac{1}{20}$
81. $\frac{3}{200}$
82. 1.7065
83. 0.778
84. 1.855
85. 946.61
86. 108.705
87. 3,257.61
88. 17.4
89. 36.46
90. 524.29
91. 229.98
92. 11.535

93. 26.44
94. 63
95. 7.85508
96. 2.38
97. 3.65
98. 0.42
99. 3.46
100. 37.5
101. 33.04
102. 1.6
103. 2.37
104. 0.5
105. 0.025
106. 0.75
107. 0.15
108. 0.375
109. 0.4
110. 2.25
111. 0.8
112. 0.875
113. 75
114. 1:100, 0.01, 1%
115. 3:4, 0.75, 75%
116. 3:50, 0.06, 6%
117. 1:5, 0.2, 20%
118. 24
119. 15
120. 42
121. $8\frac{1}{3}$
122. 2
123. 160

Chapter 1
1. IX
2. VII
3. XXVI
4. XV
5. XXIV
6. XIX
7. VIII
8. III
9. XVI
10. XXVIII
11. XXII
12. I
13. LXI
14. XI
15. XX
16. XLII
17. IV
18. XIII
19. XXXIV
20. L
21. M
22. XC
23. VI
24. CC
25. XII
26. 4
27. 7
28. 10
29. 3
30. 6
31. 19
32. 15
33. 8
34. 30
35. 11
36. 5
37. 24
38. 40
39. 13
40. 2000
41. 39
42. 35
43. 2
44. 14
45. 9
46. 12
47. 358
48. 60
49. 500
50. 100

Chapter 2
Exercise 1
1. $\frac{3}{5}$
2. $\frac{1}{2}$
3. $\frac{1}{5}$
4. $\frac{24}{49}$
5. $\frac{5}{8}$
6. $\frac{1}{4}$
7. $\frac{1}{2}$
8. $\frac{1}{2}$
9. $\frac{3}{8}$
10. $\frac{3}{4}$
11. $\frac{1}{8}$
12. $\frac{2}{9}$
13. $\frac{2}{3}$
14. $\frac{7}{8}$
15. $\frac{1}{16}$
16. $\frac{1}{2}$
17. $\frac{2}{3}$
18. $\frac{1}{3}$
19. $\frac{3}{5}$
20. $\frac{4}{5}$
21. $\frac{1}{8}$
22. $\frac{1}{20}$
23. $\frac{1}{4}$
24. $\frac{1}{4}$
25. $\frac{1}{3}$
26. 6
27. 4
28. 70
29. 20
30. 3
31. 36
32. 6
33. 14
34. 66
35. 125
36. 9
37. 4
38. 6
39. 22
40. 9
41. 3
42. 6
43. 20
44. 6
45. 40
46. 16
47. 4
48. 15
49. 70
50. 40

Exercise 2
1. 7
2. 2
3. 4
4. 4
5. $3\frac{3}{4}$
6. 9
7. 2
8. 3
9. $1\frac{1}{2}$
10. $2\frac{1}{3}$
11. $5\frac{5}{8}$
12. $3\frac{1}{2}$
13. $5\frac{3}{7}$
14. $7\frac{5}{7}$
15. $6\frac{1}{3}$
16. $1\frac{1}{4}$
17. $3\frac{2}{3}$
18. $1\frac{2}{3}$
19. $18\frac{1}{3}$
20. $6\frac{1}{4}$
21. $4\frac{3}{5}$
22. $5\frac{1}{4}$
23. $13\frac{1}{3}$
24. $6\frac{9}{11}$
25. $3\frac{1}{9}$

Exercise 3
1. $\frac{22}{9}$
2. $\frac{7}{17}$
3. $\frac{15}{2}$
4. $\frac{23}{3}$
5. $\frac{13}{2}$
6. $\frac{22}{5}$
7. $\frac{61}{8}$
8. $\frac{53}{5}$
9. $\frac{57}{8}$
10. $\frac{52}{5}$
11. $\frac{44}{5}$
12. $\frac{17}{3}$
13. $\frac{34}{5}$
14. $\frac{31}{8}$
15. $\frac{93}{10}$
16. $\frac{25}{4}$
17. $\frac{35}{6}$
18. $\frac{38}{9}$
19. $\frac{48}{5}$
20. $\frac{202}{25}$

21. $\frac{407}{100}$
22. $\frac{55}{7}$
23. $\frac{11}{2}$
24. $\frac{30}{7}$
25. $\frac{91}{4}$

Exercise 4
1. $\frac{3}{49}$
2. $\frac{9}{10}$
3. $\frac{3}{25}$
4. $\frac{7}{10}$
5. $\frac{2}{5}$
6. $\frac{2}{7}$
7. $\frac{6}{7}$
8. $\frac{4}{5}$
9. $\frac{3}{125}$
10. $\frac{9}{15}$
11. $\frac{1}{100}$
12. $\frac{1}{125}$
13. $\frac{2}{5}$
14. $\frac{3}{50}$
15. $\frac{1}{6}$
16. $\frac{3}{5}$
17. $\frac{3}{24}$
18. $\frac{1}{75}$
19. $\frac{1}{150}$
20. $\frac{3}{10}$
21. $\frac{9}{70}$
22. $\frac{1}{125}$
23. $\frac{1}{150}$
24. $\frac{1}{200}$
25. $\frac{1}{12}$
26. $\frac{3}{150}$
27. $\frac{8}{9}$
28. $\frac{3}{10}$
29. $\frac{4}{5}$
30. $\frac{4}{5}$
31. $\frac{5}{9}$
32. $\frac{5}{6}$
33. $\frac{1}{25}$
34. $\frac{3}{10}$
35. $\frac{7}{9}$
36. $\frac{3}{50}$

Exercise 5
1. $1\frac{22}{27}$
2. $\frac{9}{32}$
3. $2\frac{1}{32}$
4. $1\frac{23}{40}$
5. $2\frac{9}{32}$
6. $8\frac{59}{72}$
7. $73\frac{37}{54}$
8. $1\frac{7}{45}$
9. $7\frac{1}{24}$
10. $132\frac{17}{40}$
11. $4\frac{1}{10}$
12. $51\frac{1}{2}$
13. $6\frac{53}{84}$
14. $47\frac{7}{12}$
15. $16\frac{41}{96}$
16. $16\frac{7}{8}$
17. $1\frac{4}{9}$
18. $17\frac{13}{24}$
19. $1\frac{37}{48}$
20. $1\frac{7}{32}$

Exercise 6
1. $\frac{5}{16}$
2. $\frac{3}{16}$
3. $\frac{1}{5}$
4. $\frac{7}{16}$
5. $\frac{17}{90}$
6. $\frac{3}{10}$
7. $1\frac{7}{24}$
8. $5\frac{19}{20}$
9. $5\frac{7}{15}$
10. $2\frac{11}{24}$
11. $\frac{3}{40}$
12. $4\frac{1}{8}$
13. $27\frac{13}{15}$
14. $12\frac{2}{3}$
15. $10\frac{3}{5}$
16. $10\frac{1}{4}$
17. $3\frac{1}{6}$
18. $11\frac{7}{36}$
19. $28\frac{1}{2}$
20. $17\frac{1}{12}$
21. $44\frac{9}{10}$
22. $48\frac{3}{50}$
23. $57\frac{23}{60}$
24. $24\frac{7}{10}$
25. $13\frac{1}{2}$

Exercise 7
1. $\frac{1}{16}$
2. $\frac{14}{45}$
3. $\frac{5}{18}$
4. $\frac{5}{48}$
5. $\frac{3}{40}$
6. $\frac{1}{3}$
7. $\frac{3}{8}$
8. $\frac{1}{6}$
9. $\frac{5}{18}$
10. $\frac{16}{45}$
11. $\frac{3}{16}$
12. $\frac{7}{250}$
13. $\frac{6}{25}$
14. $10\frac{5}{9}$
15. $30\frac{5}{24}$
16. $6\frac{3}{32}$
17. $16\frac{19}{32}$
18. $72\frac{4}{25}$
19. $7\frac{2}{9}$
20. 99
21. $177\frac{47}{64}$
22. $176\frac{1}{24}$
23. $5\frac{179}{392}$
24. $773\frac{1}{2}$
25. $1429\frac{7}{8}$

Exercise 8
1. 1
2. $\frac{9}{20}$
3. $\frac{1}{70}$
4. $1\frac{3}{7}$
5. $\frac{2}{3}$
6. $\frac{2}{3}$
7. $\frac{1}{75}$
8. $\frac{5}{12}$
9. $\frac{4}{5}$
10. $\frac{25}{93}$
11. 2

12. $\frac{3}{10}$
13. $1\frac{41}{85}$
14. $\frac{25}{64}$
15. $\frac{1}{3}$
16. $\frac{1}{30}$
17. $8\frac{2}{3}$
18. $14\frac{16}{21}$
19. $5\frac{1}{18}$
20. $\frac{39}{112}$
21. $17\frac{5}{7}$
22. 33
23. $\frac{38}{57}$
24. $2\frac{2}{13}$
25. $1\frac{17}{28}$

Chapter 3
Exercise 1
1. Four tenths
2. Three tenths
3. Six hundredths
4. One thousandth or one one-thousandth
5. One hundredth or one one-hundredth
6. Nine tenths
7. Seven and twenty-three hundredths
8. Three and five hundredths
9. Two and forty-two hundredths
10. One and seventy-five hundredths
11. Fifteen thousandths
12. Five tenths

Exercise 2
1. 4.5
2. 5.4
3. 6.4
4. 7.2
5. 2.5
6. 10.9
7. 9.8
8. 3.3
9. 7.6
10. 14.1
11. 8.7
12. 5.1
13. 7.35
14. 5.13
15. 8.58
16. 4.57
17. 9.35
18. 11.42
19. 2.54
20. 6.11
21. 10.20
22. 3.50
23. 4.44
24. 1.75
25. 0.33
26. 0.67

Exercise 3
1. 0.1
2. 0.005
3. 0.375
4. 0.6
5. 0.28
6. 0.007
7. 0.06
8. 0.03
9. 0.875
10. 0.2
11. 0.857
12. 0.02
13. 0.9
14. 0.6
15. 0.12
16. 0.5
17. 0.8
18. 0.625
19. 0.02
20. 0.75
21. 0.7
22. 0.889
23. 0.833
24. 0.16
25. 0.4

Exercise 4
1. $\frac{1}{10}$
2. $\frac{1}{4}$
3. $\frac{3}{25}$
4. $\frac{7}{20}$
5. $\frac{13}{20}$
6. $\frac{4}{5}$
7. $2\frac{1}{2}$
8. $\frac{1}{25}$
9. $\frac{2}{5}$
10. $\frac{3}{4}$
11. $\frac{3}{20}$
12. $\frac{22}{25}$
13. $\frac{3}{50}$
14. $1\frac{1}{2}$
15. $\frac{1}{5}$
16. $5\frac{116}{125}$
17. $\frac{18}{25}$
18. $\frac{9}{10}$
19. $\frac{6}{25}$
20. $\frac{3}{8}$
21. $\frac{33}{500}$
22. $\frac{1}{1000}$
23. $\frac{1}{5000}$
24. $\frac{1}{2000}$
25. $\frac{1}{125}$

Exercise 5
1. 32.755
2. 59.3
3. 39.5
4. 29.4
5. 22.627
6. 27.1401
7. 52.442
8. 0.31
9. 26.713
10. 311.837
11. 11.275
12. 5.314
13. 9.315
14. 67.303
15. 110.364
16. 32.775
17. 154.695
18. 22.15
19. 91.843
20. 9.424
21. 48.186
22. 13.2303
23. 11.016
24. 19.511
25. 21.755

Exercise 6
1. 47.294
2. 1.5
3. 333.838
4. 2.875
5. 3.6
6. 3.13
7. 2.7
8. 45.1
9. 3.17
10. 7.83
11. 2.72
12. 80.78
13. 17.64
14. 15.2
15. 24.75
16. 376.5
17. 26.75
18. 18.21
19. 3.11
20. 5.12
21. 264.9

22. 16.55
23. 85.665
24. 3.13
25. 3.518

Exercise 7
1. a. 60
   b. 600
   c. 6000
2. a. 0.5
   b. 5
   c. 50
3. a. 8
   b. 80
   c. 800
4. a. 0.05
   b. 0.5
   c. 5
5. a. 7
   b. 70
   c. 700
6. a. 2
   b. 20
   c. 200
7. a. 0.01
   b. 0.1
   c. 1
8. a. 0.3
   b. 3
   c. 30
9. a. 14.3
   b. 143
   c. 1430
10. a. 0.1
    b. 1
    c. 10

Exercise 8
1. 0.38
2. 291.816
3. 1.35
4. 8.375
5. 120
6. 31.132
7. 287.5
8. 46.2
9. 3.645
10. 64.12
11. 0.924
12. 5.6
13. 279
14. 0.0054

15. 0.001286
16. 27.6
17. 613.534
18. 5.152
19. 85.14
20. 56.012
21. 197.106
22. 193.18
23. 0.04588
24. 6.0
25. 10678.2

Exercise 9
1. 0.75
2. 7.273
3. 5
4. 2
5. 20
6. 3.231
7. 8
8. 1.5
9. 13.714
10. 10
11. 0.92
12. 2.574
13. 0.096
14. 0.02
15. 8.023
16. 4.306
17. 1500
18. 50
19. 5
20. 0.08
21. 0.334
22. 2.592
23. 0.503
24. 1.2
25. 0.002

Exercise 10
1. 0.25
2. 0.75
3. 0.5
4. 0.756
5. 0.85
6. 0.12
7. 0.8
8. 0.6
9. 0.75
10. 0.3
11. 0.75
12. 1.75

13. 0.015
14. 0.025
15. 0.01
16. 0.05
17. 0.65
18. 0.012
19. 0.002
20. 0.064
21. 0.325
22. 0.025
23. 0.45
24. 0.025

Chapter 4
Exercise 1
1. 0.45
2. 0.5
3. 0.99
4. 0.02
5. 0.25
6. 0.14
7. 0.82
8. 0.07
9. 0.05
10. 0.32

Exercise 2
1. 80%
2. 25%
3. 12.5 or $12\frac{1}{2}$%
4. 250%
5. 50%
6. 45.9 or $45\frac{9}{10}$%
7. 10%
8. 15%
9. 345%
10. 1.5 or $1\frac{1}{2}$%
11. 52%
12. 28%
13. 470%
14. 75%
15. 19%
16. 720%
17. 3.8%
18. 12%
19. 324.6 or $324\frac{3}{5}$%

20. 0.8 or $\frac{4}{5}$%
21. 30%
22. 7.5 or $7\frac{1}{2}$%
23. 6.5 or $6\frac{1}{2}$%
24. 0.6 or $\frac{3}{5}$%
25. 1760%

Exercise 3
1. 3
2. 18.85
3. 70
4. 57.96
5. 146.25
6. 234
7. 32
8. 165.74
9. 3
10. 32.045

Chapter 5
Exercise 1
1. $\frac{1}{50}$
2. $\frac{1}{25}$
3. $\frac{2}{5}$
4. $7\frac{27}{100}$
5. $\frac{1}{2}$
6. $\frac{1}{2}$
7. 0
8. $1\frac{5}{46}$
9. $2\frac{2}{15}$
10. $\frac{1}{10}$
11. $\frac{4}{25}$
12. $2\frac{17}{44}$
13. 0.39
14. 8.93
15. 80.725

16. 4.875
17. 1.8
18. 5.7
19. 11.7
20. 30
21. 30
22. 0.863
23. 2.0
24. 11.76

Exercise 2
Decimals:
1. 0.06
2. 0.1
3. 0.75
4. 0.27
5. 0.045
6. 0.3
7. 0.12
8. 0.15
9. 0.5
10. 0.096
11. 0.0005
12. 0.2
13. 0.8
14. 0.00005

Fractions:
1. $\frac{3}{50}$
2. $\frac{1}{10}$
3. $\frac{3}{4}$
4. $\frac{27}{100}$
5. $\frac{9}{200}$
6. $\frac{3}{10}$
7. $\frac{3}{25}$
8. $\frac{3}{20}$
9. $\frac{1}{2}$
10. $\frac{12}{125}$
11. $\frac{1}{2000}$
12. $\frac{1}{5}$
13. $\frac{4}{5}$
14. $\frac{1}{20,000}$

Chapter 6
Exercise 1
1. 1:3
2. 3:4
3. 3:4
4. 3:5
5. 1:2
6. 2:5
7. 9:25
8. 1:2
9. 7:8
10. 37:46
11. 5:9
12. 2:3
13. 2:25
14. 1:4
15. 3:4
16. 1:10
17. 1:2
18. 7:100
19. 3:5
20. 1:50
21. 9:20
22. 3:100
23. 9:100
24. 1:25
25. 9:100
26. 2:5
27. 1:5000
28. 1:125
29. 9:1000
30. 1:250
31. 7:100
32. 1:20
33. 1:10
34. 3:5000
35. 1:200
36. 17:400

Exercise 2
1. 1
2. 18
3. 11
4. 170
5. 6
6. 4.8
7. 1.8
8. 0.5
9. 0.36
10. 1.92
11. 3
12. 4
13. 1.5
14. 20
15. 2
16. 0.25
17. 15
18. 1
19. 1.2
20. 0.25
21. 0.67
22. 1.5
23. 7.5
24. 6.67
25. 0.5

Unit 1 Posttest
1. XLVI
2. CXXXII
3. XXVII
4. XIV
5. 8
6. 29
7. 91
8. 15
9. 30
10. 21
11. 32
12. 60
13. $11\frac{1}{2}$
14. $14\frac{2}{3}$
15. 4
16. $2\frac{10}{17}$
17. $\frac{27}{8}$
18. $\frac{133}{9}$
19. $\frac{5}{6}$
20. $\frac{7}{8}$
21. $\frac{2}{5}$
22. $1\frac{7}{24}$
23. $1\frac{13}{40}$
24. 1.525
25. 16.6613
26. $\frac{2}{15}$
27. $\frac{1}{2}$
28. 25.52
29. 10
30. $\frac{1}{4}$
31. $13\frac{2}{3}$
32. ratio 3:4, percentage 75, decimal 0.75
33. fraction $\frac{5}{100}$ or $\frac{1}{20}$, ratio 5:100 or 1:20, decimal 0.05
34. 7.52
35. 0.06
36. 28
37. $7\frac{7}{8}$
38. 48
39. $\frac{1}{5}$ or 0.2
40. 20
41. 15
42. 0.9
43. 0.04
44. 5
45. $\frac{1}{60}$
46. 48
47. 2
48. 0.06 or $\frac{3}{50}$
49. $\frac{1}{60}$
50. 38.636 or 38.64

Unit II Pretest

1. 1000
2. 1000
3. 1000
4. 1000
5. 1
6. 1
7. c
8. a
9. b
10. milligram
11. centimeter
12. microgram
13. kilogram
14. milliliter
15. gram
16. millimeter
17. liter
18. meter
19. 4
20. 5500
21. 0.02
22. 10
23. 4.5
24. 0.325
25. 75
26. 0.004
27. 1.5
28. 2,752,000
29. 5
30. 800
31. ℥
32. C
33. gr
34. ♏
35. O
36. lb
37. ʒ
38. L
39. 8
40. 45
41. 900 or 1000
42. $\frac{2}{5}$ or 0.4
43. 81.8
44. 2
45. 2
46. $\frac{1}{6}$
47. 500
48. 30
49. 45
50. 176
51. 16
52. 1
53. 36
54. 1
55. 1800 or 2000
56. 20
57. 99
58. 45
59. 4 or $4\frac{1}{5}$
60. 50
61. 4
62. 12.5
63. 2
64. 69
65. 2.2
66. 3.6
67. 30
68. 39.4
69. 450
70. 32
71. 0.48
72. 8
73. 18
74. 78.8
75. 180
76. 100
77. 39.1
78. 100.8
79. 37.2
80. 97.9
81. 93.3
82. 104
83. $\frac{3}{5}$ or $\frac{1}{2}$
84. 20 (or 16)
85. 15 or 16
86. iv
87. viii
88. xxx
89. 75
90. 60

91. 1 ounce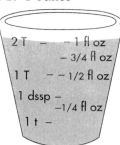

92. 4 fluidrams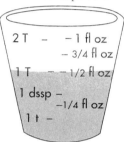

93. 1 tablespooon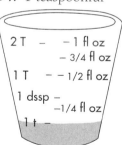

94. 1 teaspoonful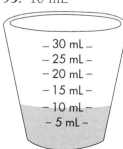

95. 10 mL

96. 5 cc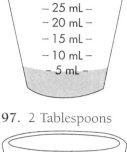

97. 2 Tablespoons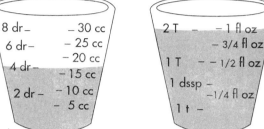

98. 2 drams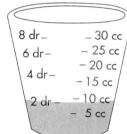

99. $\frac{1}{2}$ ounce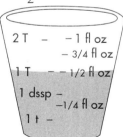

100. 25 mL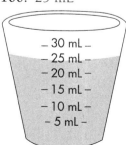

Chapter 7

Exercise 1
1. 320
2. 0.5
3. 2000
4. 500
5. 120
6. 1500
7. 32
8. 10,000
9. 100
10. 16
11. 4000
12. 600
13. 250
14. 1.5
15. 40

Exercise 2
1. 0.06
2. 0.05
3. 0.64
4. 0.008
5. 2.2
6. 0.027
7. 0.2
8. 0.006
9. 0.01
10. 0.25
11. 0.016
12. 0.012
13. 0.075
14. 0.335
15. 0.0048

Exercise 3
1. 200
2. 0.0005
3. 3000
4. 500
5. 1000
6. 0.04
7. 5
8. 0.008
9. 0.06
10. 5000
11. 0.02
12. 600
13. 0.5
14. 0.03
15. 0.025
16. 250
17. 0.015
18. 1.24
19. 1200
20. 0.0001
21. 3
22. 0.00008
23. 5700
24. 0.4
25. 2.5
26. 1.5
27. 2000
28. 0.001

Exercise 4
1. 15
2. 0.2
3. 450
4. 0.005
5. 10
6. 500
7. 1000
8. 0.04
9. 2
10. 1
11. 50
12. 0.03
13. 20
14. 0.25
15. 750
16. 0.02
17. 0.3
18. 4000
19. 900
20. 100
21. 0.25

Exercise 5
1. $\frac{1}{8}$
2. 60
3. 4
4. 2
5. 6
6. 64
7. 1
8. 8
9. 16
10. 16
11. 0.25 or $\frac{1}{4}$
12. 1
13. 0.5 or $\frac{1}{2}$
14. 128
15. 0.25 or ($\frac{1}{4}$ avoirdupois)
16. 0.5 or $\frac{1}{2}$
17. 6
18. 60
19. 0.5 or $\frac{1}{2}$
20. 120

Exercise 6
1. 8
2. 30
3. 1
4. 16
5. $\frac{1}{2}$ or 0.5
6. 2
7. 60
8. $\frac{3}{8}$ or 0.375
9. $1\frac{1}{2}$
10. 36 or (48 avoirdupois)
11. 4 or ($5\frac{1}{3}$ avoirdupois)
12. 90
13. 0.5 or $\frac{1}{2}$
14. 12
15. $\frac{2}{3}$ or ($\frac{1}{2}$ avoirdupois)
16. 4
17. $\frac{3}{4}$ or 0.75
18. 0.33 or $\frac{1}{3}$ or (0.25 or $\frac{1}{4}$ avoirdupois)
19. $\frac{1}{4}$
20. 360

Exercise 7
1. ℥
2. C or gal
3. gr
4. ♏
5. ʒ
6. O or pt.
7. lb
8. qt

Exercise 8
1. ounce
2. gallon
3. liter
4. minim
5. pint
6. pound
7. quart
8. pint
9. dram
10. grain
11. fluidounce
12. fluidram

Exercise 9
1. 15 or 16
2. 600
3. 8000
4. 15 or 16
5. 8
6. 0.227
7. 4
8. 300 or 325
9. 30
10. 1
11. 3150, 3178, 3182
12. 0.018 or 0.02
13. 59.09
14. 1440, 1500 or 1536
15. 10
16. 1200
17. 2
18. 1350 or 1440
19. 8
20. 4

Exercise 10
1. 1
2. xv or 15
3. $135\frac{3}{10}$
4. $\frac{2}{3}$
5. 30
6. viiss, $7\frac{1}{2}$ or $8\frac{1}{3}$
7. 0.4 or $\frac{2}{5}$
8. ii or 2
9. 90 or 100

10. xxx, 30, or $33\frac{1}{3}$
11. 165 or 167.67
12. 176
13. xxiiss or $22\frac{1}{2}$
14. $\frac{1}{2}$, $\frac{8}{15}$, or $\frac{12}{25}$
15. xxx or 30
16. 12.1 or 12.2
17. 1.5 or 1.7
18. 5.5 or $5\frac{1}{2}$
19. $\frac{1}{4}$ or $\frac{4}{15}$
20. 90 or 100

Chapter 8
Exercise 1
1. 15 or 12
2. 1
3. 1
4. 0.06
5. i or 1
6. ii or 2
7. 1
8. 40
9. viii or 8
10. 45 or 50
11. ii or 2 or $1\frac{7}{8}$
12. ss or $\frac{1}{2}$
13. $\frac{1}{4}$ or .25
14. 10 or 8
15. 0.8 or 1
16. 0.0625 or $\frac{1}{16}$
17. xvi or 16
18. 2
19. viii or 8
20. $\frac{3}{4}$ or .75
21. 1 or $\frac{4}{5}$
22. 2
23. 1
24. 0.25 or $\frac{1}{4}$
25. 30
26. $\frac{1}{30}$
27. i or 1
28. 30 or $37\frac{1}{2}$
29. 4 or $3\frac{1}{5}$
30. iv or 4

Exercise 2
1. a. 1 tablespoon

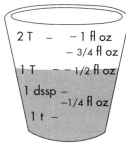

b. 4 fluidrams

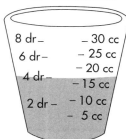

c. 15 cc

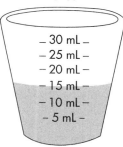

d. 15 mL

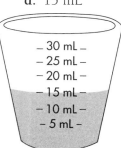

2. a. 1 teaspoonful

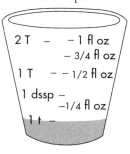

b. 5 cc

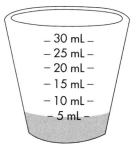

c. 5 mL

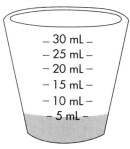

3. 2 fluidrams

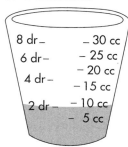

4. 10 mL

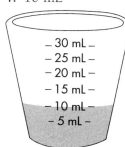

5. a. 2 tablespoonfuls

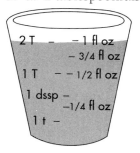

b. 8 fluidrams

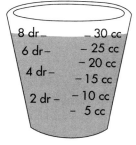

c. 15 mL

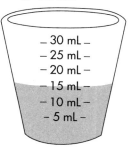

6. 1 dessert spoonful

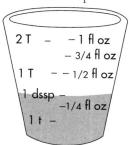

7. a. $\frac{3}{4}$ fluidounce

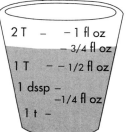

b. 6 fluidrams

Chapter 9
Exercise 1
1. 40
2. 18
3. 2
4. 1000
5. 4
6. 400
7. 180
8. 0.24
9. 6
10. 1500
11. 2
12. 50
13. 50
14. 100
15. 420
16. 132.7
17. 55
18. 5
19. 30
20. 572.5
21. (a) 2.5, (b) 2
22. 20
23. decrease
24. 340
25. 5
26. 30
27. (a) 1
    (b) lesser

Exercise 2
1. 25
2. 4
3. 135
4. 270
5. 236.4 or 240
6. 4
7. 2.7
8. 5
9. 1
10. 10
11. 2
12. 15
13. 4.8
14. 275.8
15. 8
16. 21.875
17. 6.6
18. 1.8
19. 0.56
20. 50
21. 1500
22. 22
23. 375
24. 118.2
25. 1.36
26. (a) 185
    (b) 1.85 or 1.88
27. 162.5
28. 52.5
29. 2.5
30. 3.75
31. 30
32. (a) increasing
    (b) 82.5
33. 0.6
34. 66.6
35. 800 or 833
36. 88 or 91.67
37. 155
38. (a) 4.375, (b) 7.5,
    (c) 3.125 or $3\frac{1}{8}$
39. 3.52 or 3.66
40. 3.6
41. 6.25
42. 28

Chapter 10
1. 98.9 or 99 F
2. 37.1 C
3. 100.8 F
4. 38.6 C
5. 99.7 F
6. 37.9 C
7. 98.2 F
8. 38.9 C
9. 103.3 F
10. 39.2 C
11. 102.9 F
12. 36.7 C
13. 104 F
14. 36.2 C
15. 101.1 F
16. 39.9 C
17. 100.4 F
18. 37.7 C
19. 99.3 F
20. 38.1 C
21. 103.6 F
22. 37.2 C
23. 103.6 F
24. 39.4 C
25. 96.8 F
26. 38.2 C
27. 100 F
28. 37.6 C
29. 102 F
30. 37.3 C

Unit II Posttest
1. 0.002
2. 2000
3. 4
4. 0.01
5. 15
6. 750
7. 400
8. 0.6 or $\frac{3}{5}$
9. 0.003
10. 30
11. 32
12. 76 or (96 avoirdupois)
13. 30
14. 16
15. 1
16. 1
17. $\frac{1}{2}$
18. 8
19. 150
20. 480
21. 0.05
22. 0.34
23. 54.54
24. 3.409 or 3.41
25. 300, $333\frac{1}{3}$, or 333.33
26. 600
27. 20
28. 3
29. 90 or 100
30. 77 or 77.78
31. 30 or 33.33
32. 52.5 or $52\frac{1}{2}$
33. iii or 3
34. 1
35. 7.5, $7\frac{1}{2}$, or 8.33
36. iv or 4
37. 1
38. $1\frac{1}{2}$
39. 5
40. xxx or 30
41. 45
42. 4000
43. 250
44. 0.74
45. 4
46. 30 or 31.25
47. 4.4
48. 42.5
49. 38.9
50. 101.12 or 101.1
51. 39.4
52. 100.76 or 100.8
53. a. 140 b. 1400
54. a. 6.25 b. 10
    c. 3.75
55. 3
56. a. 15 or 16 b. 4
57. a. i b. 30 or 32
58. a. 2500
    b. 1.56 or 1.6
59. a. 1080
    b. 2.16 or 2.2
60. a. 3409
    b. 3.375 or 3.4

Unit III Pretest

1. Right patient, right drug, right dosage, right time, right route of administration, right to accurate documentation, right to knowledge about prescribed drug therapy, and right to refuse medication.
2. Check the agency's written policies.
3. a. Continues in effect until cancelled.
   b. Drug is to be given when necessary, but not more often than prescribed; is a type of standing order.
   c. Is to be given one time only.
   d. Order is to be carried out immediately and only once unless specified otherwise.
   e. A written document stating physician's orders that can be carried out within the agency without first notifying the physician.
4. a. These are medications that are available for emergency use.
   b. Containers of multiple doses; each dose must be measured by the health provider.
   c. An amount of drug that supplies one dose.
5. Variations of the computerized unit dose system are used. Each dose of medicine is prepared by the pharmacy and dispensed to the health care unit. This may be done using a special conveyor system or a special drug cart.
6. a. 12 mg
   b. 3 tablets
   c. 60 mL
   d. 3000 U
7. Ask physician to clarify orders—how often and under what circumstances is the drug to be given?
8. a. qid
   b. q4h
   c. prn, sos
   d. pc
   e. ac
   f. bid
   g. stat
9. a. Take one 20 mg tablet of simvastatin (Zocor) every day with evening meal.
   b. Take 600 mg calcium carbonate orally twice a day with lunch and dinner.
   c. Take 10 mg thioridazine (Mellaril) every day at bedtime.
10. a. 0800
    b. 2130
    c. 1715
11. a. Benadryl
    b. Diphenhydramine hydrochloride
    c. Capsule
    d. 50 mg per capsule
    e. 1 capsule 3 to 4 times/day or as directed by physician
    f. Orally
    g. Parke-Davis
12. Recheck medications to be sure that the correct medications and dose have been prepared for 8 AM.
13. Verify when patient last received medication by checking chart; use information on records such as medication administration record, medication card, computerized envelope, or kardex to identify patient, drug and dose and for recording drug, check patients identification bracelets for name, room number, allergies, ask patient to state name. In some agencies, a picture of patient may be used for identification.
14. Name of drug, dose given, time given, route of administration, legal name or initials of person administering drug.
15. Medication administration record
16. a. Darryl Foster, 37 years old, Room 501
    b. Dr. Donalds
    c. Phenobarbital
    d. Prednisone, no dose given, orally, every day at 9 AM and furosemide (Lasix), 10 mg orally, given immediately (once only) at 5:30 AM
    e. CT at 9 AM on February 10
17. Name of medication; reasoning for taking it; expected effects and common side effects of the medication; how to contact physician, if necessary; times or circumstances for taking medication; amount of drug to take; how to administer drug; what to do if a dose is forgotten or omitted for health reasons.
18. 8 AM, 3 PM, or 10 PM or 0800, 1500, 2100
19. a. 0.125 mg/tab
    b. 1
    c. 7

20. a. 5200
    b. 1300
    c. 4
    d. 2
    e. 25
    f. 50
    g. Never crush or dissolve. The coating keeps the medicine from dissolving in the stomach. It will be absorbed after it passes through the stomach. Crushing the tablets will let the aspirin inside them come in contact with the stomach and may cause Mr. Swurasky to feel "sick" to his stomach.
21. Because the Procardia XL acts over a long time, it will relieve his symptoms much longer. Taking the regular tablets as he suggested will give him a very high dose initially and cause serious problems that may be much more costly than not using the 20 mg capsules. Tell him to destroy the 20 mg capsules.
22. a. 4000
    b. 1000
    c. 500
    d. 2
    e. 8
23. Use one 1 mg tablet + one 0.5 mg tablet
24. One 60 mg tablet
25. 90 or 100
26. a. 0.3
    b. Amount is very small, manufacturer suggests disguising taste with milk or orange juice. Note that some disagree with using these because patient may develop a dislike for them.
27. 10 mL
28. a. 3
    b. 500 mg
    c. 6
29. Place 9 g of NaCl in a measure. Fill to 1000 mL with water.
30. Humulin BR
31. Regular
32. a. f

b.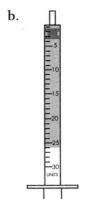
    c. a
    d. g
    e. a, d, g
33. a. Lilly
    b. NPH
    c. Iletin II
    d. Purified beef
    e. 100 U/mL
34. a. Regular, velosulin
    b. NPH, Lente
    c. Ultralente
35. a. 5 % dextrose in water
    b. Isotonic
    c. 3000 mL or 3 L
    d. Yes, 40 mEq Kcl/L
    e. 6 AM
    f. Yes, 24 h
    g. No
    h. 1 L or 1000 mL
    i. 20.8 or 21
    j. 125

36.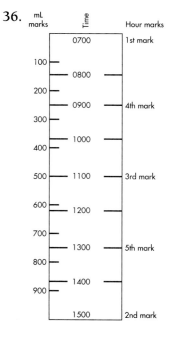

37. a. 125
    b. 31.25 or 31
    c. 156
38. a. 4.1 or 4
    b. 0.4
    c. 25
39. KO, TKO, KVO
40. a. 100
    b. 100
    c. 16.6 or approximately 17
41. a. 750
    b. 30
42. Policy and/or procedure manual
43. Hospital formulary, Physicians Desk Reference, or package insert
44. 4000
45. 12 mL
46. 48,000
47. If 1 mL or less, use a tuberculin syringe; if more than 1 mL use a regular syringe. Do *not* use insulin syringe because it is designed to measure insulin only.
48. 10,000 U/mL
49.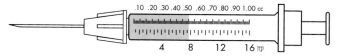
50. 0.2 mg
51. 300

52. a. 65 kg
    b. 0.25 mg/mL
    c. 250 mcg/mL
    d. 195 mcg/kg/min
    e. 0.78 mL/min
    f. 44.8 or 45 mL/h
53. a. 1500
    b. 375 mg
    c. Erythromycin (EryPed 400)
    d. 4.687 or 4.7 mL of erythromycin (EryPed 400)
54. a. 150
    b. 1.875 or 1.9 of EryPed 400 or 3.75 of EryPed 200
    c. 7.5 or 7.6 mL of EryPed 400 or 15 mL EryPed 200
55. a. 25.8
    b. 774 to 1032
    c. 387 to 516
    d. 193.5 to 258
    e. 1800-0200-1000
56. a. 35
    b. 0.7
    c. Use a syringe
57. a. 22
    b. 0.848 or 0.85
    c. 325
    d. 1
58. 216.67
59. 295 mg
60. Young's is higher and Clark's is lower.
61. Physiologic changes occur with age; may be more sensitive to drugs and changes in diet and health.
62. Gastrointestinal disturbances, expected effects do not occur, unexpected effects occur, motor incoordination, depression of central nervous system.
63. Often elderly take many drugs, misuse of drugs, self-medication.
64. Allows checking for incompatibility of prescribed drugs, correct dose.
65. Regimen is too complex or doesn't fit with lifestyle, unpleasant effects of the medicines, cost of the medicine, problems obtaining drug such as transportation, inability to read and/or understand directions on label, inability to open container or remove medication from it.

66. Possible points to include in a teaching plan:
    - Name of each medication
    - Amount of medication
    - Whether to take with food or milk
    - Specific times to take
    - Which medications can be taken at the same time
    - Reasons why not to take a dose of medicine
    - What to do if a dose is forgotten
    - How to store medicines
    - Can prescription be refilled?
    - How, when, and why to contact physician
    - Ways to remember to take medicine
67. Where it's stored and if it's stored appropriately away from heat, light, moisture. Note that supply of some drugs may require refrigeration.
68. Over the counter drug.
69. Clarify order with prescribing physician.
70. That she must not omit medication. Even though she feels well, her blood pressure could be dangerously high.
71. Consult his physician and ask if fatigue is a side effect of the medication.
72. Read labels of all drugs carefully.
73. It is a small dose of medicine that is used to determine whether the patient is sensitive to the drug.
74. Carry identification card with this information, inform family and others, wear bracelet or necklace medallions that are engraved with this information, inform health care providers of allergies.
75. Person is likely to develop a dislike for milk and refuse to drink it.
76. Blood tests are needed to tell how much the medication is lowering cholesterol; whether a change in the dosage is needed.

Chapter 11
Exercise 1
1. 400 mg
2. 1.2 g
3. 30 mg
4. 600 mg
5. 10,000 U
6. 4 capsules
7. 12 tablets
8. 2 tablets
9. 3000 mL or 3L
10. 150 mL

Exercise 2
1. Give 10 mg morphine sulfate subcutaneously every 4 hours, when necessary or if needed, for abdominal pain.
2. Give 100 mg thiamine hydrochloride orally every day.
3. Give 125 thousandths mg of digoxin (Lanoxin) every day by mouth.
4. Give 1 grain of codeine sulfate by mouth every 4 hours, if necessary.
5. Give 2 grains of caffeine sodium benzoate, hypodermically.
6. Give one 10 mg bisacodyl (Dulcolax) suppository rectally, immediately (at once).
7. Give 10 mg furosemide (Lasix) intravenously, immediately.
8. Give 60 mg terfenadine (Seldane) orally twice a day.
9. Give 2 capsules of Charcocaps PO after meals. Repeat dose in ½ hour if necessary.
10. Give ½ grain of codeine suspension every 4 to 6 hours, if necessary.
11. Instill 1 g estrogen (Premarin Cream) vaginally twice a week.
12. Twice a day, cleanse lesion on right cheek with hydrogen peroxide (H_2O_2), then apply 2% erythromycin to lesion.
13. Give 20 milliequivalents potassium chloride orally, every morning after eating.
14. Instill one metered dose of beclomethasone (Vancenase) nasal spray twice a day.
15. Give a 300 mg tablet of ferrous sulfate orally twice a day with meals.
16. Give 25 mg nortriptyline capsule orally three times a day.
17. Give 1 tablet pancrelipase (Viokase) three times a day with meals.
18. Apply one 0.2 mg patch of nitroglycerin (Trans–derm-nitro), topically, every day. Remove after 12 hours.
19. Apply 5% acyclovir ointment topically three times a day to lesion on right leg.
20. Give 0.29 mL of cyclosporin solution orally with meals and in chocolate milk.
21. Instill 2% solution of homatropine hydrobomide ophthalmic solution into both eyes four times a day.

Exercise 3
1. 0920
   zero nine twenty hundred hours
2. 1630
   sixteen thirty hundred hours
3. 0315
   zero three fifteen hundred hours
4. 0645
   zero six forty-five hundred hours
5. 2020
   twenty twenty hundred hours
6. 0900 to 1900
   zero nine hundred hours to nineteen hundred hours
7. 0600 to 1800
   zero six hundred hours to eighteen hundred hours
8. 0800 to 1600
   zero eight hundred hours to sixteen hundred hours
9. 0700—1300—1900
   zero seven hundred hours—thirteen hundred hours—nineteen hundred hours
10. 0600—1200—1800—2400
    zero six hundred hours—twelve hundred hours—eighteen hundred hours—twenty-four hundred hours

Exercise 4
1. 1000
2. 1410
3. 0300
4. 1945
5. 0400
6. 1715

Exercise 5

Label	Trade name	Generic name	Dosage unit	Strength	Usual dose	Method of administration	Amount supplied in container
1		Codeine phosfate	Tablet	60 mg	30 mg	Orally*	100 tablets
2	Keflin	Cephalothin	mL	Depends on dilution	2 to 12 g daily	IM or for IV, see literature	2 g
3	Lanoxin	Digoxin	Tablets	125 mcg (0.125 mg)	Individualized*	Orally*	1000 tablets
4	Stelazine	Trifluoperazine	mL	10 mg/mL	6 to 40 mg daily	Orally	2f℥ (59 mL)
5		Phenobarbital	Tablets	30 mg tablet		Orally*	10 × 10 (100)
6	Fero-Gradumet	Ferrous sulfate	Tablets	525 mg tablet	1-2 tablets a day	Orally*	100 tablets
7	Slow-K	Potassium chloride	Extended-release capsule	8 mEq (600 mg) capsule	Varies	Orally*	100 tablets
8	Nembutal	Pentobarbital sodium	mL	100 mg/ 2 mL single dose ampule	100 mg	IM or IV	100 mg/ 2 mL
9	Pyridium	Phenoazopyrine HCl	Tablets	200 mg tablet	1 tablet 3 times a day	Orally*	100 tablets

*This information is not given on the label but would be found in the package insert and physician's order. Unless a drug is packaged in a sterile container, it is not intended for injection. Topical medications are never given orally.

7. 2214
8. 0817
9. 0242

Exercise 6
1. a. Darryl Foster
   b. 37
   c. 501
   d. Dr. Donalds
2. Prednisone
   Lasix
3. Both orally
4. Every day
5. Once
6. 2/8, 2/9, 2/10
7. 0900 or 9 AM
8. Immediately
9. 0530 or 5:30 PM
10. a. C.T.
    b. M.J.
11. a. Cathy Tag
    b. Mary Jones
12. Phenobarbital

Exercise 7
1. Codeine
2. a. L.T.
   b. B. Wilson RN
3. a. 2/6
   b. P. Little RN
   c. 0.25 mg
   d. Every day (1 x/da)
   e. Orally
   f. On 2/6 at 9:50 AM by P. Little.
      On 2/7 at 10 AM by P. Little.
      On 2/8 at 10 AM by P. Little.
4. a. 2/7
   b. D. Gail RN
   c. 40 mg
   d. Twice a day
   e. Orally
   f. on 2/7, given at 1545 or 3:45 PM by D. Gail RN
      on 2/8, given at 1010 or 10:10 AM by T. Sax RN
5. a. 2/7
   b. D. Gail RN
   c. 1 g
   d. Every 6 hours
   e. Intravenously

   f. 1215 or 12:15 PM by P. Little, RN
      18 (1800) or 6 PM by D. Gates RN
      2345 or 11:45 PM by D. Gates RN
   g. 06 or 6 AM by M. Doerrer RN
6. a. 2/8
   b. T. Sax RN
   c. 1000 and 2200 or 10 AM and 10 PM
   d. Topical
   e. OD or right eye
   f. 1010 or 10:10 AM by T. Sax RN

Exercise 8
1. a. 1.5 mL (cc)
   b. Intramuscularly
2. a. 1
   b. 0600-1400-2200 (6-2-10)
   c. Orally
3. a. 1
   b. Subcutaneously
4. a. One tablet phenobarbital, 30 mg
   b. Four times each day
   c. According to table 11-1, p. 136, 9-1-5-9
5. a. 1 capsule propoxyphene (Darvon), Plain, 32 mg
   b. Every 6 hours
6. a. 1 capsule propoxyphene (Darvon Compound-65)
   b. 3 hours
   c. As needed, when necessary
7. a. 1 mL
   b. Intravenous
   c. Immediately
   d. No
   e. Units
   f. Check policy manual, ask your employer or instructor
8. a. 1 caplet per dose
   b. 1000-1400-1800-2200 (6-12-6-12)
9. a. 10-2-4-8-10
   b. Add one dose at 7 AM or 7-10-2-4-8-10
10. a. Rectally
    b. Do not repeat this dose
    c. $7\frac{1}{2}$ grains
11. a. Drops
    b. Right
    c. Twice daily
    d. Ou

12. Antibiotic preparations are given at equally spaced time intervals to keep the blood level constant; this prevents organisms from developing resistance to antibiotic drugs and assists in the inhibition of their growth or the killing of the organisms. She can adjust the time she takes the first capsule each day to fit her schedule, as long as she maintains the necessary equal time intervals throughout the twenty-four hours.
13. a. Taking the drug at the time intervals prescribed is necessary to maintain the right amount of drug in the blood for controlling her symptoms. The physician will schedule blood tests periodically; these tests will enable the physician to regulate the dose of the drug.
    b. Planning with Susan allows her to determine the best times for her to take the medication without her usual pattern of daily activities. For example, if she usually arises at 8 AM, this would be a natural time for her to take her first dose of medication. However, if she prefers to take the second dose of medication at 7 PM and usually sleeps until 11 AM, she may decide that she prefers to take the first dose of medication at 7 AM because she finds it easy to go back to sleep. Multiple alternatives are possible; the important consideration is finding a schedule that is compatible with the requirements of the prescribed drug therapy and the preferences of the patient.
    c. To progress from total dependence on the nurse to independence through self-medication, a plan would be devised into which Susan has input. At first, the nurse might remind Susan that it is time to take her medication and ask that she come to the nurse's station to prepare and take each dose. Before her dismissal, Susan would be asked to demonstrate complete responsibility for her own drug therapy. The use of checklists and multiple opportunities to practice this responsibility allows for corrective teaching as well as for the development of self-confidence and good habits.
    d. The nurse usually takes this responsibility.
14. Considerations might include always making certain that she carries an adequate supply of medication with her when she plans to be away from home, carrying a copy of her prescription with her, telephoning her physician, or asking a physician in private practice or who is contacted through an emergency service to contact her physician so she may obtain an emergency supply of medication.
15. One alternative is that she might consider taking the drug only after eating, if she has previously been taking the drug without eating. Another alternative is to change the time schedule so that two capsules are taken each time, instead of three capsules. With the physician's approval, she might follow a time schedule that approximates 8-hour intervals.
16. One plan might be as follows: 7:30 AM—nefedipine (Procardia), isosorbide dinitrate (Isordil), atenolol (Tenormin), nitroglycerin (Trans-derm), and ducosate (Colace); 1 PM—Nefedipine, Isordil; 5 PM—Isordil; 10 PM—Nefedipine, Isordil. Other variations could be planned according to the time the patient usually awakens and retires.
17. a. one
    b. propoxyphene (Darvon N-100)
    c. every 3 to 4 hours as needed
18. If the medication wrapper has not been opened.
19. a. 1000
    b. 1600
    c. 2145
    d. 2400
    e. 3 AM
    f. 2 PM
    g. 10 PM
    h. 3:15 PM

Chapter 12
Exercise 1
1. a. 90 mg
   b. Three 30 mg capsules
   c. Nine 30 mg capsules
   d. Sixty-three 30 mg capsules

2. a. 250 mcg or 0.25 mg tablet
   b. One 250 mcg tablet
3. Two 325 mg tablets
4. a. 200 mg strength
   b. One 200 mg tablet
   c. 400 mg
5. a. 600 mg
   b. 600 mg
   c. Four 600 mg tablets
   d. One 600 mg tablet
6. a. 50 mcg (0.05 mg)
   b. One 50 mcg tablet
7. a. 10 mg tablet
   b. One 10 mg tablet
8. a. 25 mg
   b. 4
   c. 28
9. Two 30 mg capsules
10. a. 10 mg
    b. Two 10 mg tablets
11. a. 20 mg tablet
    b. One 20 mg tablet
12. a. 5 mg tablet
    b. One 5 mg tablet
13. a. 20 mg capsules
    b. 60 mg
    c. 90 capsules
14. No. The dose is the same, but the drug is released over time when the extended-release type tablet is used and is released more rapidly when nifedipine (Procardia) is used. He should obtain 30 mg tablets.
15. a. 1 mg tablet
    b. One 1 mg tablet
    c. 2 mg
16. a. 150 mg capsule
    b. 4 capsules
    c. 600 mg
17. a. Aspirin (Ecotrin), 325 mg
    b. One 325 mg tablet
18. a. Procainamide (Procan SR) 500 mg
    b. One 500 mg capsule
    c. 30 capsules
19. a. Acetaminophen (Regular Strength Tylenol), 325 mg
    b. Two 325 mg tablets
20. 1000 mg or 1 g

Exercise 2
1. a. 1000 mg
   b. Two 500 mg capsules
   c. Eight 500 mg capsules
2. a. Two 250 mg capsules
   b. Four 500 mg capsules
3. a. 500 mg capsule
   b. One 500 mg capsule
4. Four 250 mg capsules
5. a. Three 250 mg capsules
   b. Six 250 mg capsules
6. a. 500 mg capsule
   b. One 500 mg capsule
   c. Four 500 mg capsules
   d. Twenty 500 mg capsules
7. a. 50 mg tablet
   b. Two 50 mg tablets
   c. Six 50 mg tablets
   d. Sixty 50 mg tablets
8. a. 50 mcg or 0.05 mg tablet
   b. Two 50 mcg tablets
9. a. 250 mg capsule
   b. One 250 mg capsule
10. a. Sulfisoxazole (Gantrisin)
    b. 2 g
    c. Four 0.5 g tablets
    d. 160 tablets

Exercise 3
1. a. 4 mg
   b. Give one 4 mg tablet
2. One 6 mg tablet and one 4 mg tablet
3. a. 2 mg tablet and 5 mg tablet
   b. One 2 mg tablet and one 5 mg tablet
4. One 5 mg tablet, (b)
5. One 2 mg tablet and one 2½ mg tablet
6. a. 75 mg tablet and 150 mg tablet
   b. One 75 mg tablet and one 150 mg tablet
7. a. 25 mg tablet and 50 mg tablet
   b. One 25 mg tablet and one 50 mg tablet
8. a. 10 mg tablet and 25 mg tablet
   b. One 10 mg tablet and one 25 mg tablet
9. a. 50 mg tablet and 10 mg tablet
   b. One 50 mg tablet and one 10 mg tablet
10. a. 15 mg tablet and 30 mg tablet
    b. One 15 mg tablet and one 30 mg tablet

Exercise 4
1. 90 or 100 mg
2. 1 tablet
3. 0.6 mg
4. 1 tablet
5. 1 tablet
6. 3 tablets
7. 1 tablet
8. 2 tablets
9. 1 tablet
10. 1 capsule
11. 2 tablets
12. 1 tablet
13. 1 capsule
14. 1 tablet
15. 1 tablet
16. 2 tablets
17. 1 tablet
18. a. 200 mg tablet
    b. 1 tablet
19. 1 capsule
20. 1 tablet
21. 2 tablets

Chapter 13
Exercise 1
1. 8 mL
2. 3.6, 3.8, 3.9, or 4 mL
3. 5 mL
4. a. 20 mL
   b. 4 teaspoonfuls
   c. Six 500 mg doses
5. a. 10 mL
   b. Oral
   c.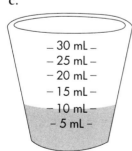
   d. 50
6. a. 60 mg
   b. 100 doses
   c. 25 days
7. a. 4 f℥
   b. 1 tablespoonful
   c. $\frac{1}{2}$ ounce
8. a. 90
   b. 90 mL
9. a. Use Penicillin V 250 mg (Pen-Vee K)
   b. 5 mL
10. 15 mL
11. 10 mL
12. a. 5 mg
    b. 3 tablets per day
    c. 7.5 mL
13. a. 20 mg capsule
    b. 10 mg capsule
    c. No
14. a. 0.3 mL
    b. See art
15. a. 15 mL
    b. 237 mL
16. 3 containers of lithium citrate 8 mEq lithium per 5 mL
17. a. 20 mL
    b. 4 teaspoonfuls (5 mL = 1 t)
    c. 6 doses (1 f℥ = 30 mL)
18. a. 30 mL
    b. 8 teaspoonfuls
    c. 2 doses
19. a. 0.6 mL
    b. See art
20. a. 20 mL
    b. 10 mL

Exercise 2
1. 2 mL
2. 3 mL
3.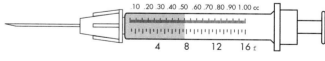
4. 0.5 mL
5. a. 1 mL
   b.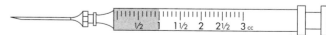

6. a. 1 mg/mL
   b. 1 mL
   c.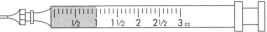
7. a. 0.4 mg/mL
   b. 0.5 mL
   c. 0.75 mL if 0.4 mg/mL
8. a. Codeine 30
   b. 1 mL
9. a. 0.5 mL
   b. 0.5 mL
10. a. 15 mg/mL
    b. 1 mL
11. a. 10 mg/mL
    b. 0.6 mL
12. a. 15 mg/mL
    b. 1 mL
13. a. 0.75 mL
    b.
14. a. 1 mg/mL
    b. 1 mL of 1 mg/mL
    c. 0.5 mL
15. a. 0.5 mL
    b. 0.2 mL
16. 1 mL (30 mg) unit dose
17. 1.5 mL (45 mg)
18. a. 0.5 mL
    b. 1 mL
19. a. 1 mL containing 1.5 mg/mL
    b. 1 mL

Exercise 3

1. a. 0.75
   b. 2.5 mL
   c. 0.75 mL
2. a. 1000
   b. 1 g

Chapter 14
Exercise 1
1. a. C
   b. Beef
   c. Short action
   d. See art

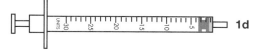

2. a. W
   b. Human
   c. Short
   d. See art
   e. External infusion pump

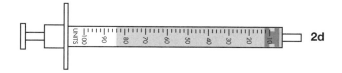

3. a. X
   b. Pork
   c. Intermediate action
   d. See art

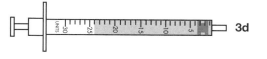

4. a. M
   b. Beef-pork
   c. Intermediate action
   d. See art

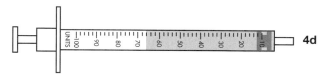

5. a. T
   b. Human
   c. Intermediate action
   d. See art

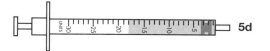

6. a. E
   b. Pork
   c. Short action
   d. See art

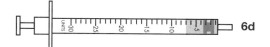

7. a. G
   b. Beef-Pork
   c. Long action
   d. See art

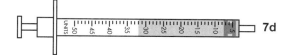

8. a. O
   b. Beef
   c. Long action
   d. See art

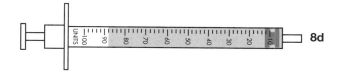

9. a. R
   b. Human
   c. Both short and intermediate action
   d. See art

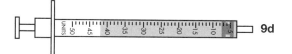

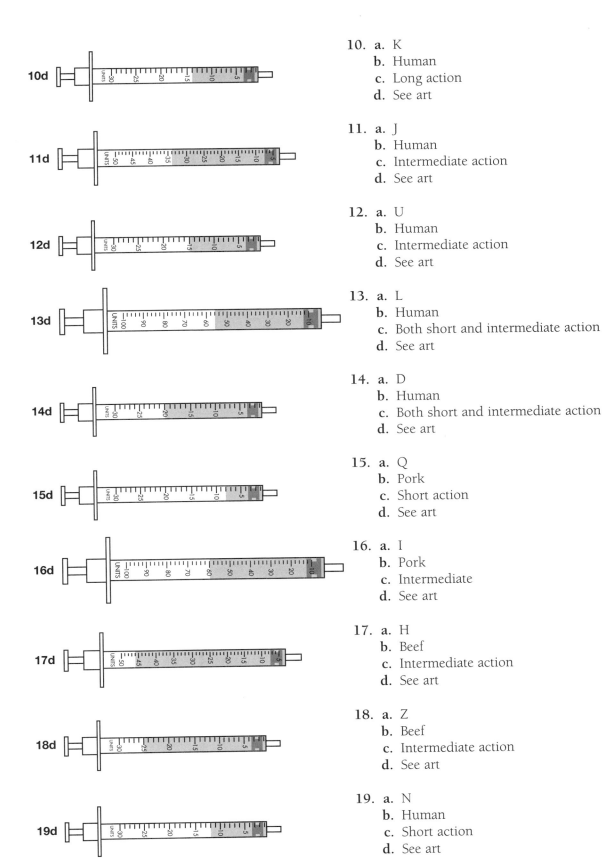

10. a. K
    b. Human
    c. Long action
    d. See art

11. a. J
    b. Human
    c. Intermediate action
    d. See art

12. a. U
    b. Human
    c. Intermediate action
    d. See art

13. a. L
    b. Human
    c. Both short and intermediate action
    d. See art

14. a. D
    b. Human
    c. Both short and intermediate action
    d. See art

15. a. Q
    b. Pork
    c. Short action
    d. See art

16. a. I
    b. Pork
    c. Intermediate
    d. See art

17. a. H
    b. Beef
    c. Intermediate action
    d. See art

18. a. Z
    b. Beef
    c. Intermediate action
    d. See art

19. a. N
    b. Human
    c. Short action
    d. See art

20. a. V
    b. Beef
    c. Intermediate action
    d. See art

21. a. F
    b. Beef
    c. Intermediate action
    d. See art

22. a. S
    b. Human
    c. Short action
    d. See art

23. a. P
    b. Pork
    c. Intermediate action
    d. See art

24. a. A
    b. Human
    c. Intermediate action
    d. See art

25. a. Y
    b. Human
    c. Both short and intermediate actions
    d. See art

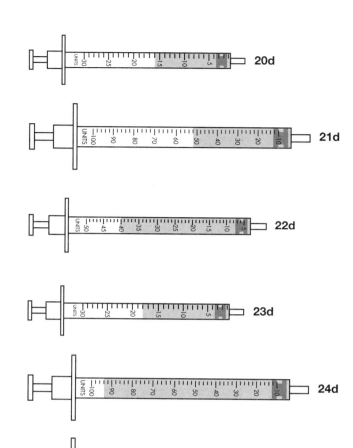

26. a. Humulin BR, Velosulin BR
    b. B, W
27. a. 0.6 mL

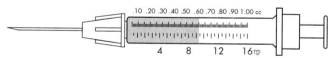

    b. 0.3 mL

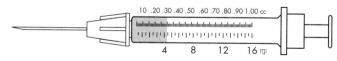

Chapter 15
Exercise 1
1. a. 5% dextrose in water
   b. Isotonic
   c. 1000 mL
   d. No
   e. 8 AM
   f. Yes, 8 hours
   g. No
2. a. 5% dextrose in water
   b. Isotonic
   c. 2000 mL
   d. No
   e. Postop
   f. Yes, 24 hours
   g. No
3. a. 5% dextrose in water
   b. Isotonic
   c. 100 mL
   d. Yes, 900 mg clindamycin
   e. Postsurgery
   f. 30 minutes
   g. q12h
   h. No
4. a. Ringer's lactate in 5% dextrose
   b. Hypertonic
   c. 1000 mL
   d. No
   e. 9 AM
   f. Yes, 8 hours
   g. No
5. a. 5% dextrose in 0.45% NaCl
   b. Hypertonic
   c. 1000 mL
   d. Yes, 20 mEq KCl
   e. Doesn't say
   f. Yes, 12 hours
   g. No
6. a. Lactated Ringer's solution in 5% dextrose
   b. Hypertonic
   c. 1000 mL
   d. No
   e. 1700 hours or 5 PM
   f. Yes, 8 hours
   g. No
7. a. Lactated Ringer's solution in 5% dextrose
   b. Hypertonic
   c. Amount needed to replace nasogastric output (mL/mL)
   d. No
   e. No time given (will depend upon schedule for monitoring urinary output)
   f. No
   g. No
8. a. 5% dextrose in water
   b. Isotonic
   c. 3000 mL
   d. Yes, 40 mEq KCl in each 1000 mL
   e. No time given
   f. Yes, 24 hours
   g. No
9. a. 0.45% NaCl
   b. Hypotonic
   c. 250 mL
   d. Yes, 2500 U heparin
   e. No time given
   f. No, not stated directly, but does this indirectly by giving rate
   g. Yes, 10 mL

Exercise 2
1. a. Lactated Ringer's in 5% dextrose in water
   b. Hypertonic
   c. 1000 mL
   d. No
   e. 1800 hours or 6 PM January 21
   f. Yes, until 2 AM on January 22
   g. Yes, 125 mL/h
2. a. 5% dextrose in 0.45% NaCl
   b. Hypertonic
   c. 1000 mL
   d. Yes, 20 mEq KCl
   e. 1830 or 6:30 PM on April 27
   f. Yes, until 0230 or 2:30 AM on April 28 or 8 hours
   g. No
3. a. 5% normal serum albumin
   b. 500 mL
   c. No
   d. 1300 hours or 1 PM on June 23
   e. Yes, stop at 1400 hours or 2 PM on June 23 (same day) = 1 hour
   f. Yes, 500 mL per hour, 8.3 mL/min

4. a. 0.9% NaCl
   b. Isotonic
   c. 50 mL
   d. Yes, 20 mg famotidine
   e. 1900 hours or 7 PM on May 4
   f. Yes, 15 minutes
   g. Yes, 200 mL/h or 3.3 mL/min
   h. Yes, (1) in 8 h (2) 2 times or 2 doses
5. a. 5% dextrose
   b. Isotonic
   c. 50 mL
   d. Yes, 1 g cefazolin (Ancef)
   e. 2100 hours or 9 PM
   f. Yes, 15 minutes
   g. Yes, 200 mL/h or 3.3 mL/minute (Note that $\frac{1}{4}$ of 200 is 50 mL and $\frac{1}{4}$ hour = 15 minutes)
6. a. 0.45% NaCl
   b. Hypotonic
   c. 250 mL
   d. Yes, 25,000 U heparin
   e. 0900 hours or 9 AM on September 18
   f. 0900 hours or 9 AM on September 19
   g. Yes, 24 hours
   h. Yes, 10 mL/h or 0.17 mL/min
7. a. 5% dextrose in water
   b. Isotonic
   c. 500 mL
   d. Yes, 10,000 U of heparin
   e. 1000 hours or 10 AM on December 23
   f. 1000 hours or 10 AM on December 14
   g. Yes, 10 hours
   h. Yes, 50 mL/h or 0.8 mL/min
8. a. 5% dextrose in water
   b. Isotonic
   c. 50 mL
   d. Yes, 1 g aztreonam
   e. 1100 hours or 11 AM on October 14
   f. 1 hour
   g. Yes, 100 mL/h or 1.7 mL/min
   h. Yes, every 12 hours
9. a. 5% dextrose in water
   b. Isotonic
   c. 50 mL
   d. Yes, 10 mg prochlorperazine
   e. 1100 hours or 11 AM on November 2
   f. 15 minutes
   g. Yes, 200 mL/h or 3.3 mL/min
   h. Order is "open" and is to be continued until stopped
10. a. 5% dextrose in water
    b. Isotonic
    c. 100 mL
    d. Yes, 500 mg vancomycin
    e. 1100 hours or 11 AM on November 2
    f. Yes, 1 hour
    g. Yes, 100 mL/h or 1.7 mL/min
    h. Undetermined

Exercise 3
1. 125 mL/h
2. 100 mL/h
3. 500 mL/h
4. 83.3 mL/h
5. 125 mL/h
6. 125 mL/h
7. 125 mL/h
8. 200 mL/h
9. 300 mL/h
10. 200 mL/h

Exercise 4
Approximately is used whenever the answer yields part of a drop. This alerts the health professional that the rate is not exact but is close to the rate needed to deliver the solution in the time allowed.

1. a. 2.08 or 2.1 mL/min
   b. Approximately 21 gtts/min
2. a. 3.3 mL/min
   b. Approximately 33 gtts/min
3. a. 1.66 or 1.7 mL/min
   b. Approximately 102 gtts/min (Note: use minidropper to get rate of 60)
4. a. 1.66 or 1.7 mL/min
   b. 25.5 or approximately 26 drops/minute
5. a. 4.16 or 4.2 mL/min
   b. Approximately 50 gtts/min
6. a. 5.55 or 5.6 mL/min
   b. Approximately 112 gtts/min
7. a. 1.3 mL/min
   b. Approximately 78 drops/minute
8. a. 1 mL/min
   b. 60 gtts/min

Exercise 5
1. 20.83, $20\frac{5}{6}$, or 21

2. 31.25, $31\frac{1}{4}$, or 31

3. 41.66, 41.7, $41\frac{2}{3}$, or 42

4. 62.5, $62\frac{1}{2}$, or 63

5. 46.87, 46.9, $46\frac{7}{8}$, or 47

6. 41.66, $41\frac{2}{3}$, or 42

7. 125

8. 24.3, $24\frac{3}{10}$, or 24

9. 23.8, $23\frac{4}{5}$, or 24

10. 166.66, $166\frac{2}{3}$, or 167

11. 166.66, $166\frac{2}{3}$, or 167

12. 16.66, $16\frac{2}{3}$, or 17

13. 20.8, $20\frac{4}{5}$, 21

14. 83.3, $83\frac{3}{10}$, 83

15. 41.66, $41\frac{2}{3}$, or 42

16. 27.77, $27\frac{7}{9}$, or 28

Exercise 6
1. a. 15
   b. 75
   c. 75
   d. 90
   e. 90
2. a. 12.5
   b. 62.5 or 63
   c. 62.5 or 63
   d. 75
   e. 75
3. a. 25
   b. 125
   c. 31.25 or 31
   d. 150
   e. 37.5 or 38
4. a. 50
   b. 250
   c. 41.66 or 42
   d. 300
   e. 50
5. a. 31.25 or 31
   b. 156.25 or 156
   c. 26.04 or 26
   d. 187.5 or 188
   e. 31.25, $31\frac{1}{4}$ or 31
6. a. 31.25 or 31
   b. 156.25 or 156
   c. 156
   d. 187.5 or 188
   e. 187.5 or 188
7. a. 20.8 or 21
   b. 104.1 or 104
   c. 26
   d. 124.8 or 125 mL
   e. 31.25 or 31
8. a. 37.5
   b. 187.5 or 188
   c. 31.25 or 31
   d. 225
   e. 37.5 or 38
9. a. 18.75 or 19
   b. 93.75 or 94
   c. 93.75 or 94
   d. 112.5 or 113
   e. 112.5 or 113

Exercise 7
1. 24 mEq
2. 0.75 million U
3. a. 37.5 or 38 gtts/min
   b. 0.9 million U
4. a. 16 mEq
   b. 64 mEq

Chapter 16
Exercise 1
1. 10,000
2. 40,000
3. 30,000
4. a. 1000
   b. 3000
5. a. 5000 U/mL, either 1 mL or 10 mL vial can be used for correct dose. There is less risk of solution being contaminated by others if 1 mL vial is used.
   b. 5000 U/0.5 mL and 5000 U/mL
6. a.

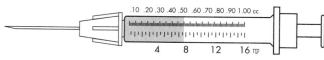

   b.

7. 0.5 mL

8. 25 U/mL, because it is the exact dose
9. 40 U/mL
10. 25 mL/h
11. 30 mL/h
12. a. 80 U/mL
    b. 13.75 or 14 mL/h
    c. 26,880 U is within the normal range of dosage
13. a. 45 mL/h
    b. 21,600 U is within the normal range of dosage
14. 2 mL of heparin (5,000 U/mL)
15. 20 mL of heparin (5000 U/mL)

Chapter 17
Exercise 1
a. 0.2 mg   b. 200 mcg/mL   c. 61 mL/min

Exercise 2
1.
Nipride 100 mg in 500 mL of D_5W* (Concentration: 1 mL = 200 mcg)

mcg/min	Weight in kilograms							
	54		56		58		60	
0.5	$\frac{27}{1620}$	8.1	$\frac{28}{1680}$	8.4	$\frac{29}{1740}$	8.7	$\frac{30}{1800}$	9
1	$\frac{54}{3240}$	16.2	$\frac{56}{3360}$	16.8	$\frac{58}{3480}$	17.4	$\frac{60}{3600}$	18
2	$\frac{108}{6480}$	32.4	$\frac{112}{6720}$	33.6	$\frac{116}{6960}$	34.8	$\frac{120}{7200}$	36
3	$\frac{162}{9720}$	48.6	$\frac{168}{10,080}$	50.4	$\frac{174}{10,440}$	52.2	$\frac{180}{10,800}$	54

*The flow rate (mL/hour) will change if the strength changes. This table is for a concentration of 1 mL = 200 mcg only. Mixtures are usually standardized to avoid confusion.

2. 34.8 or 35
3. 52.2 or 52
4. Yes, 33.6 or 34 mL/h is the correct rate.
5. 50 mg

Exercise 3
1. 0.8 mg/mL
2. 800 mcg/mL
3. 60 kg
4. 240 mcg/min
5. 0.3 mL/min
6. 18 mL/h

Exercise 4
1. 24 mL/h
2. 30 mL/h
3. 15 mL/h
4. a. No
   b. 50 mL/h

Chapter 18
Exercise 1
1. a. 20-28
   b. 10-14
   c. 1.2 mL
   d. No, it exceeds the normal range of 10-14 mg
2. a. 100 mg
   b. 33.3 mg
   c. 2 mL
   d. 0.666 or 0.7 mL
   e. 1 mL of 250 mg/5 mL suspension
3. a. 400 mg
   b. 100 mg
   c. 25 mL
   d. EryPed 200
4. a. 4500-6000 mg
   b. 1500 mg
   c. 3 t
5. a. 62.5 mg
   b. 15.6 mg
   c. 0.3 mL
6. a. 19.3
   b. 579 mg/day
   c. 193 mg/dose
   d. 7 AM-3 PM-10 PM
7. a. 21.8
   b. 654 and 872
   c. 327 to 436
   d. 163.5 and 213 mcg (μg)
   e. 7
   f. 1400 and 2200 hours
   g. 6 AM-2 PM-10 PM
8. 240 mg
9. a. 60 kg
   b. 30 mg/dose
10. a. 77
    b. 38.5 to 60
    c. Yes, 50 mg falls between 38.5 and 61.6
    d. Consult with physician before giving medicine.
11. a. 125 mg/dose
    b. 500 mg/day
    c. 6 hours
12. 500 to 1000 mg/day
13. a. 30 kg
    b. 2250 to 3000 mg/kg/day
    c. 562.5 to 750 mg/dose
    d. 1800-2400-0600-1200
14. a. 20.9 kg
    b. 500 to 1000 mg
    c. 125 to 250 mg
    d. 5 to 10 mL of 125 mg/5 mL
15. a. 17.27 or 17.3
    b. 432.5 to 865 mg
    c. 216.25 to 432.5
    d. Yes, 250 is between 216.25 and 422.5 mg
    e. 10 mL
16. a. 6 mL
    b. 10 mL
17. a. 34.5
    b. 276 to 414
    c. 69 to 103.5
    d. Yes
    e. 6
18. a. 2
    b. 8
    c. 22.5 mg/day
    d. 45 mg
    e. 2.25 mL
    f. 9
19. a. 300 mg
    b. 300 mg
    c. One 300 mg capsule

Exercise 2
1. 15 or 15.3 mL
2. 0.34 or 0.35 mL

3. 6.76, 6.8, or 7 gr
4. 0.9 or 0.92 mg
5. 15.9 or 16 mcg (μg)
6. 12.44 or 12.4 mL
7. 7, 7.05, or 7.1 mcg (μg)
8. 0.9 or 0.92
9. 0.51 or 0.5 g
10. 700 mg

Exercise 3
1. 10 mL
2. 1.17 or 1.2 mL
3. 5.86 or 5.87 mcg (μg)

Exercise 4
1. $3.3\ (3\frac{1}{3})$ mg
2. gr viii g or gr 8
3. gr v or 5

Chapter 19
Exercise 1
1. a. Indomethacin (Indocin) 50 mg
   b. 1 tablet
   c. 3 times a day after meals
2. 10 mL of oral suspension 25 mg/5 mL
3. a. 100 mg
   b. Ninety 100 mg tablets
4. 20 mg tablet
5. a. Twice a day
   b. 250 mg
   c. 5 mL
6. a. 15 mg capsule
   b. Twenty-one 15 mg capsules
7. a. 5
   b. 50,000 USP U
   c. 150,000 USP U
   d. 150,000 USP U
8. a. Two 20 mg tablets
   b. One 20 mg tablet + one 40 mg tablet or three 20 mg tablets
9. a. Four 200 mg capsules
   Two 400 mg tablets
   One 800 mg tablet
   b. 800
   c. 50

   d. 4 t or 20 mL
   e. 1000 mL or 1 L

Chapter 20
Exercise 1
1. a, b, c, only
2. b, c, d; a is incorrect—It is common practice to avoid using a challenge dose after near-fatal reactions.
3. b, c, d
4. Heat, moisture, and light. Also, it is possible for children to retrieve medication from this location.
5. That the medicine will cause this kind of skin discoloration, that it can be lessened or covered completely with special makeup, why it is important for her to take this medicine (i.e., what this medicine will do for her state of health).
6. Advise him that if people are allergic to a drug in any form, they will be allergic to all other forms of the drug. He should avoid all preparations containing the drug(s) to which he is allergic.
7. Some of the methods include compartmentalized pill boxes, alarms (wristwatch, clocks), marking on a calendar (write it in or cross it off) when a dose is taken, keeping a daily diary of drugs taken, or using a mechanical dispenser.
8. He can ask the pharmacist to use regular caps on his medicine (i.e., those that are not childproof) but then he must keep his medicines out of the reach of children.
9. The term *prn* means whenever necessary but never more frequently than every 4 to 6 hours and then only for severe headache. You might explain that the medicine cannot be taken more often than every 4 to 6 hours.
10. He should avoid operating dangerous equipment such as motorized vehicles or electrical tools such as power saws. Ask him about other tools and appliances he uses that require coordination.

Unit III Posttest

1. 2 tablets
2. 2 tablets
3. a. 500 mcg (μg) (0.5 mg)
   b. 1 tablet (500 mcg)
4. 2 tablets
5. Two 250 mg capsules
6. a. 30 mg
   b. 1 tablet
7. a. 325 mg
   b. 2
8. 1.5 or $1\frac{1}{2}$ mL
9. 16 mL
10. 125 mg
11. 0.5 or $\frac{1}{2}$
12. a. 600 mg
    b. 100 mg/dose
13. 1.10 or 1.11
14. 125 gtts/min
15. 41.66 or 42
16. 60 mEq
17. a. 125 mL/h
    b. 0.625 g or 625 mg
18. 200 mL of 5% sodium bicarbonate
19. 2.25 g NaCl; add water to make 250 mL
20. 40 mL of 1:4 solution

Comprehensive Posttest

1. XIII
2. IX
3. 16
4. 4
5. 49
6. 15
7. $\frac{7}{10}$
8. $\frac{1}{4}$
9. $4\frac{2}{3}$
10. $9\frac{5}{8}$
11. $\frac{23}{8}$
12. $\frac{38}{7}$
13. $\frac{8}{40}$
14. $\frac{3}{10}$
15. $\frac{2}{3}$
16. $\frac{5}{8}$
17. $2\frac{3}{8}$
18. $10\frac{16}{21}$
19. $4\frac{1}{9}$
20. $\frac{29}{32}$
21. $34\frac{1}{2}$
22. $1\frac{23}{32}$
23. Four and seventeen hundredths
24. Two hundred thirty-five thousandths
25. 0.89
26. 0.6
27. $\frac{1}{40}$
28. $\frac{1}{2000}$
29. 6.687
30. 22.4343
31. 6.711

32. 8.746
33. 36.5408
34. 8424
35. $1\frac{13}{33}$
36. $\frac{30}{47}$
37. 1153.85
38. 17.24
39. 0.2
40. 0.125
41. 7.125
42. 16.429
43. Ratio 3:4
    Decimal 0.75
    Percentage 75%
44. Ratio 7:8
    Decimal 0.875
    Percentage 87.5 or $87\frac{1}{2}$
45. 32.11
46. 10.56
47. 40
48. 66
49. 0.005
50. 2
51. 0.4
52. 30 or 32
53. 2200 or 2205
54. 81.82
55. 80
56. 3.3
57. 37.8
58. 98.2
59. 10
60. 2
61. 1500
62. 0230
63. 4 PM
64. 10 PM
65. a. Pyridium
    b. Phenazopyridine
    c. Tablet
    d. 100 mg
    e. 2 tablets 3 times a day
    f. Orally
    g. Store at controlled room temperature of 15° to 30° C (59° to 86° F), dispense in tight container, keep this and all drugs out of the reach of children, requires prescription

66. a. both 2 mg and 5 mg tablet
    b. One 2 mg tablet and one 5 mg tablet
67. a. 50 mg
    b. 2
    c. 28
68. Use one 200 mg tablet
69. a. 500 mcg (0.5 g) tablet
    b. 1 tablet
70. a. Once a day (every day)
    b. 10 mL
    c. By mouth or orally
    d. 12 doses
    e.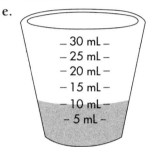
71. a. Choose 125 mg
    b. 5 mL
    c.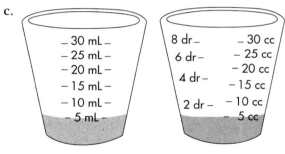
72. a. 10 mL of 8 mEq/5 mL or 5 mL of 16 mEq/15 mL
    b. 2
73. a. $1\frac{1}{2}$ mL
    b.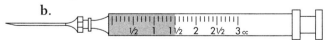
74. a. 0.5 mg/mL
    b. 1 mL
    c.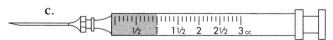
75. a. 10 mg/mL
    b. 1 mL
    c.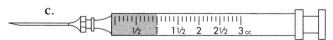

76. a. 2 g
    b. 2 g
    c. 20 to 40 mL
77. a. 825 mg
    b. 0.825 g
    c. 2.06 or 2 mL
78. 36 g
79. a. 4
    b. 2.16 g
    c. $\frac{1}{2}$ t
    d. Place salt in glass, fill with water of desired temperature and stir until dissolved.
80. a. NPH Iletin I
    b. Beef-pork
    c. Intermediate
    d.
81. a. Humulin L
    b. Recombinant DNA
    c. Intermediate
    d. 0.3 mL/30 unit syringe
82. a. 5% dextrose in 0.45 NaCl
    b. Hypotonic
    c. 1000 mL
    d. Yes, 20 mEq KCl
    e. 1800 or 6 PM
    f. Yes, 12 hours
    g. No
83. a. 5% dextrose
    b. Isotonic
    c. 50 mL
    d. Yes, 1 g cefazolin (Ancef)
    e. Yes, 12 hours
    f. Yes, 15 minutes
    g. Yes, 200 mL/h or 3.3 mL/min
84. 125 mL/h
85. 60
86. 20.8 or 21
87. 16.6 or $16\frac{2}{3}$
88. a. 31.25 mL/h
    b. 156.25
    c. 52
    d. 187.5
    e. 62.5 or 63
89. 0.75 million U
90. 28
91. 40,000 U
92. 30 mL
93. 20,000 to 40,000 U/day
94. 40
95. 24
96. a. 3000 to 4000 mg/day
    b. 1000 mg
    c. 10 mL
97. a. 30
    b. 240 to 360 mg/kg/day
    c. 90 mg/kg/day
    d. 24 mL
    e. 16 mL
98. The following schedule is satisfactory. Take estrogen (Premarin), pravastatin (Pravachol), benazepril (Lotensin), and aspirin (Ecotrin) at breakfast time. Take one calcium and one multivitamin tablet after lunch or dinner time. Taking psyllium (Metamucil) before the evening meal it may decrease her appetite.
99. a. 5 kg
    b. 0.28
    c. 98,823
100. a. 10 mg
     b. $1\frac{1}{2}$
     c. $4\frac{1}{2}$
     d. A device called a pill splitter that can be obtained at most pharmacies.

Index

A

Abbreviation
  insulin, 205
  in intravenous therapy, 214-215
  in medication orders, 134, 136
Acetaminophen, 169
  body surface calculation, 121
  pediatric dosage, 254
  prepackaged unit dose, 155
Activity time span of insulin, 206
Acyclovir
  geriatric dosage, 268
  pediatric dosage, 253
Albumin, 218
Aldomet; see Methyldopa
Allopurinol, 267
Aluminum hydroxide, 154
Aminophylline
  critical care dosage, 250
  suppositories, 154
Amoxicillin
  gram dosage, 177
  milligram dosage, 113, 171
  oral suspension, 114
  pediatric dosage, 253
  solution, 185, 197
Amphojel; see Aluminum hydroxide
Ampicillin, 172, 239
Amrinone lactate, 250
Ancef; see Cefazolin
Anspor; see Cephradine
Apothecaries' system, 76-82
  equivalents in, 79-82
Arabic numbers, 9-11
Arithmetic, 1-62
  Arabic numbers, 9-11
  decimals in, 33-46, 51-53
  fractions in, 13-31, 51-53
  percentage in, 47-49
  posttest, 60-62
  pretest, 2-8
  proportion in, 58-59
  ratio in, 55-57
  Roman numerals, 9-11
Aspirin
  divided doses, 112

Aspirin—cont'd
  enteric-coated, 168
  milligram dosage, 163
Ativan; see Lorazepam
Atropine, 153, 191
Aztreonam, 220

B

Beef insulin, 204
Blood tests, 276-277
Body surface area, child dosages, 257-258

C

Calibrated dropper in household measure, 84, 85
Capsule
  delayed-release, 159
  in oral dosage computation, 158-159
  single-dose, 128
  size, 173-177
Card, medication, 133-134
Carpuject syringe, 129
Cart, medication, 132-133
Cartridge of medication, 129
Cefazolin, 150
  injectable, 195
  intravenous, 219
Cefoperazone, 196
Celsius, 96-100
Centi-, 69
Centigrade, 96-100
Centimeter, 90, 93
Cephalexin, 254-255
Cephalothin, 198
Cephradine, 173
Child dosages, 251-260
  calculation based on body surface area, 257-258
  calculation based on weight in kilograms, 251-257
  Clark's formula, 260
  West nomogram, 259
  Young's formula, 260
Chlorpromazine, 165, 172, 177
Clark's formula, 260
Cleocin; see Clindamycin
Clindamycin
  capsule, 168
  milligram dosage, 176

327

Clindamycin—cont'd
  pediatric dosage, 255-256
Codeine
  gram dosage, 114
  solution, 191
Common denominator, 22, 26
Compatibility of medications
  geriatric dosages, 262
  intravenous solutions, 233-235
Compliance
  geriatric considerations, 262-264
  home care considerations, 274-276
CompuMed automated medication dispenser, 275
Computerized infusion pump, 222-223
Computerized label, 232
Computerized order, 217-220
Computerized unit dose system, 128-133
Container
  cylindrical graduate, 73
  single-dose, 128
Continuous infusion of heparin, 240
Controlled Substances Act, 152
Coumadin; see Warfarin
Critical care dosages, 245-250
Cross products in oral dosage computation, 157
Cyanocobalamin, 192
Cylindrical graduate container, 73

D

Dalmane; see Flurazepam
Darvon; see Propoxyphene hydrochloride
Deci-, 69
Decimals, 33-46
  adding, 38-39
  comparing, 45-46
  dividing, 43-45
  fractions and, 35, 37, 51-53
  multiplying, 40-43
  percentage to, 47-49, 51-53
  to ratio, 56
  rounding of, 34-38
  subtracting, 39-40
  in temperature conversion, 97
Deka-, 69
Delayed-release capsule, 159
Demerol; see Meperidine
Denominator, 13-14
Dexamethasone, 174, 175
Dextrose in water, 219
Diabetes insipidus, insulin dosage
  activity time span, 206
  labels, 205, 206, 207-208
Diabetes mellitus, insulin dosage, 202-212
  hypoglycemia and hyperglycemia, 202-204
  sources of insulin, 204
  strength of, 204
  syringes for, 204-205
Diazepam, 166
Dicloxacillin sodium, 172

Diet, home care considerations, 271
Digoxin
  interpretation of physician's order, 150
  milligram dosage, 112, 163
  patient weight and, 120
  pediatric dosage, 254
Dilantin; see Phenytoin
Dilaudid; see Hydromorphone
Diluent for reconstituted solution, 193
Diluted solutions, 193-201
  external, 199-201
  reconstitution of, 193-199
Dilution, of external solution, 199-201
Diphenhydramine, 165, 185
Disposal of drugs, 265
Dosage, 105-201
  critical care, 245-250
  formula
    Clark's, 260
    in injectable solutions, 189
    in oral solutions, 183
    Young's, 260
  geriatric, 261-268
    compliance, 262-264
    computation of, 265-266
    drug compatibility, 262
    drug interactions, 261-262
    nursing interventions to reduce drug therapy, 265
    physiologic factors, 261
    storage and disposal, 265
  heparin, 119, 153, 219, 240-244
  insulin, 116-117, 202-212
    activity time span, 206
    hypoglycemia and hyperglycemia, 202-204
    labels, 205, 206, 207-208
    sources of insulin, 204
    strength of, 204
    syringes for, 204-205
  intravenous fluids and medications, 118, 213-239
    calculating rate of flow, 221-227
    compatibility of medications with each other and intravenous solutions, 233-235
    determining amount of administered drug in particular amount of solution, 239
    determining flow rate for specific amount in specified amount of time, 238-239
    estimating rate of flow, 227-228
    flushing intravenous lines, 238
    heparin, 240, 241-244
    heparin lock, 237
    home care considerations, 276
    increasing rate of flow by specified percent, 228-231
    intermittent administration of, 235-236
    keep open rate of flow, 231
    reading orders for, 214-220
    volume control chambers, 236
  oral, 156-180
    assessment in, 162-169
    calculation methods, 159-162

Dosage—cont'd
  oral—cont'd
    checking calculations, 157
    metric size, 170-173
    ratio and proportion, 156-157
    systems in, 178-180
    tablet size, 173-177
    tablets and capsules, 158-159
  pediatric, 251-260
    calculation based on body surface area, 257-258
    calculation based on weight in kilograms, 251-257
    Clark's formula, 260
    West nomogram, 259
    Young's formula, 260
  physician's orders, 123-155
    administration of drug, 144-151
    administration times, 136-138
    checking of, 141
    components of, 135-136
    drugs and, 127-133
    identification cards for, 133-134
    interpreting, 134-135
    for intravenous therapy, 214-220
    legal aspects of, 124
    medication labels in, 142-144
    military time, 138-140
    patient education, 151-152
    storage and control of drugs, 152-155
    transcription of, 140-141
    types of, 126-127
  pretest, 107-122
  from solutions, 181-201
Dose
  preparation of, 144
  single, 128, 129
  unit, 129-132
Dram, 76, 77
Drip factor, 221, 225-226
Drip rate, 224
Drop as household measure, 83
Drop factor, 221
Dropper, calibrated, 84, 85
Drug allergy, 273
Drug compatibility
  geriatric considerations, 262
  intravenous solutions, 233-235
Drug history, 270
Drug interactions
  geriatric dosages and, 261-262
  over-the-counter drugs, 270-271
Drug profile sheet, 130-131
Drugs
  administration of, 144-151
    documentation and observation in, 146-151
    heparin, 237, 240-244
    intravenous, 213-239; *see also* Intravenous fluids and medications
    times of, 136-138
  critical care dosages, 245-250

Drugs—cont'd
  emergency supply of, 127
  geriatric dosages, 261-268
    compliance, 262-264
    computation of, 265-266
    drug compatibility, 262
    drug interactions, 261-262
    nursing interventions to reduce drug therapy, 265
    physiologic factors, 261
    storage and disposal, 265
  heparin, 219
    dosage and administration, 119, 240-244
    physician's order, 153
  home care considerations, 269-279
    basic medication information, 271-274
    compliance, 274-276
    obtaining medications, 278
    over-the-counter drugs, 277
    patient teaching, 269-270
    psychology of medicating, 270-271
    safeguarding welfare of patient, 276-277
  individual supply of, 127
  insulin, 202-212
    activity time span, 206
    labels, 205, 206, 207-208
    sources of insulin, 204
    strength of, 204
    syringes for, 204-205
  intravenous fluids and medications, 118, 213-239
    calculating rate of flow, 221-227
    compatibility of medications with each other and intravenous solutions, 233-235
    determining amount of administered drug in particular amount of solution, 239
    determining flow rate for specific amount in specified amount of time, 238-239
    estimating rate of flow, 227-228
    flushing intravenous lines, 238
    heparin, 240, 241-244
    heparin lock, 237
    home care considerations, 276
    increasing rate of flow by specified percent, 228-231
    intermittent administration of, 235-236
    keep open rate of flow, 231
    reading orders for, 214-220
    volume control chambers, 236
  labels, 142-144
  legal aspects of therapy, 124
  pediatric dosages, 251-260
    calculation based on body surface area, 257-258
    calculation based on weight in kilograms, 251-257
    Clark's formula, 260
    West nomogram, 259
    Young's formula, 260
  reconstitution of, 193-199
  single dose of, 128, 129
  stock, 127
  storage and control of, 152-155
  supplies and storage of, 127-133

Drugs—cont'd
  systems, 128-133
Dynapen; see Dicloxacillin sodium

E

Enteric-coated tablet, 158, 159
Epinephrine, 193
Erythromycin
  oral suspension, 120, 184
  pediatric dosage, 253
Extended-release capsule, 159

F

Fahrenheit, 96-100
Famotodine, 219
Fluids and medications, intravenous, 213-239
  calculating rate of flow, 221-227
  compatibility of medications with each other and intravenous solutions, 233-235
  determining amount of administered drug in particular amount of solution, 239
  determining flow rate for specific amount in specified amount of time, 238-239
  estimating rate of flow, 227-228
  flushing intravenous lines, 238
  heparin lock, 237
  increasing rate of flow by specified percent, 228-231
  intermittent administration of, 235-236
  keep open rate of flow, 231
  reading orders for, 214-220
  volume control chambers, 236
Fluoxetine hydrochloride, 186
Flurazepam, 267
Flushing intravenous line, 238
Foot, linear, 93
Formula
  Clark's, 260
  in injectable solutions, 189
  in oral dosage computation, 161
  in oral solutions, 183
  Young's, 260
Fractions
  adding, 22-26
  changing mixed numbers, 17-19
  comparing size of, 19-22
  to decimals, 35
  decimals and percentage, 51-53
  decimals to, 37
  dividing, 30-31
  expressing, 14-17
  improper, 17-19
  multiplying, 28-30
  subtracting, 26-28
  in temperature conversion, 98-99
  types of, 14
Furazolidone, 187
Furosemide, 150
  geriatric dosage, 268
  pediatric dosage, 254

Furoxone; see Furazolidone

G

Gallon, 83
Gantrisin; see Sulfisoxazole
Gemini Infusion System, 222
Geriatric dosages, 261-268
  compliance, 262-264
  computation of, 265-266
  drug compatibility, 262
  drug interactions, 261-262
  nursing interventions to reduce drug therapy, 265
  physiologic factors, 261
  storage and disposal, 265
Glassful as household measures, 83
Glycerol elixir, 185
Graduate container, 73
Grains, 76, 178-179
Gram, 69
  metric equivalents, 70
  in oral dosage computation, 178-179
Griseofulvin, 184, 187

H

Haldol; see Haloperidol
Haloperidol, 186
Hecto-, 69
Heparin, 219
  dosage and administration, 119, 240-244
  physician's order, 153
Heparin flush, 237, 240
Heparin lock, 237
Heparinization, 237
Home care, 269-279
  basic medication information, 271-274
  compliance, 274-276
  obtaining medications, 278
  over-the-counter drugs, 277
  patient teaching, 269-270
  psychology of medicating, 270-271
  safeguarding welfare of patient, 276-277
  storage of medications, 278
Household measures, 83-88
Human insulin, 204
Humulin, 203
Hydromorphone, 192
Hyperglycemia, 202-204
Hypertonic solution, intravenous, 214
Hypoglycemia, 202-204
Hypotonic solution, intravenous, 214

I

Ibuprofen, 164
Identification card for medication orders, 133-134
Imodium; see Loperamide hydrochloride
Inch, 93
Individual supply of medicine, 127
Indocin; see Indomethacin
Indomethacin, 266-267

Infusion pump, 222-223
Injectable solution, 188-193
   heparin lock, 237
   home care considerations, 275-276
   reconstituted, 193-195
Inocor; *see* Amrinone lactate
Insulin dosage, 116-117, 202-212
   activity time span, 206
   labels, 205, 206, 207-208
   sources of insulin, 204
   strength of, 204
   syringes for, 204-205
Intermediate-action insulin preparation, 206
Intermittent infusion
   of heparin, 240
   of intravenous medications, 235-236
Intramuscular injection, 188-193
Intravenous fluids and medications, 118, 213-239
   calculating rate of flow, 221-227
   compatibility of medications with each other and intravenous solutions, 233-235
   determining amount of administered drug in particular amount of solution, 239
   determining flow rate for specific amount in specified amount of time, 238-239
   estimating rate of flow, 227-228
   flushing intravenous lines, 238
   heparin, 240, 241-244
   heparin lock, 237
   home care considerations, 276
   increasing rate of flow by specified percent, 228-231
   intermittent administration of, 235-236
   keep open rate of flow, 231
   reading orders for, 214-220
   volume control chambers, 236
Intravenous piggyback, 233, 234
Intravenous tubing, 221
   compatibility of medications and intravenous solutions, 233-234
   flushing, 238
   volume control chamber, 236
Iodinated glycerol elixir, 185
Isotonic solution, intravenous, 214

K

Keep open rate of flow, 231
Keflin; *see* Cephalothin
Kilo-, 69
Kilogram, 245
   pediatric dosages based on, 251-257

L

Label
   computerized, 232
   insulin, 205, 206, 207-208
   intravenous solution, 213
   medication, 142-144
Lactated Ringer's solution, 215, 216
Lanoxin; *see* Digoxin
Lasix; *see* Furosemide
Legal aspects of drug therapy, 124
Length, metric units of, 89-90
Levothyroxine, 164, 173
Lidocaine, 250
Lifeshield Connector and Docking Station, 233
Linear measure, 89-95
   English conversions of, 93-95
   metric/SI system of, 89-93
Liquid, household measure of, 84, 85
Liter, 69, 70
Lithium, 154-155, 187
Long-action insulin preparation, 206
Loperamide hydrochloride, 188
Lorazepam, 113, 167
Lovastatin, 166

M

Macrodrip intravenous tubing, 221
MAR; *see* Medication administration record
Measurement systems in oral dosage computation, 178-180
Medic Alert, 272, 273
Medication administration record, 146, 147-149
Medication cart, 132-133
Medication orders, 124-141
   administration times, 136-138
   checking of, 141
   components of, 135-136
   drug supplies and storage, 127-133
   identification cards for, 133-134
   interpreting, 134-135
   military time and, 138-140
   transcribing, 140-141
   types of, 126-127
Medications
   administration of, 144-151
      documentation and observation in, 146-151
      heparin, 237, 240-244
      intravenous, 213-239; *see also* Intravenous fluids and medications
      times of, 136-138
   critical care dosages, 245-250
   emergency supply of, 127
   geriatric dosages, 261-268
      compliance, 262-264
      computation of, 265-266
      drug compatibility, 262
      drug interactions, 261-262
      nursing interventions to reduce drug therapy, 265
      physiologic factors, 261
      storage and disposal, 265
   heparin, 219
      dosage and administration, 119, 240-244
      physician's order, 153
   home care considerations, 269-279
      basic medication information, 271-274
      compliance, 274-276
      obtaining medications, 278

Medications—cont'd
  home care considerations—cont'd
    over-the-counter drugs, 277
    patient teaching, 269-270
    psychology of medicating, 270-271
    safeguarding welfare of patient, 276-277
  individual supply of, 127
  insulin, 202-212
    activity time span, 206
    labels, 205, 206, 207-208
    sources of insulin, 204
    strength of, 204
    syringes for, 204-205
  intravenous, 118, 213-239
    calculating rate of flow, 221-227
    compatibility of medications with each other and intravenous solutions, 233-235
    determining amount of administered drug in particular amount of solution, 239
    determining flow rate for specific amount in specified amount of time, 238-239
    estimating rate of flow, 227-228
    flushing intravenous lines, 238
    heparin, 240, 241-244
    heparin lock, 237
    home care considerations, 276
    increasing rate of flow by specified percent, 228-231
    intermittent administration of, 235-236
    keep open rate of flow, 231
    reading orders for, 214-220
    volume control chambers, 236
  labels, 142-144
  legal aspects of therapy, 124
  pediatric dosages, 251-260
    calculation based on body surface area, 257-258
    calculation based on weight in kilograms, 251-257
    Clark's formula, 260
    West nomogram, 259
    Young's formula, 260
  reconstitution of, 193-199
  single dose of, 128, 129
  stock, 127
  storage and control of, 152-155
  supplies and storage of, 127-133
  systems, 128-133
Medicine box, 274
Medicine cup
  household measures on, 83, 84
  in millimeters, 73
Meniscus, 84, 85
Meperidine, 153
  pediatric dosage, 254
  solution, 191
Metamucil; see Psyllium
Meter, 69, 89-90
Methicillin, 198
Methyldopa, 267
Metric size in oral dosage computation, 170-173

Metric system
  changing units in, 71-73
  English conversions of, 93-95
  linear measure in, 89-95
  weight and volume in, 69-76
Mevacor; see Lovastatin
Microdrip intravenous tubing, 221
Microgram, 245
Military time, 138-140
Milli-, 69
Milligram, 245
Milliliters/hour rate of flow, 223, 224-226
Millimeter, 90
Minim, 76, 77
Morphine, 191-192
Motrin; see Ibuprofen
Mycostatin; see Nystatin

N

Nafcillin
  gram dosage, 115
  injectable, 197
Nalidixic acid, 253
NegGram; see Nalidixic acid
Nembutal; see Pentobarbital
Neosporin, 151
NeoSynephrine; see Phenylephrine hydrochloride
Nifedipine
  milligram dosage, 166, 167
  tablets, 112
Nipride; see Sodium nitroprusside
Nitroglycerin ointment, 151
Noncompliance, 262-264
Norflex; see Orphenadrine citrate
Numerator, 13-14
Numorphan; see Oxymorphone
Nursing interventions to reduce drug therapy, 265
Nystatin, 184

O

Open rate of flow, 231
Oral dosage, 156-180
  assessment in, 162-169
  calculation methods, 159-162
  checking calculations, 157
  metric size in, 170-173
  ratio and proportion in, 156-157
  systems in, 178-180
  tablet size in, 173-177
  tablets and capsules in, 158-159
Oral solution, 183-188
  reconstituted, 195-199
Orphenadrine citrate, 190
Ounce, 76, 77
Over-the-counter drugs
  actions with prescribed drugs, 270-271
  home care considerations, 277
Oxacillin, 253
Oxymorphone, 193

P

Pancrease MT, 267-268
Patient education
    home care considerations, 269-270
    of physician order, 151-152
Pediatric dosages, 251-260
    calculation based on body surface area, 257-258
    calculation based on weight in kilograms, 251-257
    Clark's formula, 260
    West nomogram, 259
    Young's formula, 260
Penicillin V, 153, 185
Pentazocine lactate, 192
Pentobarbital, 190
Percentage, 47-49
    fractions and decimals, 51-53
    as ratio, 55
Phenazopyridine, 164
Phenobarbital, 153, 177
Phenylephrine hydrochloride, 154
Phenytoin
    divided dose, 163
    milligram dosage, 165
    pediatric dosage, 252
    solution, 186
Physician order, 123-155
    drugs
        administration of, 144-151
        storage and control of, 152-155
    for intravenous therapy, 214-220
    legal aspects of, 124
    medication labels in, 142-144
    medication orders in, 124-141
        administration times of, 136-138
        checking of, 141
        components of, 135-136
        drugs and, 127-133
        identification cards for, 133-134
        interpreting, 134-135
        military time, 138-140
        transcription of, 140-141
        types of, 126-127
    patient education of, 151-152
Piggyback, 233, 234
Pill splitter, 275
Pint, 83
Piperacillin, 199
Plum Infusion System, 222
Pork insulin, 116, 204
Potassium chloride, 117, 118-119, 238, 239
Potassium iodide, 114, 186, 188
Pravachol; *see* Pravastatin
Pravastatin, 267
Prescription, 135-136
Prn order, 126
Procainamide hydrochloride, 168-169, 250
Procan SR; *see* Procainamide hydrochloride
Procardia; *see* Nifedipine
Prochlorperazine, 220
Product, cross, 157
Product of means, 156
Pronestyl; *see* Procainamide hydrochloride
Proportion, 58-59
    in household measure, 85
    in injectable solutions, 189
    in oral dosage computation, 156-157
    in oral solutions, 183
    of two ratios, 160-161
Propoxyphene hydrochloride, 153, 155
Protocol for medication, 126-127
Prozac; *see* Fluoxetine hydrochloride
Psychology of medicating, 270-271
Psyllium, 277

Q

Quart, 83

R

Ranitidine hydrochloride, 184
Rate of flow in intravenous therapy
    calculation of, 221-227
        in drops, 224
        in milliliters/hour, 223, 224-226
    determination for specific amount of drug in specified amount of time, 238-239
    estimation of, 227-228
    increasing by specified percent, 228-231
    keep open, 231
Ratio, 55-57
    of label and dose, 160-161
    in oral dosage computation, 156-157
    of size, 161-162
Refrigeration of medications, 278
Rider, 233
Rifadin; *see* Rifampin
Rifampin, 256-257
Ringer's Lactate, 215, 216
Roman numerals, 9-11

S

Saline flush, 237
Schedule in medication orders, 136
Short-action insulin preparation, 206
Signing off in medication orders, 140
Single dose order, 126
SISH, 237
Size
    in oral solutions, 183
    of two ratios, 161-162
Sodium bicarbonate, 185
Sodium nitroprusside, 246, 248, 249
Solutions
    diluted, 193-201
        external, 199-201
        reconstitution of, 193-199
    home care considerations, 275-276
    injectable, 188-193
    intravenous, 213-239

Solutions—cont'd
  intravenous—cont'd
    calculating rate of flow, 221-227
    compatibility of medications with each other and intravenous solutions, 233-235
    determining amount of administered drug in particular amount of solution, 239
    determining flow rate for specific amount in specified amount of time, 238-239
    estimating rate of flow, 227-228
    flushing intravenous lines, 238
    heparin lock, 237
    increasing rate of flow by specified percent, 228-231
    intermittent administration of, 235-236
    reading orders for, 214-220
    volume control chambers, 236
  oral, 183-188
Standing order, 126
Staphcillin; see Methicillin
Stat order, 126, 127
Stelazine; see Trifluoperazine
Stock medication, 127
Storage of medications
  geriatric considerations, 265
  home care considerations, 278
Strength
  of external solution, 199-201
  of intravenous solution, 214
Streptomycin, 198
Subcutaneous injection, 188-193
  heparin, 240
Sulfisoxazole, 173, 253
Synthroid; see Levothyroxine
Syringe
  adding medication to IV solution, 232
  Carpuject, 129
  for heparin administration, 241
  for injectable solutions, 189
  insulin, 204-205
  tuberculin, 205
Systeme International de'Unités; see Metric system

T

Tablet
  in oral dosage computation, 158-159
  size, 173-177
Talwin; see Pentazocine lactate
Taste of medicine, 276
Teaspoonful, 83
Temperature conversion, 96-100
  decimals in, 97
  fractions in, 98-99
Tetracycline, 154

Thermometer, 98-99
Thorazine; see Chlorpromazine
Timed-release capsule, 158-159
Time-strip for IV container, 217, 227
Tonicity of intravenous solution, 214
Total parenteral nutrition, 228
Trifluoperazine, 192
Tuberculin syringe, 205
Twenty-four hour time, 138-140
Tylenol; see Acetaminophen

U

Unit dose, 129-132, 204

V

Valium; see Diazepam
Vancomycin, 220
Verbal order for medication, 124-125
Vial
  adding medication to IV solution, 232
  heparin, 241
Vitamin B_{12}, 192
Volume
  apothecary units of, 76
  equivalents in, 79-80
  household measures of, 83
  metric units of, 70
Volume control chamber, 236

W

Warfarin, 164, 176
Weight
  apothecary units of, 76
  equivalents in, 80-81
  in kilograms for pediatric dosage, 251-257
  metric units of, 70
Weights and measures, 63-103
  apothecaries' system in, 76-82
  household measures in, 83-88
  linear units in, 89-95
  metric/SI in, 69-76
  posttest, 101-103
  pretest, 65-68
  temperature conversion in, 96-100
West nomogram, 259

Y

Young's formula, 260

Z

Zovirax; see Acyclovir
Zyloprim; see Allopurinol

METRIC/SI SYSTEM

Units of volume

1 liter (L) = 1000 milliliters (mL)
0.001 1 liter (L) = 1 milliliter (mL)
1 milliliter (mL) = 1 cubic centimeter (cc)

Units of weight

1 milligram = 1000 micrograms
1 gram (g) = 1000 milligrams (mg)
0.001 gram (g) = 1 milligram (mg)
1 kilogram (kg) = 1000 grams (g)
0.001 kilogram (kg) = 1 gram (g)

Metric/SI equivalents

Volume - liter (L)	Weight - gram (g)
0.001 liter = 1 milliliter	0.001 milligrams = 1 microgram
0.01 liter = 1 centiliter	0.001 gram = 1 milligram
0.1 liter = 1 deciliter	0.01 gram = 1 centigram
1 liter = 1000 milliliters	0.1 gram = 1 decigram
10 liters = 1 dekaliter	10 grams = 1 dekagram
100 liters = 1 hectoliter	100 grams = 1 hectogram
1000 liters = 1 kiloliter	1000 grams = 1 kilogram

Metric/SI units of length

1 meter (m) = 1000 millimeters (mm)
0.001 meter (m) = 1 millimeter (mm)
1 meter (m) = 100 centimeters (cm)
1 centimeter (cm) = 10 millimeters (mm)
1 millimeter (mm) = 0.1 centimeter (cm)

APPROXIMATE EQUIVALENTS
METRIC AND APOTHECARIES' SYSTEMS

Volume

Metric/SI system	Apothecaries' equivalents
1 milliliter (mL)*	= 15 minims (♏xv)
4 milliliters (mL)	= 1 fluidram (f℈i)
30 milliliters (mL)	= 1 fluidounce (f℥i)
500 milliliters (mL)	= 1 pint (O)
1000 milliliters (mL) or 1 liter (L)	= 1 quart (qt)
1 gallon (C)	= 4 quarts (qt)

Weight

Metric/SI system	Apothecaries' equivalents
0.06 gram (g) or 60 milligrams (mg)	= 1 grain (gr i)
1 gram (g) or 1000 milligrams (mg)	= 15 grains (gr xv)
4 grams (g)	= 1 dram (℈i)
30 grams (g)	= 1 ounce (℥i)
0.45 kilogram (kg) or 450 grams (g)	= 1 pound (1 lb)
1 kilogram (kg)	= 2.2 pounds (lb)

METRIC/SI - ENGLISH EQUIVALENTS

English system	Metric/SI equivalents
1 inch (in)	= 2.5 centimeters (cm)
1 foot (ft)	= 30 centimeters (cm)
1 yard (yd)	= 0.9 meters (m)
1 mile (mi)	= 1.6 kilometers (km)

Metric/SI system	English equivalents
1 kilometer (km)	= 0.6 mile (mi)
1 meter (m)	= 39.4 inches (in) or 1.1 yard (yd)
1 decimeter (dm)	= 4 centimeters (cm)
1 centimeter (cm)	= 0.4 inches (in)
1 millimeter (mm)	= 0.04 inches (in)

APOTHECARIES' SYSTEM

Volume

60 minims (♏) = 1 fluidram (f℈)
8 fluidrams (f℈) = 1 fluidounce (f℥)
16 fluidounces (f℥) = 1 pint (pt or O)
2 pints (pt or O) = 1 quart (qt)
4 quarts (qt) = 1 gallon (gal or C)

Weight (Troy)

60 grains (gr) = 1 dram (℈)
8 drams (℈) = 1 ounce (℥)
480 grains = 1 ounce
12 ounces (℥) = 1 pound (lb)*

*16 ounces equals 1 pound avoirdupois.

HOUSEHOLD MEASURES

Volume

15 drops (gtt xv) = 1 mL or 1 cc
1 teaspoonful (t) = 1 fluidram (f℈i) or 5 (4) mL*
1 tablespoonful (T) = 4 fluidrams (f℈iv)
2 tablespoonfuls (T) = 1 fluidounce (℥i)
6 fluidounces (f℥vi) = 1 teacupful
8 fluidounces (f℥viii) = 1 glassful

Household, apothecaries', and metric/SI equivalents

Household	Apothecaries'	Metric/SI
1 drop	= 1 minim	= 0.06 mL
15 drops	= 15 minims	= 1 mL
1 teaspoonful	= 1 fluidram	= 5 (4) mL*
1 tablespoonful	= 4 fluidrams	= 15 mL
2 tablespoonfuls	= 1 fluidounce	= 30 mL
1 teacupful	= 6 fluidounces	= 180 mL
1 glassful	= 8 fluidounces	= 240 mL
1 pint	= 16 fluidounces	= 480 mL
1 quart	= 32 fluidounces	= 960 mL
1 gallon	= 128 fluidounces	= 3840 mL

*mL and cc are generally accepted as equivalents.